T0202315

Depression and
Type 2 Diabetes

Depression and Type 2 Diabetes

Edited by

Khalida Ismail
Department of Psychological Medicine,
Institute of Psychiatry, Psychology and Neuroscience,
King's College London, London, UK

Andreas Barthel
Medicover Bochum, Germany and Department of Medicine III,
University Hospital Carl Gustav Carus, Dresden, Germany

Stefan R. Bornstein
Department of Medicine, and Development and
International Affairs, University of Dresden, Dresden,
Germany, and Diabetes and Nutritional Sciences, Rayne
Institute, Denmark Hill Campus, King's College London,
London,UK

Julio Licinio
College of Medicine, State University of New York,
Upstate Medical University,
Syracuse, New York, USA

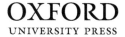

OXFORD
UNIVERSITY PRESS

Great Clarendon Street, Oxford, OX2 6DP,
United Kingdom

Oxford University Press is a department of the University of Oxford.
It furthers the University's objective of excellence in research, scholarship,
and education by publishing worldwide. Oxford is a registered trade mark of
Oxford University Press in the UK and in certain other countries

First Edition published in 2018

Impression: 2

Published in the United States of America by Oxford University Press
198 Madison Avenue, New York, NY 10016, United States of America

British Library Cataloguing in Publication Data

Data available

Library of Congress Control Number: 2018931001

ISBN 978-0-19-878928-4

Printed and bound by
CPI Group (UK) Ltd, Croydon, CR0 4YY

Oxford University Press makes no representation, express or implied, that the
drug dosages in this book are correct. Readers must therefore always check
the product information and clinical procedures with the most up-to-date
published product information and data sheets provided by the manufacturers
and the most recent codes of conduct and safety regulations. The authors and
the publishers do not accept responsibility or legal liability for any errors in the
text or for the misuse or misapplication of material in this work. Except where
otherwise stated, drug dosages and recommendations are for the non-pregnant
adult who is not breast-feeding

Links to third party websites are provided by Oxford in good faith and
for information only. Oxford disclaims any responsibility for the materials
contained in any third party website referenced in this work.

Preface

Owing to their increasing prevalence and adverse impact on quality of life, type 2 diabetes and depression are the most important comorbidities in the twenty-first century, posing a major challenge for both developed and developing nations' healthcare systems. Historically, the scientific culture and clinical care of both disorders have been segregated by a Cartesian mind–body dualism. However, over the last decades two key aspects have become more and more evident. First, patients with mental disorders—in particular with depression—frequently develop secondary metabolic problems—in particular type 2 diabetes—and vice versa. Secondly, both type 2 diabetes and depression share some common biological features and mechanisms, typically merging at the level of hormonal regulation and thereby blurring the clear-cut borders between disciplines. Based on this background it is obvious that in real world settings patients require our clinicians to have a broad and solid understanding of hormonal and metabolic as well as psychological medicine—a need that seems to be contrary to the increasing subspecialization of clinicians in today's medical practice. The increasing gulf between different specialties in medicine has not been addressed so far.

Given this situation, the purpose of this book is to cover common aspects of both depression and the metabolic syndrome in order to give clinicians, scientists, and health professionals a practical guide on hand to improve the understanding and the treatment of depressive patients with metabolic dysfunction—and diabetes patients suffering from depressive disorders and related conditions. Moreover, students who are about to enter research or clinical work will find this book a best-practice example in approaching one issue from different angles and disciplines. To accomplish this goal, the book is structured in 18 comprehensive chapters, each written by internationally recognized experts in their fields.

Many of the authors are associated with the joint transCampus based at King's College London (UK) and the Technische Universität Dresden (Germany). Their work on this book has been strongly supported by the International Network on Diabetes and Depression and the German Australian Institute for Translational Medicine, which are both funded by the German Federal Ministry of Education and Research (BMBF), our collaborative research centre (DFG 205), and the transCampus programme.

A common key aspect of all involved institutions is the integration of basic science and clinical research in the field of mental and metabolic disorders with a focus on public health. The directed flow from bench to bedside, from academia to practical medicine is nothing else than translational medicine applicable in our everyday professional life. In some way this book is a condensed extract of the shared work of these institutions over the last years and gives a summary on the international state of the art. Each of the chapters highlights a specific topic and can be read independent of each other. This will help the reader to obtain a quick and comprehensive overview in this complex field.

The realization of this book would not have been possible without the eager, continuous and indispensable assistance of the following people (in alphabetical order): Aline Günther, Felix Klee, Maria Nopper, Martin Wloszczynski, Patricia Becker, Peter Stevenson, Philipp Gussek, Rachel Goldsworthy, and Shancy Bock.

Therefore, the authors and editors wish to express a special thanks to these people 'behind the scenes'.

Contents

Abbreviations

5-HT	5-hydroxytryptamine, serotonin		HbA_{1c}	glycated haemoglobin
ACTH	adrenocorticotropic hormone		HIC	high-income country
ASD	autism spectrum disorder		HPA	hypothalamic–pituitary–adrenal
AVP	arginine–vasopressin		HPA axis	hypothalamic–pituitary–adrenal axis
BDNF	brain-derived neurotrophic factor		HRE	hormone response elements
CBG	corticosteroid-binding globulin		HSP	heat shock protein
CNS	central nervous system		IBS	inflammatory bowel disease
CRF	corticotrophin-releasing factor		IFG	impaired fasting glucose
CRH	corticotrophin-releasing hormone		K_d	dissociation constant
			K_i	ionization constant
CSF	cerebrospinal fluid		LIC	low-income country
CVD	cardiovascular disease		LPS	lipopolysaccharide
DDS	Diabetes Distress Scale		MCI	mild cognitive impairment
DEX	dexamethasone		MDD	major depressive disorder
DSM-III	diagnostic and statistical manual of mental disorders 3rd edition		MR	mineralocorticoid receptor
			NCD	non-communicable disease
DST	dexamethasone suppression test		NLRs	NODE-like receptors
			NSAID	non-steroidal anti-inflammatory drug
EEC	enteroendocrine cell		PAID	Problem Areas in Diabetes
ENS	enteric nervous system		PHQ-9	Patient Health Questionnaire-9
FFA	free fatty acids		PRRs	pattern recognition receptors
FGID	functional gastrointestinal disorder		PVN	paraventricular nucleus
GABA	gamma aminobutyric acid		PYY	peptide YY
GF	germ-free		SCN	suprachiasmatic nuclei
GI	gastrointestinal		SPF	specific-pathogen free
GLP-1	glucagon-like peptide 1		T1DM	type 1 diabetes mellitus
GR	glucocorticoid receptor		T2D	type 2 diabetes
GRE	glucocorticoid response element		TLRs	toll-like receptors
			TSST	Trier Social Stress Test
GWAS	genome-wide association studies			

Contributors

Mohamad M. Almedawar
Department of Medicine III,
University Hospital Carl Gustav
Carus, Dresden, and Faculty of
Medicine of the TU Dresden,
Dresden,
Germany

Ebaa Al-Ozairi
Faculty of Medicine,
Health Sciences Centre,
Kuwait

Clive Ballard
University of Exeter Medical School,
St Luke's Campus, Exeter,
UK

Andreas Barthel
Medicover Bochum,
Germany and Department of
Medicine III,
University Hospital Carl Gustav
Carus,
Dresden,
Germany

Michael Bauer
Department of Psychiatry and
Psychotherapy,
University Hospital Carl Gustav
Carus,
Dresden, and Faculty of Medicine of
the TU Dresden,
Dresden,
Germany

Andreas L. Birkenfeld
Department of Medicine III,
University of Dresden, Dresden,
Germany, and Diabetes and
Nutritional Sciences, Rayne Institute,
Denmark Hill Campus, King's
College London,
London,
UK

Stefan R. Bornstein
Department of Medicine, and
Development and International
Affairs, University of Dresden,
Dresden, Germany, and Diabetes and
Nutritional Sciences, Rayne Institute,
Denmark Hill Campus, King's College
London,
London,
UK

Marijke A. Bremmer
Department of Psychiatry,
VU University Medical Centre,
Amsterdam,
The Netherlands

Boon-How Chew
Department of Family Medicine,
Faculty of Medicine and Health
Sciences,
Universiti Putra Malaysia (UPM),
Serdang,
Malaysia

Andrea Danese
MRC Social, Genetic and
Developmental Psychiatry Centre
and Department of Child &
Adolescent Psychiatry,
Institute of Psychiatry, Psychology
and Neuroscience,
King's College London,
London,
UK

Christopher Garrett
Diabetes and Mental Health Group
Department of Psychological
Medicine,
Institute of Psychiatry, Psychology
and Neuroscience,
King's College London,
London,
UK

Lidia Castagneto Gissey
Surgical Sciences Department,
Medical School "Sapienza" University,
Rome,
Italy

Shlomo Ben-Haim
Hobart Healthcare Group,
UK

Norbert Hermanns
Research Institute of the Diabetes
Academy Mergentheim (FIDAM),
Bad Mergentheim,
Germany

Khalida Ismail
Department of Psychological
Medicine,
Institute of Psychiatry, Psychology
and Neuroscience,
King's College London, London,
UK

Mario F. Juruena
Centre for Affective Disorders,
Institute of Psychiatry, Psychology
and Neuroscience,
King's College London,
London,
UK

Carol Kan
Institute of Psychiatry, Psychology
and Neuroscience,
King's College London,
London,
UK

Harold E. Lebovitz
State University of New York Health
Science Center at Brooklyn,
New York,
USA

Julio Licinio
College of Medicine,
State University of New York,
Upstate Medical University,
Syracuse, New York,
USA

James R. Casella Mariolo
Surgical Sciences Department,
Medical School "Sapienza"
University,
Rome,
Italy

Geltrude Mingrone
Department of Interna Medicine
and General Surgery,
Catholic University,
Rome,
Italy, and
Diabetes and Nutritional Sciences,
Rayne Institute, Denmark Hill
Campus, King's College London,
London, UK

Henning Morawietz
Department of Medicine III,
University Hospital Carl Gustav
Carus, Dresden and Faculty of
Medicine of the TU Dresden,
Dresden,
Germany

Calum D. Moulton
Diabetes and Psychiatry
Research Group,
King's College London,
London,
UK

Giuseppe Nisticò
European Brain Research Institute,
'Rita Levi-Montalcini' Foundation,
Rome,
Italy

Robert Nisticò
European Brain Research Institute,
'Rita Levi-Montalcini' Foundation,
Rome, Italy
Department of Biology,
University of Rome 'Tor Vergata',
Rome,
Italy

Brenda W. Penninx
Department of Psychiatry,
VU University Medical Center,
Amsterdam,
The Netherlands

Frank Petrak
Department of Psychosomatic
Medicine and Psychotherapy
LWL-University Clinic Bochum,
Ruhr-University Bochum,
Bochum,
Germany

Carla Petrella
Institute of Cell Biology and
Neurobiology (IBCN),
CNR,
Rome,
Italy

John C. Pickup
Division of Diabetes and Nutritional
Sciences,
Faculty of Life Sciences and
Medicine,
King's College London,
Guy's Hospital,
London,
UK

Gregory D. M. Potter
Leeds Institute of Cardiovascular and
Metabolic Medicine,
University of Leeds,
Leeds,
UK

Bonnie Röhrig
Department of Psychosomatic
Medicine and Psychotherapy
LWL-University Clinic Bochum,
Ruhr-University Bochum,
Bochum,
Germany

Francesco Rubino
Department of Metabolic and
Bariatric Surgery,
Diabetes and Nutrition Science
Division,
King's College London,
London,
UK

Peter E. H. Schwarz
Department of Medicine III,
University Hospital Carl Gustav
Carus, Dresden, Paul Langerhans
Institute Dresden of the Helmholtz
Center Munich at The University
Hospital Carl Gustav Carus and
Faculty of Medicine of the TU
Dresden,
Dresden,
Germany

Eleanor M. Scott
Leeds Institute of Cardiovascular and
Metabolic Medicine,
University of Leeds,
Leeds,
UK

Richard C. Siow
School of Cardiovascular Medicine
& Sciences, King's British Heart
Foundation Centre of Research
Excellence,
King's College London,
London,
UK

Frank J. Snoek
Department of Medical psychology,
VU University Medical Center and
Academic Medical Center,
Amsterdam,
The Netherlands

Patrick Timpel
Department of Medicine III,
University Hospital Carl Gustav
Carus, Dresden and Faculty of
Medicine of the TU Dresden,
Dresden,
Germany

Kirsty Winkley
Florence Nightingale School of
Nursing & Midwifery,
King's College London,
London,
UK

Ma-Li Wong
College of Medicine,
State University of New York,
Upstate Medical University, Syracuse,
New York,
USA

Allan H. Young
Centre for Affective Disorders,
Institute of Psychiatry, Psychology
and Neuroscience,
King's College London,
London,
UK

Introduction

Imagine you are a little child growing up in a poor country. Money and re-sources including food are scarce, but times are peaceful. Like your peers, you're playing around, attending school and—because you're a kid and you're all in the same situation—you don't realize the economical limitations and the heavy efforts of your parents to keep things going and to improve life. Everything is normal for you, you're simply happy because life is an interesting and easy-going adventure.

Later, as a young adult, you realize that things have changed. Times were still peaceful, money wasn't that scarce any more and your parents were able to af-ford a fridge. Earlier, you had to walk or bike a lot, now you could take the bus and you started even dreaming of an own car. In the meantime your parents became old, for traditional reasons they would rather save their money—just in case that times get worse again—and they don't consume very much.

Now you're over 70 years old. Fortunately, times remained peaceful. Your parents died 20 years ago—both were old, but in good shape. And they were happy, probably because of their accomplishments over a life time. While your parents never had a car, you had several in your life. While your parents used their little garden to grow fruits and vegetables themselves, you get your supply conveniently delivered from the supermarket, and while your parents were physically hard working, you had an office job. Your parents had little leisure time, while you were able to enjoy TV every evening. Your parents were slim, while you're overweight. Most strikingly, you have some diagnoses since your fifties and your doctor prescribes you drugs to treat your diabetes and your de-pression. You can't remember that your parents had these problems, but two out of your six siblings apparently have.

This story sounds more than trivial but in fact this is what millions of people in Germany, in the UK, and in Europe remember from their own life experiences of the decades after the Second World War. Currently, the same epidemiologic development is happening with great reproducibility worldwide. In countries with robust and sustained economical growth like the BRIC countries (Brazil, Russia, India, China) as well as in most African and other Asian countries, the incidence of both type 2 diabetes and depression is dramatically increasing. Obviously, we're facing a striking challenge in the field of mental and metabolic disorders and we need to develop strategies to deal with this situation.

One of the major challenges for our healthcare systems is that patients are getting older, frequently show multimorbidity, and that disorders often have multidisciplinary aspects. Further, knowledge in medicine is growing exponentially making it difficult to keep pace even for a specialist, and for a generalist it is almost impossible to cover all facets in an individual patient with severe disorders. In order to fill in some gaps and to improve help for patients suffering from type 2 diabetes and depression, this book addresses special topics and important questions related to this complex.

Chapter 1

Global burden of diabetes and depression

Julio Licinio, Andreas L. Birkenfeld, and Stefan R. Bornstein

Introduction

According to the International Federation of Diabetes (IDF) (Table 1.1), 'diabetes is one of the largest global health emergencies of the 21st century' [1].

Diabetes is an important public health problem and one of four priority non-communicable diseases (NCDs) targeted for action by world leaders [2] due to the worldwide increasing incidence and prevalence during the last decades. The increase in numbers of diabetic patients is strongly correlated with a rapidly changing lifestyle all over the world. Fast and cheap availability of energy-dense foods and a relatively sedentary life style are major contributing factors [3]. At the same time, more than 300 million people of all ages suffer from depression globally [4]. Major depressive disorder (MDD) is a leading cause of disability worldwide, and a major contributor to the overall global burden of disease. Depression results from a complex interaction of social, psychological, and biological factors, which also predispose to diabetes. Interactions exist between depression and physical health. For instance, diabetes can lead to depression and vice versa [5,6].

Type 1 and type 2 diabetes

There are two main types of diabetes: type 1 diabetes mellitus (T1DM) and type 2 diabetes mellitus (T2DM). Gestational diabetes is diagnosed in the second or third trimester of pregnancy that was not clearly overt diabetes prior to gestation. Other types of diabetes develop due to specific causes, for example monogenic diabetes syndromes and drug- or chemical-induced diabetes, but have a lower prevalence. Although T1DM is not the focus of this collected work it is important to distinguish it from T2DM. T1DM is characterized by an autoimmune reaction targeting insulin producing β cells, resulting in an absolute

Table 1.1 Actual and estimated burden of diabetes

At a glance	2017	2045
Total world population	7.5 billion	9.5 billion
Adult population (20–79 years)	4.84 billion	6.37 billion
Diabetes global estimates		
Prevalence (20–79 years)	8.8% (7.2–11.3%)	9.9% (7.5–12.7%)
Number of people with diabetes (20–79 years)	424.9 million (346.4–545.4 million)	628.6 million (477.0–808.7 million)
Number of deaths due to diabetes (20–79 years)	4.0 (3.2–5.0) million	–
Total healthcare expenditures for diabetes (20–79 years), $R=2*$ 2017 USD	USD 727 billion	USD 776 billion
Hyperglycaemia in pregnancy (20–49 years)		
Proportion of live births affected	16.2%	–
Number of live births affected	21.3 million	–
Impaired glucose tolerance (IGT) Estimates		
Global prevalence (20–79 years)	7.3% (4.8–11.9%)	8.3% (5.6%–13.9%)
Number of people with IGT (20–79 years)	352.1 million (233.5–577.3 million)	531.6 million (353.8–883.9 million)
Type 1 diabetes (0–19 years)		
Number of children and adolescents with type 1 diabetes	1,106,500	–
Number of newly diagnosed cases each year	132,600	–

*R (from health expenditure estimates): The diabetes cost ratio, which is the ratio of health expenditures for persons with diabetes to health expenditures for age- and sex-matched persons who do not have diabetes. By comparing the total costs of matched persons with and without diabetes, the costs that diabetes causes can be isolated. The $R = 2$ estimates assume that health care expenditures for people with diabetes are on average twofold higher than people without diabetes, and the $R = 3$ estimates assume that health care expenditures for people with diabetes are on average three-fold higher than people without diabetes. See Chapter 2 for more details.

Reproduced from International Diabetes Federation. *IDF Diabetes Atlas*, 8th edn. Brussels, Belgium: International Diabetes Federation, 2017. http://www.diabetesatlas.org

loss of insulin. The reaction occurs relatively rapid and early in life with a median onset of the disease between 4 and 14 years of age [7]. T2DM is characterized by insulin resistance preceding the development of diabetes by several years. Insulin resistance is a condition in which insulin receptor activation by insulin leads to a reduced response in the insulin signalling cascade in skeletal muscle, adipose tissue and the liver. Consequently, β cells secrete more insulin to overcome the resistance. Therefore, insulin resistance is a condition with increased insulin concentrations. Once insulin-secreting β cells cannot cope with increased demand, T2DM develops. T2DM and insulin resistance are closely associated with hypercaloric food consumption and a sedentary life style in genetically predisposed persons. T2DM manifests typically at an age of 40–60 years [8]. According to the World Health Organization (WHO), International Diabetes Federation, and most National Diabetes Associations, diabetes should be diagnosed if fasting plasma glucose ≥7.0 mmol/L (126 mg/dL), 2-hour plasma glucose ≥11.1 mmol/L (200 mg/dL) following a 75-g oral glucose load, or glycated haemoglobin (HbA1c) ≥6.5%. Impaired glucose tolerance (IGT) should be diagnosed if the 2-hour plasma glucose lies between 7.8–11.1 mmol/L (140–200 mg/dL) following a 75-g oral glucose load and impaired fasting glucose (IFG) should be diagnosed if fasting plasma glucose lies between 6.1 and 6.9 mmol/L (110–125 mg/dL) and 2-hour plasma glucose < 7.8 mmol/L (140) following a 75-g oral glucose load.

Global burden of diabetes

Diabetes mellitus is among the most prevalent and severe chronic diseases, affecting the health of millions of people worldwide. According to the Global Burden of Disease (GBD) report for 2015, the prevalence of diabetes rose from approximately 333 million persons in 2005 to approximately 435 million persons in 2015, an increase of 30.6% [9]. In the same period, the annual number of deaths from diabetes rose from 1.2 million to 1.5 million [10,11]. This increase is attributed in the GBD report to population growth and aging, with small decreases in age-specific and cause-specific mortality over the same period.

In high-income countries, approximately 7% to 12% of patients with diabetes are estimated to have T1DM. The relative proportions of T1DM have not been studied in great detail in low- and middle-income countries. Globally, more than 540.000 children with an age between 0 and 14 years suffer from T1DM with 86.000 being newly diagnosed in 2015. In the USA, between 2002 and 2012, the adjusted annual incidence of T1DM increased by 1.8% per year. Among patients with T1DM, the rate of increase was highest among Hispanics [12]. In the WHO DIAMOND project [13] T1DM is most common in Scandinavian populations and in Sardinia and Kuwait, and much less common in Asia and Latin America [14]. Data are generally lacking for sub-Saharan Africa and large parts of Latin America. Over the past few decades the annual incidence appears to be rising steadily by about 3% in high-income countries [12,15].

Approximately 87% to 91% of all people with diabetes suffer from T2DM. According to the Non-communicable Disease Risk Factor Collaboration (NCD-RisC) report from 2016 [16], the number of adults with diabetes in the world was 422 million in 2014 with 28.5% due to the rise in prevalence, 39.7% due to population growth and aging, and 31.8% due to interaction of these two factors. Age-standardized adult diabetes prevalence in 2014 was lowest in northwestern Europe, and highest in Polynesia and Micronesia, at nearly 25%, followed by Melanesia, the Middle East, and north Africa. Exact numbers are given in Table 1.1.

Risk factors for T2DM

Regular physical activity reduces the risk of diabetes and raised blood glucose, and is an important contributor to overall energy balance, weight control, and obesity prevention—all risk factors linked to future diabetes. The global target of a 10% relative reduction in physical inactivity is therefore strongly associated with the global target of halting the increase in diabetes diagnoses. However, the prevalence of physical inactivity globally is of increasing concern. The most recent data from 2010 show that close to 25% of the US adult population did not meet the minimum recommendation for physical activity per week and were classified as insufficiently physically active [17]. Across all country income groups women were less active than men, with 27% of women and 20% of men classified as insufficiently physically active. Physical inactivity is alarmingly common among adolescents, with 84% of girls and 78% of boys not meeting minimum requirements for physical activity for this age. The prevalence of physical inactivity is highest in high-income countries where it is almost double that of low-income countries. The Eastern Mediterranean WHO Region showed the highest prevalence of inactivity in both adults and adolescents.

Being overweight or obese is strongly linked to diabetes. Despite the global voluntary target to halt the rise in obesity by 2025, excess weight or obesity has increased in almost all countries. In 2014, the latest year for which global estimates are available, more than one in three adults aged over 18 years were overweight and more than one in ten were obese with women being more overweight or obese than men. The prevalence of obesity was highest in the Americas and lowest in South-East Asia. The proportion of people who are overweight or obese increases with the level of income in a country. High- and middle-income countries have more than double the overweight and obesity rates of low-income countries.

Table 1.2 Age-adjusted values for major depressive disorders worldwide

	All-age DALYs (thousands)			Age-standardized rate (per 100,000)		
	2005	2015	Percentage change 2005-2015	2005	2015	Percentage change 2005-2015
Mental and substance use disorders	141,375.1 (105,843.7 to 178,447.3)	162,442.3 (121,032.0 to 205,579.7)	14.9 (14.1 to 15.7)*	2189.2 (1,646.0 to 2,762.8)	2183.3 (1,627.1 to 2,766.3)	−0.3 (−1.0 to 0.3)
Schizophrenia	13,185.0 (9,635.3 to 16 203.0	15 516.1 (11,279.2 to 19,137.0)	17.7 (16.5 to 18.8)*	210.4 (154.7 to 258.4)	207.5 (151.1 to 255.5)	−1.4 (−2.4 to −0.5)*
Alcohol use disorders	11,566.7 (9,617.6 to 13,834.9)	11,194.3 (9,136.5 to 13,870.9)	−3.2 (−7.0 to 0.6)	183.4 (153.5 to 218.3)	149.4 (122.1 to 184.8)	−18.5 (−22.0 to −15.1)*
Drug use disorders	13,671.4 (11,292.6 to 16,046.0	16 909.5 (14 037.6 to 19 871.6)	23.7 (18.6 to 27.2)*	207.2 (171.5 to 242.7)	223.5 (185.8 to 262.2)	7.9 (3.5 to 10.9)*
Opioid use disorders	9,864.0 (8,127.4 to 11,516.8)	12,068.1 (9,878.0 to 14,145.1)	22.3 (17.5 to 26.1)*	150.2 (123.7 to 175.3)	159.3 (130.7 to 186.6)	6.0 (1.8 to 9.2)*
Cocaine use disorders	729.3 (558.4 to 902.4)	999.3 (773.5 to 1,233.9)	37.0 (29.2 to 47.0)*	11.3 (8.7 to 14.0)	13.4 (10.4 to 16.6)	18.7 (12.1 to 27.3)*
Amphetamine use disorders	1,001.3 (706.2 to 1,348.3)	1,402.6 (1,025.2 to 1,846.9)	40.1 (26.1 to 55.2)*	14.6 (10.4 to 19.6)	18.4 (13.5 to 24.2)	25.8 (13.3 to 39.4)
Cannabis use disorders	548.1 (351.9 to 780.7)	577.2 (371.8 to 817.6)	5.3 (3.7 to 7.1)*	7.9 (5.0 to 11.2)	7.6 (4.9 to 10.7)	−3.7 (−5.0 to −2.3)*
Other drug use disorders	1,528.7 (1245.5 to 1,861.2)	1,862.2 (1501.6 to 2,274.2)	21.8 (15.7 to 27.5)*	23.1 (19.0 to 28.0)	24.8 (20.0 to 30.2)	7.1 (1.7 to 12.0)
Depressive disorders	45,916.0 (31,684.6 to 61,591.2)	54,255.4 (37,513.6 to 72,968.9)	18.2 (17.2 to 19.2)*	726.9 (503.8 to 975.9)	734.2 (508.2 to 986.9)	1.0 (0.5 to 1.5)*
Major depressive disorder	37,544.8 (24,983.0 to 51,134.6)	44,224.4 (29,542.6 to 60,430.5)	17.8 (16.6 to 19.0)*	590.9 (395.0 to 804.5)	597.2 (399.6 to 816.6)	1.1 (0.5 to 1.7)*
Dysthymia	8,371.3 (5,537.6 to 11,983.7)	10,031.0 (6,604.4 to 14,289.3)	19.8 (18.3 to 21.5)*	136.1 (89.8 to 194.6)	137.0 (90.0 to 195.3)	0.7 (−0.2 to 1.6)

*Percentage changes that are statistically significant.

Adapted from *The Lancet,* 388, GBD 2015 DALYs and HALE Collaborators, Global, regional, and national disability-adjusted life-years (DALYs) for 315 diseases and injuries and healthy life expectancy (HALE), 1990–2015: a systematic analysis for the Global Burden of Disease Study 2015, pp. 1603–1658, 2016. This article is available under the terms of the Creative Commons Attribution License (https://creativecommons.org/licenses/by/4.0/).

DALYs

Disability-adjusted life-years (DALYs) provide a summary measure of health. Global DALYs for diabetes increased from 50 million in 2005 to 64 million in 2015 [18]. Global age-adjusted DALY rate increased from 911 per 100,000 in 2005 to 926 per 100,000 in 2015, indicating an increase of 1.6% [18].

Complications and mortality

Diabetes, especially if not well controlled, may cause macrovascular complications which are namely cardiovascular disease (CVD), cerebrovascular disease, and peripheral vascular disease and microvascular complications, namely diabetic retinopathy leading to blindness, nephropathy leading to kidney failure, peripheral neuropathy leading to lower limb amputation, and several other long-term consequences that significantly impact quality of life. Emerging other complications include non-alcoholic fatty liver disease, cognitive impairment and dementia. There are no global estimates of diabetes-related end-stage renal disease, cardiovascular events, lower-extremity amputations, or pregnancy complications, although these conditions affect many people living with diabetes. Where data are available—mostly from high-income countries—prevalence, incidence, and trends vary hugely between countries [11,18].

Macrovascular complications

Adults with diabetes historically have a two or three times higher rate of CVD than adults without diabetes [11]. The risk of CVD increases continuously with rising fasting plasma glucose levels, even before reaching levels sufficient for a diabetes diagnosis. The few countries in north America, Scandinavia, and the UK that have studied time trends in the incidence of cardiovascular events (myocardial infarction, stroke, or CVD mortality) report large reductions over the past 20 years among people with type 1 or type 2 diabetes [11] although less than the reduction in the non-diabetic population. This decrease has been attributed to reduction in the prevalence of smoking and better management of diabetes and associated CVD risk factors.

Diabetic retinopathy

Diabetic retinopathy caused 1.9% of moderate or severe visual impairment and 2.6% of blindness globally in 2010 [19]. Studies suggest that prevalence of any retinopathy in persons with diabetes is 35% while proliferative (vision-threatening) retinopathy is 7% [20]. However, retinopathy rates are higher among people with T1DM, people with longer duration of diabetes, Caucasian populations, and possibly among people of lower socioeconomic status [20].

End-stage renal disease

Pooled data from 54 countries show that at least 80% of cases of end-stage renal disease (ESRD) are caused by diabetes, hypertension, or a combination of the two [21]. The proportion of ESRD attributable to diabetes alone ranges from 12% to 55%. The incidence of ESRD is up to ten times as high in adults with diabetes as in those without. The prevalence of ESRD is heavily dependent on access to dialysis and renal replacement therapy—both of which are highly variable between (and in some cases within) countries.

Lower extremity amputations

Diabetes appears to dramatically increase the risk of lower extremity amputation because of infected, non-healing foot ulcers [22]. Rates of amputation in populations with diagnosed diabetes are typically 10 to 20 times those of non-diabetic populations, and over the past decade have ranged from 1.5 to 3.5 events per 1,000 persons per year in populations with diagnosed diabetes. Encouragingly, several studies show a 40–60% reduction in rates of amputations among adults with diabetes during the past 10–15 years in the UK, Sweden, Denmark, Spain, the USA, and Australia [22]. No such data estimates exist for low- or middle-income countries.

In summary, the number of people in the world with diabetes has quadrupled since 1980. Population growth and aging have contributed to this increase, but are not solely responsible for it. The (age-standardized) prevalence of diabetes is growing in all regions. Global prevalence doubled from 1980 to 2014, mirroring a rise in overweight and obesity. Prevalence is growing most rapidly in low- and middle-income countries. Blood glucose levels begin to have an impact on morbidity and mortality even below the diagnostic threshold for diabetes. Diabetes and higher-than-optimal blood glucose together are responsible for 3.7 million annual deaths, many of which could be prevented.

Global burden of depression

A substantial proportion of the world's health problems in high-income countries (HICs) and low- and middle-income countries (LMICs) arises from mental, neurological, and substance use disorders [4,23] (Table 1.2). A major depressive disorder is different from usual mood fluctuations and short-lived emotional responses to challenges in everyday life. Especially when long-lasting and with moderate or severe intensity, depression may become a serious health condition. It can cause the affected person to suffer greatly and function poorly at work, at school, and in the family. At its worst, depression can lead to suicide. Close to 800 000 people die of suicide every year. Suicide is the second leading cause of death in 15–29-year-olds.

Depending on the number and severity of symptoms, a major depressive disorder is categorized as mild, moderate, or severe. Some major depressive disorders can be recurrent in nature. During major depressive episodes, the person experiences depressed mood, loss of interest and enjoyment, and reduced energy leading to diminished activity for at least 2 weeks. Many people with major depression also suffer from anxiety symptoms, disturbed sleep and appetite, may have feelings of guilt or low self-worth, poor concentration, and may even have physiologically inexplicable symptoms.

An individual with a mild depressive episode will have some difficulty in continuing with ordinary work and social activities, but will probably not cease to function completely. During a severe depressive episode, it is very unlikely that the sufferer will be able to continue with social, work, or domestic activities, except to a very limited extent. Major depressive disorder can also be part of a bipolar affective disorder. This type of major depression typically consists of both manic and depressive episodes separated by periods of normal mood. Manic episodes involve elevated or irritable mood, over-activity, pressure of speech, inflated self-esteem and a decreased need for sleep.

Contributing factors and prevention

Major depressive disorder results from a complex interaction of social, psychological, and biological factors. People who have gone through adverse life events (unemployment, bereavement, psychological trauma) are more likely to develop this disorder. Depression can, in turn, lead to more stress and dysfunction, and worsen the affected person's life situation and depression itself. Depression and physical health are interrelated: for example, diabetes and other chronic diseases can lead to depression and depression can increase the risk for developing diabetes or worsen the course of diabetes, which will be detailed in this book.

Global burden of depression

The GBD 2015 estimated the burden for 291 diseases and injuries and 67 risk factors and was the second comprehensive re-analysis of the burden since GBD 1990 and GBD 2010. Accordingly, mental and substance use disorders accounted for 162 million DALYs in 2015 an increase of 14.9% since 2005. Major depressive disorders accounted for 44 million DALYs in 2015, reflecting an increase of 17.8% since 2005 [18]. Exact numbers are given in Table 1.2.

Connection and global burden of diabetes and depression

Epidemiological studies and genetic studies observed that depression is more prevalent in people with diabetes, regardless of the fact if patients have diagnosed or undiagnosed diabetes. At the same time, anxiety disorder only seems to be present in subjects who are aware of their diabetes [5,24,25]. One explanation might be that the psychological burden of being ill plays an important role in triggering anxiety and depression. However, the fact that patients with previously undiagnosed diabetes have a higher prevalence of depression could also be explained by an unfavourable lifestyle, such as lack of physical activity, an unhealthy diet, or a stressful lifestyle, or another common background of both diseases.

Severe hypoglycaemia in patients with T2DM and without antidepressive treatment is positively associated with the severity of depressive symptoms, independent of glycaemic control, insulin therapy, lifestyle factors, and diabetic complications [26]. A meta-analysis estimating the association between depression and neuropathy in patients with T2DM could not clarify if the relationship is bidirectional or not [27]. A bidirectional interaction seems, thus, possible.

Diabetes can lead to structural changes in the brain: cerebral atrophy, as well as lacunar infarcts and blood flow changes of both hypo- and hyperperfusion. Reductions in brain volumes restricted to the hippocampus were found in patients with diabetes, while an inverse relationship between glycaemic control and hippocampal volume was present [28]. Similarly, depression is associated with neurodegenerative processes, especially at the level of the prefrontal cortex and hippocampus [29].

Vice versa, there is also an increased risk for patients with major depressive disorder to develop T2DM. Recent studies regarding the association between antidepressant use and glycaemic control show that in adults with diabetes, the use of multiple antidepressant subclasses significantly worsened blood glucose levels, suggesting that antidepressive treatment may be a risk factor for suboptimal glycaemic control [30]. In contrast, selective serotonin reuptake inhibitor treatment may improve the glycaemic control in depressed T2DM patients and is the only class of antidepressants with confirmed favourable effects on glycaemic control on both short and long term use [31].

To examine the effect of diabetes on the severity of depression, a study with over 200,000 depressed patients showed that comorbid diabetes may increase the risk of complications of depression, such as suicide and hospitalization [32].

Conclusion

The WHO and other organizations warn that there is 'a substantial gap between the burden caused by mental disorders and the resources available to prevent and treat them. It is estimated that four out of five people with serious mental disorders living in low and middle income countries do not receive the mental health services that they need' [33]. In patients with diabetes, depression remains underdiagnosed and an important aspect for the diabetic specialist is awareness of this common comorbidity. A multidisciplinary approach toward diabetic patients would help improve the outcomes of disease, decrease the number of DALYs, and even mortality.

References

1. **International Diabetes Federation**. *IDF Diabetes Atlas*, 7th edn. Brussels, Belgium: International Diabetes Federation, 2015.
2. **WHO**. *Global Report on Diabetes*. WHO: Geneva, 2016
3. **ADA**. Prevention or delay of type 2 diabetes. ADA *Diabetes Care* 2017;**40**(Suppl. 1): S44–7.
4. **WHO**. *Fact Sheet: Depression*. WHO: Geneva, 2017
5. **Kan C, Pedersen NL, Christensen K**, et al. Genetic overlap between type 2 diabetes and depression in Swedish and Danish twin registries. *Molecular Psychiatry* 2016;**21**:903–9.
6. **Mendenhall E, Kohrt BA, Norris SA, Ndetei D, Prabhakaran D**. Non-communicable disease syndemics: poverty, depression, and diabetes among low-income populations. *Lancet* 2017;**389**:951–63.
7. **Katsarou A, Gudbjörnsdottir S, Rawshani A**, et al. Type 1 diabetes mellitus. *Nature Reviews Disease Primers* 2017;**3**:17016.
8. **Hanefeld M, Pistrosch, Bornstein SR, Birkenfeld AL.** The metabolic vascular syndrome—guide to an individualized treatment *Reviews in Endocrine & Metabolic Disorders* 2016;**17**:5–17.
9. **GBD 2015 Disease and Injury Incidence and Prevalence Collaborators**. Global, regional, and national incidence, prevalence, and years live with disability for 310 diseases and injuries, 1990-2015: a systematic analysis for the Global Burden of Disease Study 2015. *Lancet* 2016;**388**:1545–602.
10. **GBD 2015 Mortality and Causes of Death Collaborators**. Global, regional, and national life expectancy, all-cause mortality, and cause-specific mortality for 249 causes of death, 1980-2015: a systematic analysis for the Global Burden of Disease Study 2015. *Lancet* 2016;**388**:1459–544.
11. **Rawshani A, Rawshani A, Franzén S**, et al. Mortality and cardiovascular disease in type 1 and type 2 diabetes. *New England Journal of Medicine* 2017;**376**:1407–18.
12. **Mayer-Davis EJ, Lawrence JM, Dabelea D**, et al. Incidence trends of type 1 and type 2 diabetes among youths, 2002-2012. *New England Journal of Medicine* 2017;**376**:1419–29.
13. **DIAMOND Project group incidence and trends of childhood type 1 diabetes worldwide, 1990-1999**. *Diabetes Medicine* 2006;**23**:857–66.

14. **Tuomilehto J.** The emerging global epidemic of type 1 diabetes. *Current Diabetes Reports* 2013;**13**:795–804.

15. **Patterson CC, Dahlquist GG, Gyurus E, Green A, Soltesz G.** EURODIAB Study Group Incidence trends for childhood type 1 diabetes in Europe during 1989–2003 and predicted new cases 2005–20: a multicentre prospective registration study. *Lancet* 2009;**373**:2027–33.

16. **NCD Risk Factor Collaboration (NCD-RisC).** Worldwide trends in diabetes since 1980: a pooled analysis of 751 population-based studies with 4.4 million participants. *Lancet* 2016;**387**:1513–30.

17. **Task Force on Community Preventive Services.** A recommendation to improve employee weight status through worksite health promotion programs targeting nutrition, physical activity or both. *American Journal of Preventive Medicine* 2009;**37**:358–9.

18. **GBD 2015 DALYs and HALE Collaborators.** Global, regional, and national disability-adjusted life-years (DALYs) for 315 diseases and injuries and healthy life expectancy (HALE), 1990-2015: a systematic analysis for the Global Burden of Disease Study 2015. *Lancet* 2016;**388**:1603–58.

19. **Bourne RR, Stevens GA, White RA**, et al. Causes of vision loss worldwide, 1990–2010: a systematic analysis. *Lancet Global Health* 2013;**1**:e339–49.

20. **Yau JW, Rogers SL, Kawasaki R**, et al. Global prevalence and major risk factors of diabetic retinopathy. *Diabetes Care* 2012;**35**:556–64.

21. **United States Renal Data System.** 2014 USRDS annual data report: epidemiology of kidney disease in the United States. National Institutes of Health, National Institute of Diabetes and Digestive and Kidney Diseases, Bethesda, MD, **2014**:188–210

22. **Moxey PW, Gogalniceanu P, Hinchliffe RJ**, et al. Lower extremity amputations—a review of global variability in incidence. *Diabetic Medicine* 2011;**28**:1144–53.

23. **Murray CJ, Vos T, Lozano R**, et al. Disability-adjusted life years (DALYs) for 291 diseases and injuries in 21 regions, 1990-2010: a systematic analysis for the Global Burden of Disease Study 2010. *Lancet* 2012;**380**:2163–96.

24. **Meurs M, Roest AM, Wolffenbuttel BH**, et al. Association of depressive and anxiety disorders with diagnosed versus undiagnosed diabetes: an epidemiological study of 90,686 participants. *Psychosomatic Medicine* 2016;**78**:233–41.

25. **Moulton CD, Pickup JC, Ismail K.** The link between depression and diabetes: the search for shared mechanisms. *Lancet Diabetes Endocrinol*ogy 2015;**3**:461–71.

26. **Kikuchi Y, Iwase M, Fujii H** et al. Association of severe hypoglycemia with depressive symptoms in patients with type 2 diabetes: the Fukuoka Diabetes Registry. *BMJ Open Diabetes Res Care* 2015;**3**:e000063.

27. **Bartoli F, Carra G, Crocamo C**, et al. Association between depression and neuropathy in people with type 2 diabetes: a meta-analysis. *International Journal of Geriatric Psychiatry* 2016;**31**:829–36.

28. **Gold SM, Dziobek I, Sweat V**, et al. Hippocampal damage and memory impairments as possible early brain complications of type 2 diabetes. *Diabetologia* 2007;**50**:711–19.

29. **Sapolsky RM.** Depression, antidepressants, and the shrinking hippocampus. *Proceedings of the National Academy of Sciences* 2001;**98**:12320–2.

30. **Rubin RR, Ma Y, Peyrot M**, et al. Antidepressant medicine use and risk of developing diabetes during the diabetes prevention program and diabetes prevention program outcomes study. *Diabetes Care* 2010;**33**:2549–51.

31. **Deuschle M.** Effects of antidepressants on glucose metabolism and diabetes mellitus type 2 in adults. *Current Opinions in Psychiatry* 2013;**26**:60–5.

32. **Kim GM, Woo JM, Jung SY**, et al. Positive association between serious psychiatric outcomes and complications of diabetes mellitus in patients with depressive disorders. *International Journal of Psychiatry in Medicine* 2015;**50**:131–46.

33. **WHO**. Mental health atlas 2015

34. **Golden SH, Lazo M, Carnethon M**, et al. Examining a bidirectional association between depressive symptoms and diabetes. *JAMA* 2008;**299**:2751–29.

Chapter 2

A life course approach to understanding the association between depression and type 2 diabetes

Khalida Ismail, Calum D. Moulton, Andrea Danese, and Brenda W. Penninx

Introduction

This chapter begins with a case scenario setting the scene as to how depression and type 2 diabetes might come to co-exist. This chapter also aims to synthesize some of the evidence, where available, for potential underlying mechanisms that are common to both depression and type 2 diabetes from gestation to end of life, and highlighting areas of poor understanding that need further elucidation through multidisciplinary research. The chapter is categorized into developmental stages along the lifespan where metabolic programming could be set or reset, especially during periods of rapid human growth such as *in utero*, the first years of life, and adolescence. The theoretical notion that metabolic programming is a dynamic and plastic process, initially set by our genetic order, and then constantly being reset, from *in utero* and early childhood experiences to adulthood, as it is being modified by stressors (biological and psychological) and protective processes, provides a life course perspective that may help to resolve the difficulties in separating the cause from the effect in the relationship between depression and type 2 diabetes. By examining the progression of metabolic programming, depression and then type 2 diabetes through the lifespan offers exciting new opportunities for innovative therapeutic directions and challenges that start early in life, which offer an optimism that perhaps the epidemic of type 2 diabetes can be stemmed.

Case scenario

Imagine the next type 2 diabetes patient in your clinic in an inner-city medical setting. There is a 1 in 10 chance that this patient will meet the criteria for depressive disorder [1]. If so, reviewing her medical records, she is likely to have presented with symptoms of depressive disorder or a related disorder in her 20s [2], to have a higher body mass index, to have been diagnosed with type 2 diabetes around 5 years earlier [3], and to have a higher level of activation of innate inflammation as measured by routine clinical tests such as C-reactive protein (CRP) than those of your patients with type 2 diabetes without a depressive disorder [3,4]. Looking further back into her early childhood medical records, her mother had gestational diabetes and probably postnatal depression that was not diagnosed. She was born as a high birthweight baby, requiring a short period of neonatal intensive care. Her childhood milieu was characterized by socioeconomic deprivation, physical abuse, and over-nutrition leading to childhood obesity. Her obesity continues into adulthood, she binged on food during adolescence and continues to comfort eat to this day. She has a sedentary desk job and persistently struggles to manage her workload. As a woman with type 2 diabetes, she is more likely to develop cardiovascular disease than males with type 2 diabetes [5].

The limitations of a bidirectional model of depression and type 2 diabetes

Over the past 10 years our understanding of the nature and construct of depression in type 2 diabetes has shifted. The bidirectional association between the two conditions is well established but the battle as to which condition is the primary causal factor and which is the outcome has not been 'won' by either; rather, it is being replaced with the notion of a vulnerability model that precedes, and is shared by both conditions.

The well-known increased prevalence of depression in type 2 diabetes used to be interpreted as a non-specific reactive psychological mechanism or response to the adjustment and burden of living with a chronic condition, as regularly observed in other long-term conditions. In the clinical scenario described earlier, the clinician would have described her depression as probably an understandable consequence of struggling to manage multiple diabetes self-care tasks. However, the epidemiological findings do not support this. Depressive symptoms at the time of onset of type 2 diabetes are not as strongly associated with worsening glycaemic control as previously thought [6]. The relative risk of developing a depressive disorder after the onset of type 2 diabetes is only 24% compared to the relative risk of developing type 2 diabetes following the onset of depressive disorder which is up to 60% [7,8] (Fig. 2.1). This repeated observation of a bidirectional association but with depression having a stronger effect suggests that the 'burden' of depression on metabolic

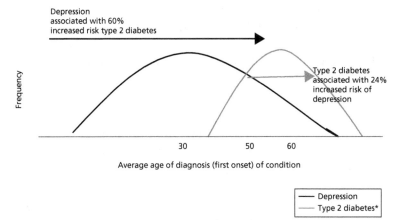

Fig. 2.1 Approximate distributions of age of onset of depression and type 2 diabetes and association between the two conditions. *The period of pre-diabetes and of symptomatic or aysmptomatic type 2 diabetes that precedes its diagnosis are not mapped in this graph.

Source data from: *Diabetes care*, 31, 12, Mezuk B, Eaton WW, Albrecht S, Golden SH., Depression and type 2 diabetes over the lifespan: a meta-analysis, pp. 2383–90, 2008; *Diabetologia*, 53, 12, Nouwen A, Winkley K, Twisk J, Lloyd CE, Peyrot M, Ismail K, et al., Type 2 diabetes mellitus as a risk factor for the onset of depression: a systematic review and meta-analysis, pp. 2480–246, 2010.

outcomes is greater and predates the 'burden' of type 2 diabetes on mental health. This is further supported by median age of onset of each condition; for depression, this is in young adult life with median ranges from the mid-20s to the mid-40s [2], which is around two decades earlier than the average age of diagnosis of type 2 diabetes.

In this second mechanism, depression, it is argued, leads to adopting diabetogenic lifestyles. However, more recent epidemiological findings go further to support the concept of third mechanism, namely a shared genetic and pathophysiological model suggesting 'starting points' earlier in the life course. For instance unhealthy lifestyles, psychosocial stress [2,9], and chronic inflammation [10] predate the onset of depressive disorders as well as of type 2 diabetes, and lifestyle and possibly anti-inflammatory interventions are effective for both [11–13].

A common inflammatory model

As described in more detail in subsequent chapters, chronic innate inflammation is a pathophysiological process that is increasingly recognized as common to depression, type 2 diabetes, and associated complications. In type 2 diabetes, chronic inflammation is well known to have wide-ranging multisystem effects such as β-cell apoptosis, insulin resistance in the periphery, and macrovascular complications [14–16]. Indeed, atherosclerosis is now viewed as a chronic inflammatory disease and inflammatory biomarkers such as CRP are used clinically and in research to help diagnose and monitor progression of cardiovascular disease [14,17].

The inflammation model of metabolism involves the initial acute stressor, which here will be circulating metabolic products released when homeostatic functioning and body's energy requirements is exceeded, followed by an acute adaptive immune response. For instance, adipocytes, which store energy, will grow as a healthy response to excess lipids initially until the endocrine system reaches its maximum load for hormesis, after which there is persistent release of excess metabolites, and the innate immunity is activated. Furthermore, increase in adipocytes triggers the secretion of pro-inflammatory cytokines. This process sets new levels for weight, blood levels of glucose, sympathetic tone, circulating levels of lipids, and ultimately manifestation in the form of cardiovascular disease and type 2 diabetes [18].

It is also possible that, in parallel and concurrently, the direction of travel of inflammation is from peripheral to central. There is now good evidence that peripheral inflammatory cytokines can communicate with the brain and lead to downregulation of serotonergic pathways, upregulation of glutamatergic pathways, and inhibition of adult neurogenesis, which may lead to subsequent depressive symptoms [19]. As in type 2 diabetes [3], elevated concentrations of circulating inflammatory cytokines are associated with increased risk of depressive symptoms in the general population [20]. Several clinical trials of anti-inflammatory medications have now reported positive effects on depressive symptoms [21]. As with atherosclerosis, inflammatory markers such as CRP have been proposed to predict clinical response to antidepressants that are known to have more potent anti-inflammatory properties [22,23].

In sum, elevated inflammation represents a promising mechanism by which both depression and type 2 diabetes could develop in parallel throughout the life course, and possible time points are explored chronologically (Fig. 2.2).

Stress versus depression

This book focuses on depression because this is what the patient suffers from clinically and this is the condition that clinicians aim to treat. It is important to consider its relationship to stress as there have been many observational studies of the relationship between stress and metabolic outcomes. For instance, in the

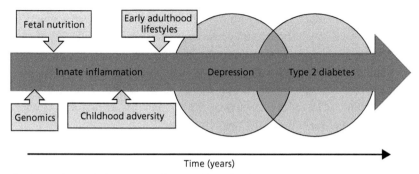

Fig. 2.2 A theoretical overview of potential mechanisms activating innate inflammation along the life course of the natural history of depression and type 2 diabetes.

Whitehall II cohort, accumulating exposure to low socioeconomic status from childhood to middle age was associated with increased risk of incident type 2 diabetes in adulthood. Nearly one-third of this was associated with chronically elevated inflammation, as measured using serum CRP and interleukin-6 [24]. A national cohort study of over 1.5 million military conscripts found that low resilience to stress in late adolescence was associated with a 1.5-fold increased risk of type 2 diabetes in later life, even after adjusting for body mass index, family history of diabetes, and socioeconomic factors [25].

There are many definitions of psychosocial stress. Here we understand psychosocial stress to be a component of the environment that contributes to the risk for developing depression. Stress is what the individual perceives based on his/her interpretation of their sensory inputs of their environment. This interpretation may be influenced by personality traits and early life modelling. Psychosocial stress is an umbrella term for many different environment stresses ranging from socioeconomic deprivation and occupational ranking, life events, abuse, and trauma. It is unclear to what extent the findings for depression and psychosocial stress are related or unrelated to each other.

Genetics

There has been momentum in the search for common genetic factors described in greater detail in Chapter 4. Current evidence suggests that there is a tentative case for common genetic basis for depression and type 2 diabetes. Twin studies have suggested a genetic overlap between type 2 diabetes and depression, implying that inherited DNA variants are important in the aetiology for this comorbidity [26]. Genome-wide association studies (GWAS) have shown that the inflammatory genetic pathways are implicated in the development of type 2 diabetes [27], although not consistently for depression [28–30]. As yet, GWAS have not detected a significant shared genetic component(s) for depression and type 2 diabetes. The reasons for the lack of evidence from GWAS may be due to heterogeneity in depression diagnoses across small studies, but with the availability of larger cohorts and new methodologies we may find stronger genetic associations between the two conditions [31].

If future research is able to identify a more robust evidence for a common genetic basis, what would be the function of these common genes? It is only speculation but potential candidate genes that have been proposed include those related to satiety and reward mechanisms, inflammatory response or clock genes controlling circadian rhythms, all of which might be common to both conditions [10]. Another mechanism that may be shared by depression and type 2 diabetes is epigenesis, which is a process that regulates the activity of DNA in the absence of induced DNA sequence change [32]. Epigenesis is likely to emerge as important as we learn more about how lifestyles and early-life stressors could affect gene expression and methylation patterns.

In utero

The rapid pace of human brain growth *in utero* is a very sensitive period vulnerable to insults at critical or sensitive periods of development, which may have lasting effects on metabolic programming. Events that trigger inflammatory processes *in utero* may impact on neurodevelopment of appetite and mood regulation setting the metabolic 'behaviour' of the young body. Extremes of birthweight outside the normal range, which is a proxy indicator of *in utero* nutrition, are known to be associated with onset of type 2 diabetes [33,34]. Whether low or high birthweight is associated with onset of depression is more controversial, although low birthweight shows an overall association with depression in later life [35].

The mechanisms by which extremes of birthweight may increase the risk for type 2 diabetes are likely to be multiple and interactive. Extremes of birthweight may alter early metabolic programming directly. For instance, babies of mothers with hyperglycaemia (gestational diabetes, type 2 diabetes, and pre-diabetes) have higher levels of circulating insulin and are more likely to experience neonatal hypoglycaemia. This could lead to wide-ranging neurodevelopmental damage (such as the satiety centre) and on pancreatic functioning [36]. Reduced breastfeeding and overfeeding from artificial supplements are common sequelae of extremes of birthweight and likely to adversely affect the setting of the metabolic pathways [37–39]. Excessive antibiotic use may change the gut microbiome [40] and may have a direct impact on neurogenesis [41]. Neonates with macrosomia are at risk of adverse physical health outcomes, including injuries and admission to intensive care [42]. Psychologically, extremes of birthweight interfere with normal maternal bonding and early attachment processes with caregivers [43].

Early childhood

Early childhood adversity, such as emotional, physical and sexual abuse, and emotional or physical neglect, bullying by peers, and other traumatic experiences are established powerful risk factors for adult depression, and a striking dose-dependent relationship between a number of adverse experiences and risk of adult depression is seen [44,45]. These childhood stressors may programme the brain towards low reward sensitivity and heightened threat reactivity, which in turn may predispose to depression [46]. In parallel, maltreatment in childhood has been shown in a number of different study designs to be associated with raised inflammation and hyperactivation of the hypothalamic–pituitary–adrenal axis in early adult life independently of other potential confounders [47,48].

Stress in children can activate an inflammatory response by triggering the sympathetic nervous system. With chronic stress, progressive reduction in the anti-inflammatory effects of glucocorticoids could maintain elevated inflammation levels [49]. As with its effects on later depression, childhood stress is associated with obesity and overweight in young adulthood and beyond [50,51]. In addition to direct physiological effects, inflammation levels may be elevated in chronically stressed children or young people because of behavioural mechanisms, including smoking, reduced exercise, and overeating [52,53]. Childhood obesity and overfeeding of children increase the risk of early-onset type 2 diabetes [54]. Obese children are more likely to be bullied, socially isolated, have low self-esteem [55], and are at greater risk for adolescence and early adulthood depression [56].

Adolescence and young adult life

The brain and the body are also rapidly developing during adolescence. Some adolescents may already carry the metabolic memory of their *in utero* and early childhood environment and may already start showing signs of pre-diabetes [57]. For other young people, it is during this stage that they experiment with their independence in their food, exercise, and substance use choices especially when under peer pressure and the food industry's marketing of readily available, energy-dense food. The peak age of onset of anxiety disorders and substance misuse disorders is in the teens [2], and unhealthy lifestyles that begin in adolescence are likely to persist and activate the chronic inflammatory response and adversely reset the metabolic programme.

Summary

The need to develop new strategies to overcome the obesity and type 2 diabetes epidemic has led scientists to study the multisystem consequences when metabolic homeostasis is breached across the life course. There is now accumulating evidence to question the construct of depression as only a psychological reaction to life events; rather, depression and type 2 diabetes may present clinically as different clinical endphenotypes but share common pathophysiological mechanisms that influence the level of activity of innate inflammation across the life course. If this is the case, then a new dawn of opportunities to deliver primary prevention at key developmental stages, namely *in utero*, early childhood and parenting, to the health of our adolescents, awaits us.

References

1. **Anderson RJ, Freedland KE, Clouse RE, Lustman PJ.** The prevalence of comorbid depression in adults with diabetes: a meta-analysis. *Diabetes Care* 2001;**24**:1069–78.
2. **Kessler RC, Amminger GP, Aguilar-Gaxiola S,** et al. Age of onset of mental disorders: a review of recent literature. *Current Opinion in Psychiatry* 2007;**20**:359–64.
3. **Laake JP, Stahl D, Amiel SA,** et al. The association between depressive symptoms and systemic inflammation in people with type 2 diabetes: findings from the South London Diabetes Study. *Diabetes Care* 2014;**37**:2186–92.
4. **Hayashino Y, Mashitani T, Tsujii S, Ishii H.** Elevated levels of hs-CRP are associated with high prevalence of depression in Japanese patients with type 2 diabetes: the Diabetes Distress and Care Registry at Tenri (DDCRT 6). *Diabetes Care* 2014;**37**:2459–65.
5. **Lyon A, Jackson EA, Kalyani RR,** et al. Sex-specific differential in risk of diabetes-related macrovascular outcomes. *Current Diabetes Reports* 2015;**15**:85.
6. **Ismail K, Moulton CD, Winkley K,** et al. The association of depressive symptoms and diabetes distress with glycaemic control and diabetes complications over 2 years in newly diagnosed type 2 diabetes: a prospective cohort study. *Diabetologia* 2017;**60**:2092–102.
7. **Mezuk B, Eaton WW, Albrecht S, Golden SH.** Depression and type 2 diabetes over the lifespan: a meta-analysis. *Diabetes Care* 2008;**31**:2383–90.
8. **Nouwen A, Winkley K, Twisk J,** et al. Type 2 diabetes mellitus as a risk factor for the onset of depression: a systematic review and meta-analysis. *Diabetologia* 2010;**53**:2480–6.
9. **Koopman RJ, Mainous AG, 3rd, Diaz VA, Geesey ME.** Changes in age at diagnosis of type 2 diabetes mellitus in the United States, 1988 to 2000. *Annals of Family Medicine* 2005;**3**:60–3.

10. **Moulton CD, Pickup JC, Ismail K.** The link between depression and diabetes: the search for shared mechanisms. *Lancet Diabetes & Endocrinology* 2015;**3**:461–71.

11. **Rimer J, Dwan K, Lawlor DA,** et al. Exercise for depression. *Cochrane Database of Systematic Reviews* 2012;**11**:CD004366.

12. **Knowler WC, Barrett-Connor E, Fowler SE,** et al. Reduction in the incidence of type 2 diabetes with lifestyle intervention or metformin. *New England Journal of Medicine* 2002;**346**:393–403.

13. **Moulton CD, Pickup JC, Amiel SA, Winkley K, Ismail K.** Investigating incretin-based therapies as a novel treatment for depression in type 2 diabetes: findings from the South London Diabetes (SOUL-D) Study. *Primary Care Diabetes* 2016;**10**:156–9.

14. **Viola J, Soehnlein O.** Atherosclerosis—a matter of unresolved inflammation. *Seminars in Immunology* 2015;**27**:184–93.

15. **Pickup JC.** Inflammation and activated innate immunity in the pathogenesis of type 2 diabetes. *Diabetes Care* 2004;**27**:813–23.

16. **Yirmiya R, Rimmerman N, Reshef R.** Depression as a microglial disease. *Trends in Neurosciences* 2015;**38**:637–58.

17. **Sabatine MS, Morrow DA, Jablonski KA,** et al. Prognostic significance of the Centers for Disease Control/American Heart Association high-sensitivity C-reactive protein cut points for cardiovascular and other outcomes in patients with stable coronary artery disease. *Circulation* 2007;**115**:1528–36.

18. **Donath MY.** Targeting inflammation in the treatment of type 2 diabetes: time to start. *Nature reviews Drug Discovery* 2014;**13**:465–76.

19. **Dantzer R, O'Connor JC, Freund GG,** et al. From inflammation to sickness and depression: when the immune system subjugates the brain. *Nature Reviews Neuroscience* 2008;**9**:46–56.

20. **Pasco JA, Nicholson GC, Williams LJ,** et al. Association of high-sensitivity C-reactive protein with *de novo* major depression. *British Journal of Psychiatry* 2010;**197**:372–7.

21. **Kohler O, Benros ME, Nordentoft M,** et al. Effect of anti-inflammatory treatment on depression, depressive symptoms, and adverse effects: a systematic review and meta-analysis of randomized clinical trials. *JAMA Psychiatry* 2014;**71**:1381–91.

22. **Uher R, Tansey KE, Dew T,** et al. An inflammatory biomarker as a differential predictor of outcome of depression treatment with escitalopram and nortriptyline. *American Journal of Psychiatry* 2014;**171**:1278–86.

23. **Strawbridge R, Arnone D, Danese A,** et al. Inflammation and clinical response to treatment in depression: a meta-analysis. *European Neuropsychopharmacology* 2015;**25**:1532–43.

24. **Stringhini S, Batty GD, Bovet P,** et al. Association of lifecourse socioeconomic status with chronic inflammation and type 2 diabetes risk: the Whitehall II prospective cohort study. *PLoS Medicine* 2013;**10**:e1001479.

25. **Crump C, Sundquist J, Winkleby MA, Sundquist K.** Stress resilience and subsequent risk of type 2 diabetes in 1.5 million young men. *Diabetologia* 2016;**59**:728–33.

26. **Kan C, Pedersen NL, Christensen K,** et al. Genetic overlap between type 2 diabetes and depression in Swedish and Danish twin registries. *Molecular Psychiatry* 2016;**21**:903–9.

27. **Mahajan A, Go MJ, Zhang W**, et al. Genome-wide trans-ancestry meta-analysis provides insight into the genetic architecture of type 2 diabetes susceptibility. *Nature Genetics* 2014;**46**:234–44.

28. **Ripke S, Wray NR, Lewis CM**, et al. A mega-analysis of genome-wide association studies for major depressive disorder. *Molecular Psychiatry* 2013;**18**:497–511.

29. Psychiatric genome-wide association study analyses implicate neuronal, immune and histone pathways. *Nature Neuroscience* 2015;**18**:199–209.

30. **Jansen R, Penninx BW, Madar V**, et al. Gene expression in major depressive disorder. *Molecular Psychiatry* 2016;**21**:339–47.

31. **Bulik-Sullivan B, Finucane HK, Anttila V**, et al. An atlas of genetic correlations across human diseases and traits. *Nature Genetics* 2015;**47**:1236–41.

32. **Yang BZ, Zhang H, Ge W**, et al. Child abuse and epigenetic mechanisms of disease risk. *American Journal of Preventive Medicine* 2013;**44**:101–7.

33. **Zimmermann E, Gamborg M, Sorensen TI, Baker JL**. sex differences in the association between birth weight and adult type 2 diabetes. *Diabetes* 2015;**64**:4220–5.

34. **Harder T, Rodekamp E, Schellong K**, et al. Birth weight and subsequent risk of type 2 diabetes: a meta-analysis. *American Journal of Epidemiology* 2007;**165**:849–57.

35. **Loret de Mola C, de Franca GV, Quevedo Lde A, Horta BL**. Low birth weight, preterm birth and small for gestational age association with adult depression: systematic review and meta-analysis. *British Journal of Psychiatry* 2014;**205**:340–7.

36. **Ross MG, Desai M**. Developmental programming of offspring obesity, adipogenesis, and appetite. *Clinical Obstetrics and Gynecology* 2013;**56**:529–36.

37. **Verd S, Barriuso L, Gich I**, et al. Risk of early breastfeeding cessation among symmetrical, small for gestational age infants. *Annals of Human Biology* 2013;**40**:146–51.

38. **Aaltonen J, Ojala T, Laitinen K**, et al. Impact of maternal diet during pregnancy and breastfeeding on infant metabolic programming: a prospective randomized controlled study. *European Journal of Clinical Nutrition* 2011;**65**:10–9.

39. **Finkelstein SA, Keely E, Feig DS**, et al. Breastfeeding in women with diabetes: lower rates despite greater rewards. A population-based study. *Diabetic Medicine* 2013;**30**:1094–101.

40. **Gibson MK, Crofts TS, Dantas G**. Antibiotics and the developing infant gut microbiota and resistome. *Current Opinion in Microbiology* 2015;**27**:51–6.

41. **Rogers GB, Keating DJ, Young RL**, et al. From gut dysbiosis to altered brain function and mental illness: mechanisms and pathways. *Molecular Psychiatry* 2016;**21**:738–48.

42. **Kc K, Shakya S, Zhang H**. Gestational diabetes mellitus and macrosomia: a literature review. *Annals of Nutrition & Metabolism* 2015;**66**(Suppl. 2):14–20.

43. **Wolke D, Eryigit-Madzwamuse S, Gutbrod T**. Very preterm/very low birthweight infants' attachment: infant and maternal characteristics. *Archives of Disease in Childhood Fetal and Neonatal Edition* 2014;**99**:F70–5.

44. **Kessler RC, McLaughlin KA, Green JG**, et al. Childhood adversities and adult psychopathology in the WHO World Mental Health Surveys. *British Journal of Psychiatry* 2010;**197**:378–85.

45. **Chapman DP, Whitfield CL, Felitti VJ**, et al. Adverse childhood experiences and the risk of depressive disorders in adulthood. *Journal of Affective Disorders* 2004;**82**:217–25.

46. **Danese A, Baldwin JR.** Hidden Wounds? Inflammatory Links Between Childhood Trauma and Psychopathology. *Annual Review of Psychology* 2017;**68**:517–44.

47. **Danese A, Pariante CM, Caspi A,** et al. Childhood maltreatment predicts adult inflammation in a life-course study. *Proceedings of the National Academy of Sciences of the United States of America* 2007;**104**:1319–24.

48. **Ouellet-Morin I, Odgers CL, Danese A,** et al. Blunted cortisol responses to stress signal social and behavioral problems among maltreated/bullied 12-year-old children. *Biological Psychiatry* 2011;**70**:1016–23.

49. **Horowitz MA, Zunszain PA, Anacker C,** et al. Glucocorticoids and inflammation: a double-headed sword in depression? How do neuroendocrine and inflammatory pathways interact during stress to contribute to the pathogenesis of depression? *Modern Trends in Pharmacopsychiatry* 2013;**28**:127–43.

50. **Baldwin JR, Arseneault L, Odgers C,** et al. Childhood bullying victimization and overweight in young adulthood: a cohort study. *Psychosomatic Medicine* 2016;**78**:1094–103.

51. **Danese A, Tan M.** Childhood maltreatment and obesity: systematic review and meta-analysis. *Molecular Psychiatry* 2014;**19**:544–54.

52. **Duivis HE, Kupper N, Vermunt JK,** et al. Depression trajectories, inflammation, and lifestyle factors in adolescence: the TRacking Adolescents' Individual Lives Survey. *Health Psychology* 2015;**34**:1047–57.

53. **Montero D, Walther G, Perez-Martin A,** et al. Endothelial dysfunction, inflammation, and oxidative stress in obese children and adolescents: markers and effect of lifestyle intervention. *Obesity Reviews* 2012;**13**:441–55.

54. **Pulgaron ER, Delamater AM.** Obesity and type 2 diabetes in children: epidemiology and treatment. *Current Diabetes Reports* 2014;**14**:508.

55. **Greenleaf C, Petrie TA, Martin SB.** Relationship of weight-based teasing and adolescents' psychological well-being and physical health. *Journal of School Health* 2014;**84**:49–55.

56. **Gibson LY, Allen KL, Davis E,** et al The psychosocial burden of childhood overweight and obesity: evidence for persisting difficulties in boys and girls. *European Journal of Pediatrics* 2017;**176**:925–33.

57. **Tam WH, Ma RC, Yang X,** et al. Glucose intolerance and cardiometabolic risk in adolescents exposed to maternal gestational diabetes: a 15-year follow-up study. *Diabetes Care* 2010;**33**:1382–4.

Chapter 3

MicroRNAs as novel biomarkers in depression, diabetes, and cardiovascular diseases

Mohamad M. Almedawar,
Richard C. Siow, and Henning Morawietz

Depression, diabetes, and cardiovascular diseases

The three leading causes of burden of disease in 2030 are projected to include depressive disorders and cardiovascular diseases (CVDs) [1]. In diabetic patients, symptoms of depression have been associated with increased clinical complications [2]. In addition, diabetes mellitus is a major risk factor of CVD [3]. The 'vascular depression' hypothesis suggests that cardiovascular disease can cause, predispose to, or aggravate depression [4]. Several studies have found a strong correlation between depression and pre-existing vascular diseases. Other studies examined vascular disease in pre-existing depression and found an increase in vascular risk factors and a negative impact on prognosis in ischaemic heart disease [5]. Recent studies implicate that microvascular dysfunction is involved in the pathophysiology of depression [6]. In addition, microRNAs (miRs) are potent regulators of gene expression in physiological and pathophysiological processes affecting the microcirculation [7]. We propose that an interaction between diabetes mellitus, depression and cardiovascular diseases involving changes in microcirculation and miR expression pattern exist (Fig. 3.1). Biomarkers would be helpful tools to identify patients at risk to develop clinical complications.

Screening for depression in pre-existing cardiovascular diseases

Screening for major depressive disorder (MDD) in CVD patients has been done mainly through diagnostic interviews or self-reporting methods such as surveys. In addition, novel biomarkers are suggested as screening tools for subjects determined to be at risk to suffer from MDD.

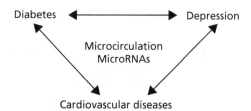

Fig. 3.1 Vicious cycle of diabetes, depression and cardiovascular diseases involving microcirculation and microRNAs.

Surveys and questionnaires

The use of self-report questionnaires to screen and diagnose MDD in CVD patients is quite common in the literature. Many validated questionnaires exist for that purpose. They vary according to sensitivity, specificity, and cut-off scores. Examples include the Patient Health Questionnaire (PHQ), Beck Depression Inventory (BDI) [8], Hospital Anxiety Depression Scale (HADS) [9], Cardiac Depression Scale (CDS) [10], and the Center for Epidemiologic Studies Depression Scale-10 (CES-D) [11]. Questionnaires that have been used in studies assessing MDD in CVD patients include the 1-year Hamilton (HAM-D) score [12], Present State Examination (PSE) [13], Diagnostic and Statistical Manual of Mental Disorders, 3rd edition (DSM-IIIR) [14], and the World Health Organization's International Classification of Diseases (ICD10) [15].

Hospital- and community-based studies also assessed the prevalence of MDD using the Diagnostic Interview Schedule (DIS). The validity of this schedule is confirmed in medical settings [16]. The DIS was used for patients with post myocardial infarction (MI) and diagnosed 16–20% of patients with MDD, a large increase compared with population rates of 3%. In fact, cardiac mortality has been both predicted and shown to be increased in MDD patients of both men and women by three and a half times even after adjusting for confounding factors. On the other hand, cardiac mortality was reduced in patients after commencing antidepressant administration [17], namely selective reuptake inhibitors [18]. Even higher rates of MDD were reported using DSM-IIIR and ICD-10 diagnostic questionnaires in patients shortly after an ischaemic stroke, with rates in hospital and community samples reaching 27% of the studied sample, and up to 40% after 4–12 months [19,20].

CVD risk factors including hypertension and diabetes have been associated with increased risk of concurrent MDD. Hypertensive patients have been found to be three times more likely to have MDD [21], whereas MDD rates in patients with diabetes ranged between 14% and 32% in cross-sectional, case-controlled studies [22]. It is also worth noting that although it has been theorized that lower cholesterol levels might lead to depression through a reduction of serotonergic receptors, studies couldn't find a positive clinical association made between low cholesterol and MDD.

Although these questionnaires have been validated, discrepancies and weak agreement have risen ever since they have been compared with clinical diagnoses by psychiatrists using the Schedules for Clinical Assessment in Neuropsychiatry (SCAN) [23]. Hence, screening for MDD requires novel objective assessments and biomarkers.

Novel biomarkers

Serum proteins, extracellular vesicles, and nucleotides in the blood are easily accessible potential biomarkers for disease diagnosis and prognosis. An established link exists between serum markers of systemic inflammation and diabetes mellitus [24] and CVD [25]. Systemic inflammation has also been associated with MDD leading to the inflammation hypothesis of depression. It explains the association of MDD with an increased level of serum pro-inflammatory cytokines and acute-phase proteins due to chronic activation of the innate immune system [26]. A recent cumulative meta-analysis by Haapakoski et al. [21] confirmed that increased levels of circulating interleukin (IL)-6 and C-reactive protein (CRP) are significantly associated with depression, based on 51 independent studies with moderate heterogeneity. Studies examining the inflammatory markers IL-1β and tumor necrosis factor (TNF)-α had high to excessive heterogeneity and hence no significant association was made between their serum levels and the incidence of MDD. In these cohort studies, persistent high concentrations of IL-6 and CRP in the blood were associated with a high risk of developing mental disorders and MDD [27]. For example, Kivimäki et al. [28] measured serum IL-6 in 4,630 adults from the Whitehall II cohort study 3 times over a period of 11 years in parallel with three psychiatric evaluations based on the General Health Questionnaire (GHQ). The evaluations ended 16 years after the initial assessment. The initial cross-sectional analysis from the first assessment showed IL-6 not to be associated with common mental disorder (a broad term including depression). However, when the 10-year risk of common mental disorder was later assessed in 2,757 participants without the disorder at the first GHQ assessment, they found that those who had a high IL-6 blood distribution (>2.0 pg/mL), had an odds ratio (OR) of 1.40 to develop common mental disorder. What's more interesting is that those patients who had chronic inflammation, high IL-6 levels in two and three consecutive assessments, had higher ORs of 1.61 and 1.75, respectively. Adjustments for acute inflammation, obesity, smoking, and drug treatments did not affect the association between the 5-year average level of IL-6 and the 10-year risk of common mental disorder. In addition, no gender-specific statistical difference was detected. It is also important to note that the study is limited by the use of questionnaires to assess common mental disorder instead of a clinical diagnosis of depression [28]. In an earlier report, the same group demonstrated the ability of CRP and IL-6 levels to predict cognitive symptoms of depression, but not vice versa [29]. Similar associations for IL-6 were found in young adults in the Avon Longitudinal Study of Parents and Children (ALSPAC). High serum IL-6 levels at the age of 9 years could predict the participants who would suffer from MDD at an age of 18 years [30]. Although these markers have been repeatedly used as predictors of MDD, they are also increased due to acute inflammation and might bias the screening if not assessed along with multiple measurements to confirm the chronic aspect. In addition, elevated aldosterone levels have been described in diabetes and cardiovascular diseases in experimental and clinical studies [31]. Mineralocorticoid receptor antagonists are beneficial in cardiovascular diseases, but their value in the treatment of diabetes is under discussion [32]. Hence, additional screening of other MDD-specific biomarkers such as miRs would help to improve the detection of patients at risk.

MicroRNAs

MiRs are a class of short non-coding RNAs that regulate the expression of genes by binding to the 3′-untranslated region or mRNAs and either inhibiting translation or initiating the degradation of the bound mRNA. Several studies detected dysregulated expression levels of miRs in the brain of MDD patients [33,34], whereas others have suggested using several miRs as prospective MDD biomarkers that are dysregulated in the serum and cerebrospinal fluid (CSF) of MDD patients including elevated miR-221-3p, miR-34a-5p, and let-7d-3p, and reduced miR-451a levels [35]. In the brain, miR-124 is the most abundantly expressed miR [36] and can be mainly found in neurons [37]. It has also been found to be expressed in microglia and to play an anti-inflammatory role by inducing microglia quiescence and inhibiting the production of pro-inflammatory cytokines. More specifically, miR-124 targets the signal transducer and activator of transcription 3 (STAT3), causing a decrease in IL-6 production [38]. Inhibition of miR-124a, however, has been found to mediate antidepressant-like effects in rat models of MDD [39]. In addition, a recent study designated miR-124-3p as a putative epigenetic signature of MDD [40]. In that study, a rat model of MDD showed an upregulation of miR-124-3p in the prefrontal cortex (PFC) and a consequent downregulation of eight of its target genes relevant to the pathogenesis of MDD. They include heat shock protein 90ab1 (*Hsp90ab1*), *Akt1* substrate1 (*Akt1s1*), glucocorticoid receptor (*Nr3c1*), mineralocorticoid receptor (*Nr3c2*), *Gria3*, *Gria4* (members of AMPA receptor family), and *Grin2a* and *Grin2b*

(NMDA receptor family members). The increased expression of miR-124-3p was attributed to hypomethylation of its gene promoter. These results were confirmed by post-mortem analysis of the PFC of MDD subjects. The authors also found that antidepressants had no impact on the expression of miR-124-3p or target genes. More interestingly, expression of serum miR-124-3p was ~3.5-fold higher in MDD patients than in controls, making it a desirable biomarker for MDD screening [41]. In fact, miR-30a-5p, miR-34a-5p, and miR-221 are three of 16 miRs reported to be downregulated in the hippocampus of MDD patients after chronic administration of antidepressant medications (lithium and valproate) [42]. These miRs target serotonin receptors (HTR2C), corticotrophin-releasing hormone receptor (CRHR1), and glutamate transporters (SCL1A2) which play pivotal roles in MDD pathology. In another study, the serum and brain expression level of miR-1202 has been shown to be decreased in MDD with implications for the response of patients to antidepressants. The decrease in miR-1202 leads to an increase in its target gene, the metabotropic glutamate receptor-4 (GRM4). The expression of GRM4 is found in the whole brain and mainly situated in the pre- and post-synapses. It regulates dopaminergic, glutamatergic, GABAergic, and serotonergic neurotransmission, making it an essential regulator of mood disorders and anxiety-related behaviours [43] and an appealing therapeutic target [44]. Serum miRs can be found either bound to the argonaute (ago2) or nucleophosmin (NPM) proteins, inside apoptotic bodies, high-density lipoproteins (HDL), or extracellular vesicles (EVs) such as microvesicles and exosomes. The role of miRs in the stress-related pathology of depressive disorders is summarized in Fig. 3.2.

The microglia and neurons have been also recently shown to release EVs that carry proteins, mRNA, and miRs. EVs play a dual role: as biomarkers of disease states and in cell–cell communication [45]. The microglia is a key structure in the brain, and its abnormal activation and increase in cell number, as well as decrease, has been associated with depression [46]. In fact, depression has been recently classified as a microglia-associated disorder, supporting the important role these cells play in the pathology of disease. Activated microglia having a proinflammatory phenotype release inflammatory cytokines that contribute to neuro-inflammation and activate compensatory tissue repair [47]. Microvesicles secreted by activated microglia after induction with ATP have been recently shown to play a role in neuro-inflammation by disseminating inflammatory factors such as IL-1β, caspase-1, and the P2X7 receptor [45,48]. One study revealed that exposure of microglia to serotonin from neurons activated the microglia and induced the release of exosomes, although that study did not explore the functional relevance of this release [50]. Low serotonin levels in patients are associated with MDD [51] and are involved in the mechanisms

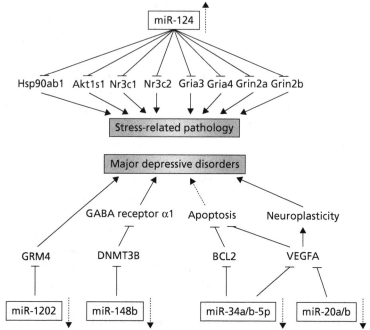

Fig. 3.2 Role of microRNAs in the stress-related pathology of depressive disorders. The proposed scheme is based on findings in references [34,49,64–68]. Akt1s1, AKT1 substrate 1; BCL2, B-cell lymphoma 2; DNMT3B, DNA methyltransferase 3 beta; GABA, gamma-aminobutyric acid; Gria, glutamate ionotropic receptor AMPA type subunit; GRM4, Glutamate receptor 4, metabotropic; Hsp90ab1, heat shock protein 90 alpha family class B member 1; MiR, microRNA; Nr3c, Nuclear receptor subfamily 3 group C member; VEGFA, vascular endothelial growth factor A.

of depression [52]. It is possible that the M2 phenotype of activated microglia is induced by serotonin and inhibits inflammation while restoring homeostasis. Hence, the lower levels of serotonin in MDD patients reduce the release of exosomes from the microglia, disrupting intracellular protein and RNA homeostasis and inducing pathological outcomes [53]. Taken together, these studies promise a variety of screening possibilities to improve the detection of MDD in CVD patients, especially in a combined assessment of psychological and clinical symptoms.

Screening for vascular disease in pre-existing depression

Prospective studies have examined the risk of CVD morbidity and mortality in patients with diagnosed MDD and found it to be two to three times higher than subjects not suffering from MDD [54]. Similarly, the risk for developing diabetes mellitus was also higher among patients suffering from MDD [55]. This underlines the importance of screening for vascular disease in patients with MDD, which has been mainly done through clinical examinations, neuroimaging, and neuropathology, as listed in order of increasing sensitivity of detecting vascular disease.

Clinical examinations

Evidence from the literature regarding increased vascular risk factors in patients with depression has been contradictory. However, several studies reporting no significant association between vascular risk factors and depression did not examine differences in the age at onset of disease and did not follow up the subjects after baseline assessment [56]. The importance of these factors is illustrated in two studies. The first by Baldwin and Tomenson [57] reported a 4.5-fold increase in vascular disease risk factors in patients with late-onset versus early-onset depression, even after adjustment for age . In another study, no association was detected between patients with depression and cerebrovascular risk factors and scores at the baseline assessment, but a significant and independent association of vascular risk factors with depression and sub-syndromic depression was found after a 1-year follow-up [58]. Still, the vascular risk factors examined in these studies were all related to stroke risk and not sensitive to other cerebrovascular or hypotensive diseases that have been associated with cognitive decline [59].

Neuroimaging

One symptom often detected with magnetic resonance imaging in patients with depression is an increase in signal hyperintensities in the white and grey matter, accompanied by lesions in the basal ganglia and frontal cortex. These symptoms appear to result from cardiovascular disease, whereby vascular risk factors and diseases including ischaemia could predict the severity of these hyperintensities. The studies examining white and grey matter hyperintensities found a severe increase primarily in the basal ganglia, in addition to a higher number of lesions in patients diagnosed with depression, especially in the late-onset group [60]. However, in most studies, periventricular lesions didn't correlate with depression. These associations have also been confirmed in community studies [61].

Neuropathology

Inflammation is a hallmark of vascular disease and inflammatory markers have also been found to be increased in the vessels of patients with depression. A post-mortem study found an increase in intracellular adhesion molecule-1 (ICAM-1) and vascular cell adhesion molecule-1 (VCAM-1) in cerebral vessels indicating post-ischaemic inflammation [62]. These findings were subclinical as the subjects didn't show vascular risk factors, suggesting a higher detection rate when examining inflammatory markers.

Implications for therapy

According to the 'vascular depression' hypothesis, the therapy for MDD itself could reduce the burden of CVD outcomes. However, in a recent meta-analysis, the changes in CVD outcomes were not significant after screening and treatment of patients with MDD [63]. Therefore, improvement of CVD outcomes in MDD patients must be approached with a combined therapy of MDD and CVD guided by multidisciplinary screening modules. MiRs might be novel biomarkers and helpful tools to identify MDD patients at risk to develop clinical complications. Moreover, identification of novel therapeutic targets to modulate miRs may represent a strategy for reducing the incidence and severity of both CVD and MDD.

References

1. **Mathers CD, Loncar D.** Projections of global mortality and burden of disease from 2002 to 2030. *PLoS Medicine* 2006;**3**:e442.

2. **Reichel A, Schwarz J, Schulze J**, et al. Depression and anxiety symptoms in diabetic patients on continuous subcutaneous insulin infusion (CSII). *Molecular Psychiatry* 2005;**10**:975–6.

3. **Nathan DM.** Diabetes: advances in diagnosis and treatment. *Journal of the American Medical Association* 2015;**314**:1052–62.

4. **Taylor WD, Aizenstein HJ, Alexopoulos GS.** The vascular depression hypothesis: mechanisms linking vascular disease with depression. *Molecular Psychiatry* 2013;**18**:963–74.

5. **Whiteford HA, Degenhardt L, Rehm J**, et al. Global burden of disease attributable to mental and substance use disorders: findings from the Global Burden of Disease Study 2010. *Lancet* 2013;**382**:1575–86.

6. **van Agtmaal MJM, Houben A, Pouwer F**, et al. Association of microvascular dysfunction with late-life depression: a systematic review and meta-analysis. *JAMA Psychiatry* 2017;**74**:729–39.

7. **Siow RC, Clough GF.** Spotlight issue: microRNAs in the microcirculation-from cellular mechanisms to clinical markers. *Microcirculation* 2012;**19**:193–5.

8. **Beck AT, Ward CH, Mendelson M**, et al. An inventory for measuring depression. *Archives of General Psychiatry* 1961;**4**:561–71.

9. **Zigmond AS, Snaith RP.** The hospital anxiety and depression scale. *Acta Psychiatrica Scandinavica* 1983;**67**:361–70.

10. **Shi WY, Stewart AG, Hare DL.** Major depression in cardiac patients is accurately assessed using the cardiac depression scale. *Psychotherapy and Psychosomatics* 2010;**79**:391–2.

11. **Andresen EM, Malmgren JA, Carter WB, Patrick DL.** Screening for depression in well older adults: evaluation of a short form of the CES-D (Center for Epidemiologic Studies Depression Scale). *American Journal of Preventive Medicine* 1994;**10**:77–84.

12. **Hamilton M.** A rating scale for depression. *Journal of Neurology, Neurosurgery, and Psychiatry* 1960;**23**:56–62.

13. **Wing J, Cooper J, Sartorius N.** *The Measurement and Classification of Psychiatric Syndromes.* Cambridge, UK: Cambridge University Press, 1974.

14. **Kendell RE.** Diagnostic and Statistical Manual of Mental-Disorders, 3rd Edition *American Journal of Psychiatry* 1980;**137**(12):1630–1.

15. **WHO.** *International Classification of Diseases and Health Related Problems.* WHO: Geneva, 1992. http://www.who.int/classifications/icd/en/ (accessed 10 April 2017).

16. **Robins LN, Helzer JE, Croughan J, Ratcliff KS.** National institute of mental health diagnostic interview schedule: its history, characteristics, and validity. *Archives of General Psychiatry* 1981;**38**:381–9.

17. **Weeke A, Juel K, Vaeth M.** Cardiovascular death and manic-depressive psychosis. *Journal of Affective Disorders* 1987;**13**:287–92.

18. **Sauer WH, Berlin JA, Kimmel SE.** Selective serotonin reuptake inhibitors and myocardial infarction. *Circulation* 2001;**104**:1894–8.

19. **Pohjasvaara T, Leppavuori A, Siira I,** et al. Frequency and clinical determinants of poststroke depression. *Stroke* 1998;**29**:2311–7.

20. **Vataja R, Pohjasvaara T, Leppavuori A,** et al. Magnetic resonance imaging correlates of depression after ischemic stroke. *Archives of General Psychiatry* 2001;**58**:925–31.

21. **Rabkin JG, Charles E, Kass F.** Hypertension and DSM-III depression in psychiatric outpatients. *American Journal of Psychiatry* 1983;**140**:1072–4.

22. **Gavard JA, Lustman PJ, Clouse RE.** Prevalence of depression in adults with diabetes. An epidemiological evaluation. *Diabetes Care* 1993;**16**:1167–78.

23. **Eaton WW, Neufeld K, Chen LS, Cai G.** A comparison of self-report and clinical diagnostic interviews for depression: diagnostic interview schedule and schedules for clinical assessment in neuropsychiatry in the Baltimore epidemiologic catchment area follow-up. *Archives of General Psychiatry* 2000;**57**:217–22.

24. **Pradhan AD, Manson JE, Rifai N,** et al. C-reactive protein, interleukin 6, and risk of developing type 2 diabetes mellitus. *Journal of the American Medical Association* 2001;**286**:327–34.

25. **Danesh J, Kaptoge S, Mann AG,** et al. Long-term interleukin-6 levels and subsequent risk of coronary heart disease: two new prospective studies and a systematic review. *PLoS Medicine* 2008;**5**:e78.

26. **Maes M.** Evidence for an immune response in major depression: a review and hypothesis. *Progress in Neuro-Psychopharmacology & Biological Psychiatry* 1995;**19**:11–38.

27. **Haapakoski R, Mathieu J, Ebmeier KP,** et al. Cumulative meta-analysis of interleukins 6 and 1beta, tumour necrosis factor alpha and C-reactive protein in patients with major depressive disorder. *Brain, Behavior, and Immunity* 2015;**49**:206–15.

28. **Kivimaki M, Shipley MJ, Batty GD,** et al. Long-term inflammation increases risk of common mental disorder: a cohort study. *Molecular Psychiatry* 2014;**19**:149–50.

29. **Gimeno D, Kivimaki M, Brunner EJ**, et al. Associations of C-reactive protein and interleukin-6 with cognitive symptoms of depression: 12-year follow-up of the Whitehall II study. *Psychological Medicine* 2009;**39**:413–23.

30. **Khandaker GM, Pearson RM, Zammit S**, et al. Association of serum interleukin 6 and C-reactive protein in childhood with depression and psychosis in young adult life: a population-based longitudinal study. *JAMA Psychiatry* 2014;**71**:1121–8.

31. **Hofmann A, Peitzsch M, Brunssen C**, et al. Elevated steroid hormone production in the db/db mouse model of obesity and type 2 diabetes. *Hormone and Metabolic Research* 2017;**49**:43–9.

32. **Hofmann A, Brunssen C, Peitzsch M**, et al. Aldosterone synthase inhibition improves glucose tolerance in Zucker Diabetic Fatty (ZDF) rats. *Endocrinology* 2016;**157**:3844–55.

33. **Smalheiser NR, Zhang H, Dwivedi Y**. Enoxacin elevates microRNA levels in rat frontal cortex and prevents learned helplessness. *Frontiers in Psychiatry* 2014;**5**:6.

34. **Lopez JP, Lim R, Cruceanu C**, et al. miR-1202 is a primate-specific and brain-enriched microRNA involved in major depression and antidepressant treatment. *Nature Medicine* 2014;**20**:764–8.

35. **Wan Y, Liu Y, Wang X, Wu J**, et al. Identification of differential microRNAs in cerebrospinal fluid and serum of patients with major depressive disorder. *PLoS One* 2015;**10**:e0121975.

36. **Sempere LF, Freemantle S, Pitha-Rowe I**, et al. Expression profiling of mammalian microRNAs uncovers a subset of brain-expressed microRNAs with possible roles in murine and human neuronal differentiation. *Genome Biology* 2004;**5**:R13.

37. **Jovicic A, Roshan R, Moisoi N**, et al. Comprehensive expression analyses of neural cell-type-specific miRNAs identify new determinants of the specification and maintenance of neuronal phenotypes. *Journal of Neuroscience* 2013;**33**:5127–37.

38. **Sun Y, Li Q, Gui H**, et al. MicroRNA-124 mediates the cholinergic anti-inflammatory action through inhibiting the production of pro-inflammatory cytokines. *Cell Research* 2013;**23**:1270–83.

39. **Bahi A, Chandrasekar V, Dreyer JL**. Selective lentiviral-mediated suppression of microRNA124a in the hippocampus evokes antidepressants-like effects in rats. *Psychoneuroendocrinology* 2014;**46**:78–87.

40. **Dwivedi Y, Roy B, Lugli G**, et al. Chronic corticosterone-mediated dysregulation of microRNA network in prefrontal cortex of rats: relevance to depression pathophysiology. *Translational Psychiatry* 2015;**5**:e682.

41. **Roy B, Dunbar M, Shelton RC, Dwivedi Y**. Identification of MicroRNA-124-3p as a putative epigenetic signature of major depressive disorder. *Neuropsychopharmacology* 2017;**42**:864–75.

42. **Zhou R, Yuan P, Wang Y**, et al. Evidence for selective microRNAs and their effectors as common long-term targets for the actions of mood stabilizers. *Neuropsychopharmacology* 2009; **34**:1395–405.

43. **Davis MJ, Iancu OD, Acher FC**, et al. Role of mGluR4 in acquisition of fear learning and memory. *Neuropharmacology* 2013;**66**:365–72.

44. **Celanire S, Campo B**. Recent advances in the drug discovery of metabotropic glutamate receptor 4 (mGluR4) activators for the treatment of CNS and non-CNS disorders. *Expert Opinion on Drug Discovery* 2012;**7**:261–80.

45. **Pegtel DM, Peferoen L, Amor S.** Extracellular vesicles as modulators of cell-to-cell communication in the healthy and diseased brain. *Philosophical Transactions of the Royal Society of London Series B* 2014;**369**:20130516.

46. **Yirmiya R, Rimmerman N, Reshef R.** Depression as a microglial disease. *Trends in Neurosciences* 2015;**38**:637–58.

47. **Rajkowska G, Miguel-Hidalgo JJ.** Gliogenesis and glial pathology in depression. *CNS & Neurological Disorders Drug Targets* 2007;**6**:219–33.

48. **Fruhbeis C, Frohlich D, Kuo WP, et al.** Neurotransmitter-triggered transfer of exosomes mediates oligodendrocyte-neuron communication. *PLoS Biology* 2013;**11**:e1001604.

49. **Warner-Schmidt JL, Duman RS.** VEGF is an essential mediator of the neurogenic and behavioral actions of antidepressants. *Proceedings of the National Academy of Sciences of the United States of America* 2007;**104**:4647–52.

50. **Glebov K, Lochner M, Jabs R, et al.** Serotonin stimulates secretion of exosomes from microglia cells. *Glia* 2015;**63**:626–34.

51. **Paul-Savoie E, Potvin S, Daigle K, et al.** A deficit in peripheral serotonin levels in major depressive disorder but not in chronic widespread pain. *Clinical Journal of Pain* 2011;**27**:529–34.

52. **Albert PR, Benkelfat C, Descarries L.** The neurobiology of depression-revisiting the serotonin hypothesis. I. Cellular and molecular mechanisms. *Philosophical Transactions of the Royal Society of London* 2012;**367**:2378–81.

53. **Brites D, Fernandes A.** Neuroinflammation and depression: microglia activation, extracellular microvesicles and microRNA dysregulation. *Frontiers in Cellular Neuroscience* 2015;**9**:476.

54. **Ariyo AA, Haan M, Tangen CM, et al.** Depressive symptoms and risks of coronary heart disease and mortality in elderly Americans. Cardiovascular Health Study Collaborative Research Group. *Circulation* 2000;**102**:1773–9.

55. **Mezuk B, Eaton WW, Albrecht S, Golden SH.** Depression and type 2 diabetes over the lifespan: a meta-analysis. *Diabetes Care* 2008;**31**:2383–90.

56. **Greenwald BS, Kramer-Ginsberg E, Krishnan KR, et al.** Neuroanatomic localization of magnetic resonance imaging signal hyperintensities in geriatric depression. *Stroke* 1998;**29**:613–7.

57. **Baldwin RC, Tomenson B.** Depression in later life. A comparison of symptoms and risk factors in early and late onset cases. *British Journal of Psychiatry* 1995;**167**:649–52.

58. **Lyness JM, Caine ED, Cox C, et al** Cerebrovascular risk factors and later-life major depression. Testing a small-vessel brain disease model. *American Journal of Geriatric Psychiatry* 1998;**6**:5–13.

59. **Kenny RA.** *Syncope in the Older Patient: Causes, Investigations and Consequeneces of Syncope and Falls.* London: Chapman and Hall; 1996.

60. **Figiel GS, Krishnan KR, Doraiswamy PM, et al.** Subcortical hyperintensities on brain magnetic resonance imaging: a comparison between late age onset and early onset elderly depressed subjects. *Neurobiology of Aging* 1991;**12**:245–7.

61. **Rabins PV, Pearlson GD, Aylward E, et al.** Cortical magnetic resonance imaging changes in elderly inpatients with major depression. *American Journal of Psychiatry* 1991;**148**:617–20.

62. Thomas AJ, Ferrier IN, Kalaria RN, et al. Cell adhesion molecule expression in the dorsolateral prefrontal cortex and anterior cingulate cortex in major depression in the elderly. *British Journal of Psychiatry* 2002;**181**:129–34.

63. Thombs BD, de Jonge P, Coyne JC, et al. Depression screening and patient outcomes in cardiovascular care: a systematic review. *Journal of the American Medical Association* 2008;**300**:2161–71.

64. Castren E, Rantamaki T. The role of BDNF and its receptors in depression and antidepressant drug action: reactivation of developmental plasticity. *Developmental Neurobiology* 2010;**70**:289–97.

65. Evans SJ, Choudary PV, Neal CR, et al. Dysregulation of the fibroblast growth factor system in major depression. *Proceedings of the National Academy of Sciences* 2004;**101**:15506–11.

66. Poulter MO, Du L, Weaver IC, et al. GABAA receptor promoter hypermethylation in suicide brain: implications for the involvement of epigenetic processes. *Biological Psychiatry* 2008;**64**:645–52.

67. Smalheiser NR, Lugli G, Rizavi HS, et al. MicroRNA expression is down-regulated and reorganized in prefrontal cortex of depressed suicide subjects. *PLoS One* 2012;**7**:e33201.

68. Takebayashi M, Hisaoka K, Nishida A, et al. Decreased levels of whole blood glial cell line-derived neurotrophic factor (GDNF) in remitted patients with mood disorders. *International Journal of Neuropsychopharmacology* 2006;**9**:607–12.

Chapter 4

Genetics

Carol Kan and Ma-Li Wong

Introduction

Both cross-sectional and longitudinal studies have reported bidirectional association between type 2 diabetes mellitus (T2DM) and depression [1,2]. The mechanisms underlying the T2DM–depression link remain unclear (see Chapter 5), with current evidence tentatively suggesting a common biological pathway for both disorders. For example, increased levels of inflammation and hyperactivity in the hypothalamic–pituitary–adrenal (HPA) axis and sympathetic nervous system have been observed in people with T2DM and depression respectively.

The natural development of T2DM is a progressive metabolic dysregulation, starting from obesity to insulin resistance and a pre-diabetes stage, which finally results in a clinical diagnosis of diabetes. A small but significant association between insulin resistance and depression has recently been reported ($r = 0.19$; 95% CI 0.11–0.27) [3]. Furthermore, a tryptophan hydroxylase polymorphism has been associated with insulin resistance in individuals with depression [4]. Inflammatory markers, such as C-reactive protein, have also been associated with depressive symptoms in individuals with newly diagnosed T2DM [5].

The underlying pathogenesis of the T2DM-depression link is therefore likely to be complex and can arise from interplay of both genetic and environmental factors. A question of interest is whether the association between T2DM and depression is predominantly due to shared genetic or environmental vulnerability.

The evidence for a genetic component to T2DM is well-established, including observations from twin studies, linkage studies, and genome-wide association studies (GWAS) [6,7]. A recent meta-analysis estimates heritability for T2DM to be 72% (95% CI 61–78% [8]).

The genetic basis of depression is more difficult to determine, with twin studies estimating the heritability at about 37% (95% CI 31–42% [9]). Two studies have reported higher heritability in females than in males (40% versus 30%; 42% versus 29% respectively) and sex-specific genetic effects [10,11]. Depression is further complicated by its high clinical heterogeneity. There is a suggestion that gene–environment interaction may influence the risk for depression, although this effect was not found in a meta-analysis [12].

T2DM and depression are global public health concerns. Finding a genetic overlap between T2DM and depression would provide more direct evidence that the epidemiological association observed was due to shared biological factors. It would also advance our knowledge of their pathogenesis, contribute to the search for subtypes of depression, and adapt epidemiological methods for multimorbid conditions. Although predicting genetic liability for complex traits is currently of limited clinical value, genetic profiling may one day allow us to cluster patients based on treatment. For example, identifying individuals with T2DM who are at high risk for developing depression would enable the physician to recommend appropriate interventions. In the long term, a greater knowledge base about T2DM and depression will allow us to develop more effective treatments for patients with both conditions and to study why depression is common in other chronic conditions such as obesity. It is therefore important to review the current literature on the genetic basis of the T2DM–depression association.

Evidence from family studies

Family history is a useful first approach in capturing the joint contribution of genetic and environmental factors to a condition, or the comorbidity between conditions (familial effects). To date, one family study of T2DM and depression has been published [13]. The study was based on an Indian cohort, with a sample of 50 patients with T2DM and 481 of their first-degree relatives. The risk for depression in first-degree relatives of patients with T2DM was found to be similar to the general population in other studies. There was, however, no control group, and individuals with any lifetime history of psychiatric disorders were excluded, leading to a low prevalence of depression (1.0%). A similar study reported the number of generations of diabetes in the family as a good predictor of child depressive symptoms [14]. Family studies do not, however, differentiate which factors contribute to the similarity of first-degree family members, since relatives share both genes and environment. Any familial effect observed could therefore be due to both genetic and/or environmental influences.

Evidence from twin studies

Twin studies provide a unique approach in investigating genetic influences on complex traits or disorders, as twins are matched for age, genetic factors, and a range of covariates in their shared environment, such as parenting style and education. Twin studies make use of the ratio of disease concordance between monozygotic (MZ) and dizygotic (DZ) twins to estimate the most likely effects of (genetic) heritability and common and individual-specific environmental factors. In simple terms, the method uses the ratio of cross-disorder concordance between MZ and DZ twins to approximate the genetic and environmental correlations between disorders. Genetic correlation estimates the degree to which genetic factors affect both disorders. It is independent of their individual heritability estimates. Therefore, a high genetic correlation does not imply a high impact of genes on the observed correlation between the conditions and the actual heritability estimate for each disorder needs to be taken into account.

There have been three twin studies investigating common genetic and environmental vulnerability to diabetes and depression. The Vietnam Era Twin Study of Aging consists of MZ and DZ twins who served in the US military during the Vietnam era (1965–1975; $n = 1237$) [15]. A small genetic correlation between T2DM and depression was reported, with a broad confidence interval (0.19; 95% CI 0–0.46). The finding is difficult to generalize at a population-level, given the sample was highly selected with participants being restricted to males aged 50–59 years who were involved in military service. The Screening Across the Lifespan Twin Study consists of MZ and DZ twins aged 40 years or older recruited from the Swedish Twin Registry ($n = 37043$) and it concluded that there was significant environmental correlation of moderate magnitude (0.54; 95% CI 0.02–0.88) between T2DM and depression [16]. Both studies do not support a common genetic pathway hypothesis. Higher rates of comorbid T2DM and depression have been observed in females than in males [17–19], with a meta-analysis reporting a higher prevalence of depression in females with T2DM (23.8%) than males (12.8%) [17]. Clearly, twin modelling incorporating sex differences is needed. A recent study reported quantitative and qualitative sex differences in the genetic overlap between depression and T2DM in two large Scandinavian populations. Replication in non-Western populations is needed to examine the generalizability of the finding [20].

Evidence from molecular genetic studies

The revolution in genomics—the ability to rapidly sequence DNA and conduct GWAS—has uncovered many genetic contributions to the development and progression of complex traits. To date, over 120 single nucleotide polymorphisms (SNPs) predisposing to T2DM and diabetes-related traits have been discovered [21]. These variants are associated with a small risk of developing T2DM (odds ratio (OR) 1.0–1.2), and in sum capture a small proportion of the genetic component of the disease. The strongest association is observed in the wnt signalling pathway member TCF7L2 (transcription factor-7-like 2) on chromosome 10 [22–24]. It is 1.5 times more common in patients than in controls, conferring an approximately 40% increased risk for T2DM. Rare variants have been associated with T2DM, but a recent analysis using empirical and simulated data suggests that compared with common variants, rare variants are unlikely to be an important source of contribution to the heritability of T2DM [7].

For depression, GWAS have been unable to identify any reproducible association signal. A meta-analysis did not identify any genome-wide findings [25], with the authors attributing the negative result to the inherent heterogeneity of the phenotypes, and insufficient power because of the high prevalence rate of depression in the general population. Fifteen novel SNPs for depression have since been identified in individuals of European descent using self-report data [26], whereas a study in Chinese females with severe depression has identified two loci that are rare in Europeans [27]. In addition, a rare mutation in the endothelial lipase gene (missense Asn396Ser) has recently been implicated in the pathogenesis of depressive symptoms in a large population-based cohort [28]. If replicable by several independent studies, this kind of association suggests how some depressive symptoms may be an epiphenomenon of atherosclerosis, which is a common pathology in type 2 diabetes.

A range of T2DM-related SNPs have been suggested to be associated with depression. For example, the Pro12Ala variant of the PPAR γ2 gene (peroxisome proliferative-activated receptor) has been implicated in inflammation, depression, and type 1 and 2 diabetes [29,30]. A locus involved in the circadian gene CRY2 (cryptochrome circadian clock 2) has been associated with both T2DM [31] and major depressive disorder with seasonal pattern [32]. A small case–control study has found individuals with depression have reduced expression of FADS1 (fatty acid desaturase), a gene involved in long-chain polyunsaturated fatty acid biosynthesis and T2DM [33]. Depressive behaviours have also been observed in adult mice lacking insulin-like growth factor (IGF)-1, a gene also implicated in T2DM [34]. In addition, SNPs associated with leptin, a peptide hormone from adipose tissue, have been linked with response to antidepressant treatment [35] and T2DM [36].

Genotypes for α-2A adrenoceptor (ADRA2A) and melatonin receptor 1B (MTNR1B) have been associated with raised plasma glucose, a T2DM-related trait [31,37]. The ADRA2A genotype has been suggested as a predictor of treatment outcome in people with depression [38]. In addition, sex-differences have been reported in the activity of the HPA axis and the ADRA2A genotype [39]. On the other hand, genetic polymorphisms and mRNA expression of MTNR1B have been demonstrated to play a significant role in patients with recurrent depression [40]. Studies have also indicated a role of the FTO (fat mass and obesity-associated) genes in T2DM and body mass index (BMI) [41,42] and a meta-analysis showed a significant inverse association between the FTO rs9939609 A variant and depression [43]. These findings from molecular genetic studies provide some evidence of the potential influence of T2DM-predisposing genes on depression.

Evidence from statistical genetics using GWAS

Both T2DM and depression are likely to be polygenetic in nature, with hundreds of susceptible alleles showing small effects. T2DM risk alleles may contribute small increments in depression risk, and vice versa. A polygenic score approach allows the cumulative effect of multiple T2DM genetic risk variants on depression status to be analysed, clarifying whether a genetic predisposition to T2DM might be related to depression or the other way around. The T2DM–depression link was examined in two GWAS datasets [44,45]. Both concluded that there is little evidence of a genetic overlap between T2DM and depression. The EpiDREAM study is a multinational, longitudinal study of individuals who were at risk for developing T2DM [44]. It examined the unidirectional association between 20 T2DM SNPs and depression case status in 17,404 individuals who were at risk for developing T2DM [45]. The Generation Scotland study is a family and population-based study with participants recruited from General Practitioners throughout Scotland, with the aim of developing more effective treatments for complex diseases based on genetic knowledge. It examined the shared aetiology between T2DM and depression using polygenic scores and Mendelian Randomization in a population cohort of 21,516 individuals [44].

There are, however, caveats with both studies, making their findings difficult to generalize. The EpiDREAM study only examined 20 SNPs associated with T2DM, and over 120 SNPs have been identified with T2DM and related traits at the GWAS significant level [21]. Thus, 20 SNPs are likely to capture only a very small proportion of the genetic component of T2DM. The Generation Scotland study, on the other hand, only had a small sample size ($n = 915$) of individuals with T2DM. Further research needs to be conducted in cohorts with a larger sample size and non-Western populations. In addition, a recent study has demonstrated a genetic overlap between BMI polygenic scores and atypical depression, defined by increased appetite or weight, but not typical depression [46]. Given the heterogeneity of depression, the degree of variance in depression subtypes, which can be explained by the additive effects of common SNPs associated with T2DM, needs to be explored.

Linkage disequilibrium score regression has been applied in one study to estimate genetic correlations among 24 complex traits, including T2DM and depression [47]. For T2DM, it uses the summary statistics from Diabetes Genetic Replication And Meta-analysis Consortium (DIAGRAM). DIAGRAM comprises 12 cohorts, with 12,171 diabetes cases and 56,862 controls [48]. It consists of individuals of European origin, drawn from Europe, the USA, and Australia. Cases were individuals with a clinical diagnosis of T2DM according to the American Diabetes Association or World Health Organization criteria. For depression, it uses the summary statistics from Psychiatric Genomics Consortium-Major Depressive Disorder Stage 1 (PGC-MDD-1). PGC-MDD-1 comprises 9240 depression cases and 9519 controls [25]. All subjects were of European ancestry, and cases were individuals with a lifetime diagnosis of depression according to the DSM-IV criteria. Using linkage disequilibrium score regression, the study did not find a statistically significant correlation between T2DM and depression [47]. If there is genetic heterogeneity between cohorts, estimates from linkage disequilibrium score regression analysis can be biased downwards. Given both DIAGRAM and PGC-MDD-1 consist of multiple cohorts, it will be useful to apply the linkage disequilibrium score regression in one large population cohort to estimate the genetic correlation between T2DM and depression.

Summary

Twin studies have suggested a genetic overlap between T2DM and depression, implying that inherited DNA variants are important in the aetiology for this comorbidity. The genetic correlations observed from twin studies indicate that only a small magnitude of the variance in liability attributes to genetic factors for the T2DM-depression link. It does not, however, indicate the genetic underpinning of the disorders in terms of causal variants. Identifying specific genetic variants will be a future research goal for gaining further insight into the aetiology.

Estimating the shared heritability between these two complex traits using larger GWAS datasets is an important next step in understanding and defining the shared genetic architectures. Gene–environment interaction is another area that needs to be explored, given genotypes can affect an individual's responses to the environment whereas environment can differentially affect the expression of genotypes. Research in the emerging epigenetic and microbiome fields might hold the key in unlocking the complex interactions between genetic and environmental factors in the T2DM–depression link.

T2DM and depression are among the leading causes of morbidity and mortality globally. The resultant societal costs of medical care and lost productivity have major public health impacts. A better understanding of the mechanisms underlying the association is therefore of high scientific, clinical, and public relevance. This research field offers real opportunities for developing novel therapeutic modalities, for example facilitating the development of stratified medicine for people with T2DM and depression or T2DM with a worse prognosis. In addition, substantial heterogeneity is observed in depression with regard to symptom manifestations, clinical course, and response to pharmacological treatment [49]. It has been suggested that specific depression subtypes are associated with different biological correlates [50]. Unravelling the genetic predisposition to T2DM and depression is a major challenge but presents an exciting opportunity to further increase our understanding of the mechanisms underlying T2DM and depression.

References

1. Chen PC, Chan YT, Chen HF, et al. Population-based cohort analyses of the bidirectional relationship between type 2 diabetes and depression. *Diabetes Care* 2013;**36**:376–82.
2. Golden SH, Lazo M, Carnethon M, et al. Examining a bidirectional association between depressive symptoms and diabetes. *JAMA* 2008;**18**;299:2751–9.
3. Kan C, Silva N, Golden SH, et al. A systematic review and meta-analysis of the association between depression and insulin resistance. *Diabetes Care* 2013;**36**:480–9.
4. Chiba M, Suzuki S, Hinokio Y, et al. Tyrosine hydroxylase gene microsatellite polymorphism associated with insulin resistance in depressive disorder. *Metabolism* 2000;**49**:1145–9.
5. Laake JP, Stahl D, Amiel SA, et al. The association between depressive symptoms and systemic inflammation in people with type 2 diabetes: findings from the South London Diabetes Study. *Diabetes Care* 2014;**37**:2186–92.
6. Barroso I. Genetics of type 2 diabetes. *Diabetic Medicine* 2005;**22**:517–35.
7. Fuchsberger C, Flannick J, Teslovich TM, The genetic architecture of type 2 diabetes. *Nature* 2016;**4**;536:41–7.
8. Willemsen G, Ward KJ, Bell CG, et al. The concordance and heritability of type 2 diabetes in 34,166 twin pairs from international twin registers: the Discordant Twin (DISCOTWIN) Consortium. *Twin Research and Human Genetics* 2015;**18**:762–71.
9. Sullivan PF, Neale MC, Kendler KS. Genetic epidemiology of major depression: review and meta-analysis. *American Journal of Psychiatry* 2000;**157**:1552–62.
10. Kendler KS, Gardner CO, Neale MC, Prescott CA. Genetic risk factors for major depression in men and women: similar or different heritabilities and same or partly distinct genes? *Psychological Medicine* 2001;**31**:605–16.
11. Kendler KS, Gatz M, Gardner CO, Pedersen NL. A Swedish national twin study of lifetime major depression. *American Journal of Psychiatry* 2006;**163**:109–14.
12. Risch N, Herrell R, Lehner T, et al. Interaction between the serotonin transporter gene (5-HTTLPR), stressful life events, and risk of depression a meta-analysis. *Journal of the American Medical Association* 2009;**301**: 2462–71.
13. Pravin D, Malhotra S, Chakrabarti S, Dash RJ. Frequency of major affective disorders in first-degree relatives of patients with type 2 diabetes mellitus. *Indian Journal of Medical Research* 2006;**124**:291–8.
14. Irving RR, Mills JL, Choo-Kang EG, et al. Diabetes and psychological co-morbidity in children with a family history of early-onset type 2 diabetes. *International Journal of Psychology* 2008;**43**:937–42.

15. Scherrer JF, Xian H, Lustman PJ, et al. A test for common genetic and environmental vulnerability to depression and diabetes. *Twin Research and Human Genetics* 2011;**14**:169–72.

16. Mezuk B, Heh V, Prom-Wormley E, et al. Association between major depression and type 2 diabetes in midlife: findings from the screening across the lifespan twin Study. *Psychosomatic Medicine* 2015;**77**:559–66.

17. Ali S, Stone MA, Peters JL, et al. The prevalence of co-morbid depression in adults with Type 2 diabetes: a systematic review and meta-analysis. *Diabetic Medicine* 2006;**23**:1165–73.

18. Alonso-Moran E, Satylganova A, Orueta J, Nuno-Solinis R. Prevalence of depression in adults with type 2 diabetes in the Basque Country: relationship with glycaemic control and health care costs. *BMC Public Health* 2014;**14**:769.

19. Anderson RJ, Freedland KE, Clouse RE, Lustman PJ. The prevalence of comorbid depression in adults with diabetes: a meta-analysis. *Diabetes Care* 2001;**24**:1069–78.

20. Kan C, Pedersen NL, Christensen K, et al. Genetic overlap between type 2 diabetes and depression in Swedish and Danish twin registries. *Molecular Psychiatry* 2016;**21**(7):903–9.

21. Prasad RB, Groop L. Genetics of type 2 diabetes-pitfalls and possibilities. *Genes* 2015;**6**:87–123.

22. Grant SF, Thorleifsson G, Reynisdottir I, et al. Variant of transcription factor 7-like 2 (TCF7L2) gene confers risk of type 2 diabetes. *Nature Genetics* 2006;**38**:320–3.

23. Kildemoes HW, Sorensen HT, Hallas J. The Danish National Prescription Registry. *Scandanavian Journal of Public Health* 2011;**39**(Suppl.):38–41.

24. Purcell, S. Variance components models for gene-environment interaction in twin analysis. *Twin Research and Human Genetics* 2002;**5**:554–71.

25. Ripke S, Wray NR, Lewis CM, et al. A mega-analysis of genome-wide association studies for major depressive disorder. *Molecular Psychiatry* 2013;**18**:497–511.

26. Hyde CL, Nagle NW, Tian C, et al. Identification of 15 genetic loci associated with risk of major depression in individuals of European descent. *Nature Genetics* 2016;**48**:1031–6.

27. CONVERGE consortium. Sparse whole-genome sequencing identifies two loci for major depressive disorder. *Nature* 2015;**523**:588–91.

28. Amin N, Jovanova O, Adams HH, et al. Exome-sequencing in a large population-based study reveals a rare Asn396Ser variant in the LIPG gene associated with depressive symptoms. *Molecular Psychiatry* 2017;**22**:537–43.

29. Eftychi C, Howson JM, Barratt BJ, et al. Analysis of the type 2 diabetes-associated single nucleotide polymorphisms in the genes IRS1, KCNJ11, and PPARG2 in type 1 diabetes. *Diabetes* 2004;**53**: 870–3.

30. Ji-Rong Y, Bi-Rong D, Chang-Quan H, et al. Pro12Ala polymorphism in PPARgamma2 associated with depression in Chinese nonagenarians/centenarians. *Archives of Medical Research* 2009;**40**:411–5.

31. Dupuis J, Langenberg C, Prokopenko I, et al. New genetic loci implicated in fasting glucose homeostasis and their impact on type 2 diabetes risk. *Nature Genetics* 2010;**42**:105–16.

32. Lavebratt C, Sjoholm LK, Soronen P, et al. CRY2 is associated with depression. *PLoS One* 2010;**24**;5:e9407.

33. **McNamara RK, Liu Y.** Reduced expression of fatty acid biosynthesis genes in the prefrontal cortex of patients with major depressive disorder. *Journal of Affective Disorders* 2011;**129**:359–63.

34. **Mitschelen M, Yan H, Farley JA,** et al. Long-term deficiency of circulating and hippocampal insulin-like growth factor I induces depressive behavior in adult mice: a potential model of geriatric depression. *Neuroscience* 2011;**185**:50–60.

35. **Kloiber S, Ripke S, Kohli MA,** et al. Resistance to antidepressant treatment is associated with polymorphisms in the leptin gene, decreased leptin mRNA expression, and decreased leptin serum levels. *European Neuropsychopharmacology* 2013;**23**:653–62.

36. **Hara K, Fujita H, Johnson TA,** et al. Genome-wide association study identifies three novel loci for type 2 diabetes. *Human Molecular Genetics* 2014;**23**:239–46.

37. **Manning AK, Hivert MF, Scott RA,** et al. A genome-wide approach accounting for body mass index identifies genetic variants influencing fasting glycemic traits and insulin resistance. *Nature Genetics* 2012;**44**:659–69.

38. **Kato M, Serretti A, Nonen S,** et al. Genetic variants in combination with early partial improvement as a clinical utility predictor of treatment outcome in major depressive disorder: the result of two pooled RCTs. *Translational Psychiatry* 2015;**24;5**:e513.

39. **Haefner S, Baghai TC, Schule C,** et al. Impact of gene-gender effects of adrenergic polymorphisms on hypothalamic-pituitary-adrenal axis activity in depressed patients. *Neuropsychobiology* 2008;**58**:154–62.

40. **Galecka E, Szemraj J, Florkowski A,** et al. Single nucleotide polymorphisms and mRNA expression for melatonin MT(2) receptor in depression. *Psychiatry Research* 2011;**189**:472–4.

41. **Frayling TM, Timpson NJ, Weedon MN,** et al. A common variant in the FTO gene is associated with body mass index and predisposes to childhood and adult obesity. *Science* 2007;**316**:889–94.

42. **Mahajan A, Go MJ, Zhang W,** et al. Genome-wide trans-ancestry meta-analysis provides insight into the genetic architecture of type 2 diabetes susceptibility. *Nature Genetics* 2014;**46**:234–44.

43. **Samaan Z, Anand SS, Zhang X,** et al. The protective effect of the obesity-associated rs9939609 A variant in fat mass- and obesity-associated gene on depression. *Molecular Psychiatry* 2013;**18**:1281–6.

44. **Clarke TK, Obsteter J, Hall LS,** et al. Investigating shared aetiology between type 2 diabetes and major depressive disorder in a population based cohort. *American Journal of Medical Genetics Part B* 2017;**174**:227–34.

45. **Samaan Z, Garasia S, Gerstein HC,** et al. Lack of association between type 2 diabetes and major depression: epidemiologic and genetic evidence in a multiethnic population. *Translational Psychiatry* 2015;**11**:e618.

46. **Milaneschi Y, Lamers F, Peyrot WJ,** et al. Polygenic dissection of major depression clinical heterogeneity. *Molecular Psychiatry* 2015;**21**:516–22.

47. **Bulik-Sullivan B, Finucane HK, Anttila V,** et al. An atlas of genetic correlations across human diseases and traits. *Nature Genetics* 2015;**47**:1236–41.

48. **Morris AP, Voight BF, Teslovich TM,** et al. Large-scale association analysis provides insights into the genetic architecture and pathophysiology of type 2 diabetes. *Nature Genetics* 2012;**44**:981–90.

49. **Ghaemi SN, Vohringer PA.** The heterogeneity of depression: an old debate renewed. *Acta Psychiatrica Scandinavica* 2011;**124**:497.
50. **Lamers F, Vogelzangs N, Merikangas KR**, et al. Evidence for a differential role of HPA-axis function, inflammation and metabolic syndrome in melancholic versus atypical depression. *Molecular Psychiatry* 2013;**18**:692–9.

Chapter 5

Innate immunity and inflammation in type 2 diabetes-associated depression

Calum D. Moulton and John C. Pickup

Introduction

Between 10% and 20% of patients with type 2 diabetes mellitus (T2DM) also have depression, twice as many as the general population [1]. Patients with comorbid T2DM and depression are at twofold increased risk of microvascular and macrovascular complications [2], dementia [3], and premature mortality [4] compared with those with T2DM alone. There is therefore a pressing need to understand the mechanisms underlying the link between depression and T2DM, in order to improve treatments and outcomes in this high-risk comorbid group.

Although psychological and behavioural factors (depression as a response to the burden of diabetes) are thought to have an important role in the link between depression and T2DM, there is strong evidence that such factors do not adequately or completely explain the association. In neuroimaging research, the brain grey matter changes that occur in T2DM have been found to be similar to those seen in depression [5]. The cross-sectional association between depression and glycaemic control is modest [6] and even weaker when tested prospectively [7]. Conventional treatment for depression is frequently effective in the treatment of depression itself in patients with T2DM [8], but this does not translate consistently into improvements in diabetes outcomes [9,10]. Moreover, the link between depression and T2DM is bidirectional: T2DM is associated with an approximately 20% increased risk of incident depression [11,12], whereas depression is associated with a 60% increased risk of incident T2DM [11]. Collectively, this suggests that shared biological mechanisms may underpin the link between depression, T2DM, and possibly associated adverse outcomes like macrovascular disease.

Low-grade systemic inflammation because of activated innate immunity has emerged as a promising candidate in this regard. Although strongly associated with depression and T2DM separately, recent population-based research has suggested that inflammation could be an important mechanism in their comorbidity. If so, reduction in inflammation provides a novel pharmacological mechanism by which to treat depression and T2DM simultaneously, as well as reducing associated long-term morbidity and mortality.

This chapter will firstly review the evidence for a pathogenic role for inflammation in both depression and T2DM, respectively. The chapter will then review the research that has tested inflammation as a common link between depression and T2DM, including evidence into its aetiology, mechanistic effects, and potential modifiability. Finally, the translational implications of this will be discussed, including recommendations for future research.

Inflammation and innate immunity

Innate immunity is the body's first-line defence against external threats such as infection, physical and chemical injury, and psychological stress [13]. These systems function to repair damage to tissues, to prevent potential injury, and to restore homeostasis. Pattern-recognition receptors cause a wide variety of immunological 'trouble-shooting', while sentinel cells (e.g. macrophages, adipocytes, and endothelium) sense threats and release cytokines such as interleukin (IL)-1, IL-6, and tumour necrosis factor (TNF)-α, which have both paracrine and systemic effects. Acting on the liver, for example, cytokines mediate the production of large amounts of proteins that are released into the bloodstream (called the 'acute-phase response' [14]), such as C-reactive protein (CRP) and fibrinogen, while stimulating triglyceride-rich very-low-density lipoprotein (VLDL) production and reduced circulating levels of high-density lipoprotein (HDL) ('dyslipidaemia'). It is for this reason that mediators such as CRP, IL-6, and TNF-α are known as 'inflammatory markers'. Cytokines also act on many other tissues throughout the body to produce a pattern of responses typical of injury, for example endothelium (increased capillary permeability), muscle (insulin resistance), pancreatic islets (decreased insulin secretion), and brain (behavioural changes) [15].

Despite the beneficial short-term effects of innate immunity in combating external threats and restoring homeostasis, there is now compelling evidence that chronic elevation of the innate inflammatory response has deleterious effects on multiple systems in the body. In particular, elevated inflammation is strongly implicated in the pathogenesis of depression, T2DM, and some associated diabetes complications, reviewed in detail below.

Inflammation in depression

Diagnosis of depression

The gold standard in diagnosis of depression is a clinical diagnostic interview based on established diagnostic criteria, such as the Schedules of Clinical Assessment in Neuropsychiatry [16]. However, such an interview is time-consuming and often unfeasible for epidemiological studies. As such, the majority of research into depression in T2DM has instead used self-report questionnaires, which frequently define 'caseness' for depression using a validated cut-off (e.g. a score of 10 or more on the Patient Health Questionnaire (PHQ-9)) [17]. Unsurprisingly, validation studies have reported high rates of false-positive depression cases using this approach [17]. This is partly due to the frequent endorsement of somatic symptoms (e.g. fatigue, and sleep and appetite disturbance) in patients with T2DM, whose aetiology may or may not be related to a depressive disorder.

Although using diagnostic criteria to define depression provides greater precision, there is growing evidence that this approach may itself have important limitations in the context of inflammation and T2DM. In cross-sectional research in the general population, somatic symptoms, such as fatigue and sleep disturbance, have been found to be more strongly associated with elevated inflammation than are more cognitive symptoms, such as low mood and poor concentration [18]. Induction of a pro-inflammatory state using interferon therapy may specifically worsen somatic symptoms [19], but anti-inflammatory treatments may have more beneficial effects on somatic symptoms [20]. In a validity study of the PHQ-9 in patients with T2DM, somatic symptoms were reported with equal frequency in patents with or without a clinical diagnosis of depression [17]. In other populations at high risk of cardiovascular disease, somatic symptoms have been found to be most predictive of mortality [21]. Collectively, this suggests that somatic symptoms may provide an important biomarker of inflammation and future mortality that may be missed by diagnostic assessment. As such, this review will include self-report questionnaires along with clinical diagnosis under the umbrella of depression.

Pathogenesis: from inflammation to depressive symptoms

In the general population, meta-analyses have found that patients with depression have consistently higher circulating concentrations of cytokines, including TNF-α and IL-6 [22,23] than non-depressed controls. Such elevated inflammatory markers have been found to predict increased incidence of depressive symptoms over time [24,25], suggesting a possible role in the pathogenesis of depressive symptoms. Moreover, in patients undergoing pro-inflammatory-associated treatment with interferon therapy, high rates of clinical depression are consistently observed [26].

The mechanisms by which elevated inflammation could lead to depressive symptoms, however, are incompletely understood. Increased cytokine serum concentrations have been found to activate the hypothalamic–pituitary–adrenal axis and increase oxidative stress in the brain [27,28]. Inflammatory cytokines may also activate the tryptophan–kynurenine pathway through activation of the enzyme indoleamine-2,3-dioxygenase (IDO) [29]. This may result both in reduced production of serotonin and increased production of tryptophan catabolites that have neurotoxic properties, such as kynurenine and quinolinic acid [29]. Cross-sectional studies have reported an association between smaller hippocampal volumes—a biomarker of persistent depression [30]—and ratios of neurotoxic kynurenine metabolites [27].

Treatment

Up to 50% of patients do not respond to the first antidepressant treatment, such as antidepressant tablets [31]. Inflammation has been suggested as one such barrier to treatment response. In a secondary analysis of the Genome-based Therapeutic Drugs for Depression study of 241 adults with major depressive disorder, elevated concentrations of CRP predicted treatment response to nortriptyline (a tricyclic antidepressant) rather than escitalopram, a selective serotonin reuptake inhibitor (SSRI) [32]. Whereas nortriptyline has also been found to inhibit migration of polymorphonuclear white blood cells towards an inflammation site, escitalopram has no such effect [33].

To date, a small number of clinical trials have tested the efficacy of anti-inflammatory agents in the treatment of depression in the general population. A meta-analysis of four studies reported that adjunctive therapy with the non-steroidal anti-inflammatory drug (NSAID) celecoxib reduced depressive symptoms, although a total of only 150 patients were included [34]. In patients with interferon-induced depression, 2 weeks of treatment with omega-3-fatty acids was found to reduce the risk of incident depression compared with placebo [35]. In a placebo-controlled trial of 60 patients, inhibition of TNF with infliximab did not improve depressive symptoms after 12 weeks. However, in the subset ($n = 21$) with high baseline CRP concentrations, the remission rate was greater in the infliximab group [36]. Building on positive results from animal studies, the antibiotic minocycline has demonstrated promise in small-scale open-label studies in depression [37] and larger randomized controlled trials (RCTs) are ongoing [38].

Inflammation in type 2 diabetes

Pathogenesis

In 1993, Pickup and colleagues [39] observed that a marker of the acute-phase response, serum sialic acid, was elevated in a group of T2DM subjects but not in a group with type 1 diabetes, matched for age, sex, and glycaemic control. Subsequently, several established acute-phase reactants have also been reported as abnormal in diabetes, including elevated white blood cell count, increased circulating cortisol and complement levels [15]. Many known risk factors for T2DM are also associated with activated innate immunity and inflammation, including inactivity, obesity, smoking, psychological stress, and sleep deprivation [15]. In recent meta-analyses, elevated levels of IL-1β, IL-6, and CRP have been found to be consistently predictive of T2DM onset [40], further suggesting a pathogenic mechanism.

At a cellular level, inflammation is thought to exert diabetogenic effects both in the pancreas and the periphery. In the pancreas, for example, human islet amyloid polypeptide interacts with immune cells to promote synthesis of IL-1β, leading resident islet macrophages to adopt a pro-inflammatory phenotype that induces islet dysfunction [41]. In the periphery, stress to the endoplasmic reticulum (ER) of adipocytes drives the production of cytokines and chemokines [42]. Taken together, the major cellular mechanisms thought to be involved in T2DM, including oxidative stress, ER stress, and the formation of islet amyloid deposits, are all associated with inflammatory responses [42].

Inflammation is likewise thought to be important in the pathogenesis of diabetes-related complications. For example, in the Lewisham Diabetes Study, elevated levels of the inflammatory marker sialic acid was a stronger risk factor for 12-year cardiovascular mortality than glycaemic control, blood pressure, cholesterol, body mass index (BMI), or smoking [43]. Mechanisms by which a cytokine-induced inflammatory response accelerates atherosclerosis may include the promotion of leucocyte recruitment to the endothelium and enhancing the procoagulant state via increased fibrinogen production [15,44].

Treatment

If innate inflammation is involved in the pathogenesis of T2DM, inflammatory pathways may provide novel targets for disease-modifying therapies. In a three-arm RCT of 89 patients with T2DM, inhibition of monocyte chemotactic protein-1 action was been found to improve glycaemia after 4 weeks [45]. In two multicentre placebo-controlled studies ($n = 108$ and $n = 286$ respectively), salsalate—a prodrug of salicylic acid that has broad-based anti-inflammatory actions via inhibition of the nuclear factor kappa light-chain enhancer of activated B-cells pathway—led to short-term and sustained improvement in glycaemic control compared to placebo [46,47]. In another placebo-controlled RCT of 70 patients with T2DM, IL-1 blockade with anakinra (recombinant human IL-1 receptor antagonist) was found to improve glycaemia and β-cell secretory function and to reduce markers of systemic inflammation compared with placebo after 12 weeks [48]. This effect was preserved at 1-year follow-up, even after withdrawal of anakinra [49].

Inflammation in comorbid depression and type 2 diabetes

Epidemiology

In contrast to the volume of research examining inflammation in depression and T2DM respectively, studies measuring inflammation in patients with the two conditions together have been sparse and almost all cross-sectional in design. In a secondary analysis of the Health ABC Study, patients with comorbid depression and T2DM were found to have elevated concentrations of IL-6 compared with those with either condition alone [50]. However, participant numbers were low (14 patients with depression and T2DM). In a Japanese cohort of 3573 people with T2DM, those with comorbid depression—defined using the PHQ-9—had higher concentrations of CRP, although the association only remained robust to confounding in patients with BMI >25 kg/m^2 [51]. In the South London Diabetes (SOUL-D) study of 1790 primary care patients with newly diagnosed T2DM, those with comorbid depression—again defined using the PHQ-9—had higher concentrations of CRP, IL-1RA, and white cell count than non-depressed controls [52]. These differences persisted after controlling for a range of pro-inflammatory confounders. This suggests that elevated inflammation may have a role in the pathogenesis of depression in T2DM, and moreover, could lead to associated complications such as cardiovascular disease.

Aetiology

We have previously suggested that an elevated inflammatory response could result from accumulation of pro-inflammatory stressors across the whole life course. Against a background of genetic predisposition in some individuals, maltreatment in childhood, low socioeconomic status, work stress, and adverse lifestyle behaviours—among other stressors—may collectively act as 'toxins' to activate the inflammatory response [15,53–55]. We have proposed that this may lead to the subsequent development of depression and T2DM disorders in parallel [54]. However, no epidemiological study to date has examined the temporal relationship between inflammation, depression, and T2DM in order to test this hypothesis.

Treatment

Most available diabetes treatments have some anti-inflammatory effect and a handful have been tested for their effects on depressive symptoms in T2DM. In an uncontrolled study, pioglitazone was shown to improve depressive symptoms in patients with bipolar depression [56]. Notably, this improvement was predicted by increased baseline concentrations of interleukin. A study of 118 post-stroke patients with T2DM found that pioglitazone improved depressive symptoms more than metformin, although no measures of inflammation were collected [57].

The incretin-based therapies—a class that includes both glucagon-like peptide-1 receptor agonists and dipeptidyl peptidase-IV inhibitors—have established anti-inflammatory properties in humans [58,59]. In a secondary analysis of the SOUL-D study, treatment with incretin-based therapies was found to be associated with greater reduction in depressive symptoms after 1 year than other diabetes therapies [60]. Moreover, depressive symptoms correlated significantly with reduction in CRP but not the measure of long-term glycaemic control, glycated haemoglobin (HbA1c), suggesting that a reduction in inflammation, rather than glycaemia, may mediate this effect.

Although no study to date has attempted to modify the tryptophan-kynurenine pathway in the treatment of depression in patients with T2DM, there is promise from animal models to support such an approach. In one experiment, rats with streptozotocin-induced diabetes treated with minocycline, an indirect inhibitor of IDO, showed a reduction in depressive-like behaviours and reduction in hippocampal IDO expression following treatment [61]. Replication of these findings in humans is now awaited.

Future directions

Current treatments for depression in T2DM are limited both by their high failure rate and by their inconsistency in improving diabetes-related outcomes. In this context, inflammation provides a promising target for disease-modifying therapies that could both improve treatment response and reduce risk of diabetes-related complications.

At a mechanistic level, there is a need for future *in vivo* and *in vitro* research to test the mechanisms by which inflammation could lead to depressive symptoms in T2DM, including candidate pathways such as tryptophan-kynurenine metabolism. In epidemiology, there is a need for high-quality prospective cohort studies to examine the aetiology of elevated inflammation in the depression in T2DM. Such research could provide subsequent opportunities for the primary prevention of depression, T2DM, or even both.

There is mounting evidence that clinical criteria for depression may exclude a large number of patients with 'sub-threshold' depressive symptoms that also have important prognostic implications. In particular, inflammation appears to be strongly associated with somatic symptoms of depression, which are reported with similar frequency in patients with and without clinical depression. Prospective cohort studies should now test whether subtypes of depression can be identified in patients with T2DM, and moreover, how such subtypes relate both to inflammation and to longer-term morbidity and mortality.

In interventional research, future experimental studies of anti-inflammatory treatments should test whether inflammation is indeed a modifiable target to treat depression in T2DM. If so, adequately powered clinical trials are needed to test the efficacy of different candidate treatments. Trials should test both specific anti-inflammatory therapies, including those with a broad-based anti-inflammatory mechanism (e.g. NSAIDs), and more targeted immune modulating therapies (e.g. specific cytokine or chemokine inhibitors). Repurposing of already-available treatments for diabetes, such as incretin-based therapies, is another promising strategy that has the added advantages of reducing treatment burden and enabling more rapid translation to the clinic.

Conclusion

Building on compelling evidence that inflammation has an aetiological role in both depression and T2DM, respectively, there is now evidence that inflammation has a role in their comorbidity. However, research into the aetiology, effects, and modifiability of inflammation in patients with depression and T2DM remains at an early stage. Multidisciplinary research is now needed to define whether inflammation has a pathogenic role in the depression of T2DM and whether it can be modified to improve outcomes. If so, biomarkers of inflammation may then be used to direct precision medicine interventions to improve depressive symptoms and glycaemic control simultaneously, while reducing long-term morbidity and mortality. Moreover, research into the aetiology of inflammation across the life-course may provide opportunities for the primary prevention of depression, T2DM, or even both conditions together.

References

1. **Anderson RJ, Freedland KE, Clouse RE, Lustman PJ.** The prevalence of comorbid depression in adults with diabetes: a meta analysis. *Diabetes Care* 2001;**24**:1069–78.

2. **de Groot M, Anderson R, Freedland KE**, et al. Association of depression and diabetes complications: a meta-analysis. *Psychosomatic Medicine* 2001;**63**:619–30.

3. **Sullivan MD, Katon WJ, Lovato LC**, et al. Association of depression with accelerated cognitive decline among patients with type 2 diabetes in the ACCORD-MIND trial. *JAMA Psychiatry* 2013;**70**:1041–7.

4. **Katon WJ, Rutter C, Simon G**, et al. The association of comorbid depression with mortality in patients with type 2 diabetes. *Diabetes Care* 2005;**28**:2668–72.

5. **Moulton CD, Costafreda SG, Horton P**, et al. Meta-analyses of structural regional cerebral effects in type 1 and type 2 diabetes. *Brain Imaging and Behavior* 2015;**9**:651–62.

6. **Lustman PJ, Anderson RJ, Freedland KE**, et al. Depression and poor glycemic control: a meta-analytic review of the literature. *Diabetes Care* 2000;**23**:934–42.

7. **Fisher L, Mullan J, Arean P**, et al. Diabetes distress but not clinical depression or depressive symptoms is associated with glycemic control in both cross-sectional and longitudinal analyses. *Diabetes Care* 2010;**33**:23–8.

8. **Petrak F, Baumeister H, Skinner TC**, et al. Depression and diabetes: treatment and health-care delivery. *Lancet Diabetes & Endocrinology* 2015;**3**(6):472–85.

9. **Safren SA, Gonzalez JS, Wexler DJ**, et al. A randomized controlled trial of cognitive behavioral therapy for adherence and depression (CBT-AD) in patients with uncontrolled type 2 diabetes. *Diabetes Care* 2014;**37**:625–33.

10. **Katon WJ, Von Korff M, Lin EH**, et al. The Pathways Study: a randomized trial of collaborative care in patients with diabetes and depression. *Archives of General Psychiatry* 2004;**61**:1042–9.

11. **Mezuk B, Eaton WW, Albrecht S, Golden SH.** Depression and type 2 diabetes over the lifespan: a meta-analysis. *Diabetes Care* 2008;**31**:2383–90.

12. **Nouwen A, Winkley K, Twisk J**, et al; **European Depression in Diabetes (EDID) Research Consortium.** Type 2 diabetes mellitus as a risk factor for the onset of depression: a systematic review and meta-analysis. *Diabetologia* 2010;**53**:2480–6.

13. **Medzhitov R, Janeway C.** Innate immunity. *New England Journal of Medicine* 2000;**343**:338–44.

14. **Baumann H, Gauldie J.** The acute phase response. *Immunology Today* 1994;**15**:74–80.

15. **Pickup JC.** Inflammation and activated innate immunity in the pathogenesis of type 2 diabetes. *Diabetes Care* 2004;**27**:813–23.

16. **Wing JK, Babor T, Brugha T**, et al. SCAN. Schedules for clinical assessment in neuropsychiatry. *Archives of General Psychiatry* 1990;**47**:589–93.

17. **Twist K, Stahl D, Amiel SA**, et al. Comparison of depressive symptoms in type 2 diabetes using a two-stage survey design. *Psychosomatic Medicine* 2013;**75**:791–7.

18. **Duivis HE, Vogelzangs N, Kupper N**, et al. Differential association of somatic and cognitive symptoms of depression and anxiety with inflammation. *Psychoneuroendocrinology* 2013;**38**:1573–85

19. **Loftis JM, Patterson AL, Wilhelm CJ**, et al. Vulnerability to somatic symptoms of depression during interferon-alpha therapy for hepatitis C: a 16-week prospective study. *Journal of Psychosomatic Research* 2013;**74**:57–63.

20. **Cavelti-Weder C, Furrer R, Keller C**, et al. Inhibition of IL-1beta improves fatigue in type 2 diabetes. *Diabetes Care* 2011;**34**:e158.

21. **Hwang B, Moser DK, Pelter MM**, et al. Changes in depressive symptoms and mortality in patients with heart failure: effects of cognitive-affective and somatic symptoms. *Psychosomatic Medicine* 2015;**77**:798–807.

22. **Dowlati Y, Herrmann N, Swardfager W**, et al. A meta-analysis of cytokines in major depression. *Biological Psychiatry* 2010;**67**:446–57.

23. **Liu Y, Ho RC, Mak A.** Interleukin (IL)-6, tumour necrosis factor alpha (TNF-α) and soluble interleukin-2 receptors (sIL-2R) are elevated in patients with major depressive disorder: a meta-analysis and meta-regression. *Journal of Affective Disorders* 2012;**139**:230–9.

24. **Khandaker GM, Pearson RM, Zammit S, Lewis G, Jones PB.** Association of serum interleukin 6 and C-reactive protein in childhood with depression and psychosis in young adult life: a population-based longitudinal study. *JAMA Psychiatry* 2014;**71**:1121–8.

25. **Pasco JA, Nicholson GC, Williams LJ**, et al. Association of high-sensitivity C-reactive protein with *de novo* major depression. *British Journal of Psychiatry* 2010;**197**:372–7.

26. **Udina M, Castellví P, Moreno-España J**, et al. Interferon-induced depression in chronic hepatitis C: a systematic review and meta-analysis. *Journal of Clinical Psychiatry* 2012;**73**:1128–38.

27. **Savitz J, Drevets WC, Smith CM**, et al. Putative neuroprotective and neurotoxic kynurenine pathway metabolites are associated with hippocampal and amygdalar volumes in subjects with major depressive disorder. *Neuropsychopharmacology* 2015;**40**:463–71.

28. **Silverman MN, Sternberg EM.** Glucocorticoid regulation of inflammation and its functional correlates: from HPA axis to glucocorticoidreceptor dysfunction. *Annals of the New York Academy of Sciences* 2012;**1261**:55–63.

29. **Maes M, Leonard BE, Myint AM**, et al. The new '5-HT' hypothesis of depression: cell-mediated immune activation induces indoleamine 2,3-dioxygenase. *Progress in Neuro-Psychopharmacology & Biological Psychiatry* 2011;**35**:702–21.

30. **Phillips JL, Batten LA, Tremblay P**, et al. A prospective, longitudinal study of the effect of remission on cortical thickness and hippocampal volume in patients with treatment resistant depression. *International Journal of Neuropsychopharmacology* 2015;**30**:18.

31. **Rush AJ, Trivedi MH, Wisniewski SR**, et al. Bupropion-SR, sertraline, or venlafaxine-XR after failure of SSRIs for depression. *New England Journal of Medicine* 2006;**354**:1231–42.

32. **Uher R, Tansey KE, Dew T**, et al. An inflammatory biomarker as a differential predictor of outcome of depression treatment with escitalopram and nortriptyline. *American Journal of Psychiatry* 2014;**171**:1278–86.

33. **Sacerdote P, Bianchi M, Panerai AE.** Chlorimipramine and nortriptyline but not fluoxetine and fluvoxamine inhibit human polymorphonuclear cell chemotaxis in vitro. *General Pharmacology* 1994;**25**:409–12.

34. **Na KS, Lee KJ, Lee JS**, et al. Efficacy of adjunctive celecoxib treatment for patients with major depressive disorder: a meta-analysis. *Progress in Neuro-Psychopharmacology & Biological Psychiatry* 2014;**48**:79–85.

35. **Su KP, Lai HC, Yang HT**, et al. Omega-3 fatty acids in the prevention of interferon-alpha-induced depression: results from a randomized, controlled trial. *Biological Psychiatry* 2014;**76**:559–66.

36. Raison CL, Rutherford RE, Woolwine BJ, et al. A randomized controlled trial of the tumor necrosis factor antagonist infliximab for treatment-resistant depression: the role of baseline inflammatory biomarkers. *JAMA Psychiatry* 2013;**70**:31–41

37. Miyaoka T, Wake R, Furuya M, et al. Minocycline as adjunctive therapy for patients with unipolar psychotic depression: an open-label study. *Progress in Neuro-Psychopharmacology & Biological Psychiatry* 2012;**37**:222–6.

38. Husain MI, Chaudhry IB, Rahman RR, et al. Minocycline as an adjunct for treatment-resistant depressive symptoms: study protocol for a pilot randomised controlled trial. *Trials* 2015;**16**:410.

39. Crook MA, Tutt P, Simpson H, Pickup JC. Serum sialic acid and acute phase proteins in type 1 and 2 diabetes. *Clinica Chimica Acta* 1993;**219**:131–8.

40. Wang X, Bao W, Liu J, et al. Inflammatory markers and risk of type 2 diabetes: a systematic review and meta-analysis. *Diabetes Care* 2013;**36**:166–75.

41. Westwell-Roper CY, Ehses JA, Verchere CB, et al. Resident macrophages mediate islet amyloid polypeptide-induced islet IL-1β production and β cell dysfunction. *Diabetes* 2014;**63**:1698–711.

42. Donath MY. Targeting inflammation in the treatment of type 2 diabetes: time to start. *Nature Reviews Drug Discovery* 2014;**13**:465–76.

43. Pickup JC, Mattock MB. Activation of the innate immune system as a predictor of cardiovascular mortality in type 2 diabetes mellitus. *Diabetic Medicine* 2003;**20**:723–6.

44. Libby P, Ridker PM, Maseri A. Inflammation and atheroslerosis. *Circulation* 2002;**105**:1135–43.

45. Di Prospero NA, Artis E, Andrade-Gordon P, et al. CCR2 antagonism in patients with type 2 diabetes mellitus: a randomized, placebo-controlled study. *Diabetes, Obesity and Metabolism* 2014;**16**:1055–64.

46. Goldfine AB, Fonseca V, Jablonski KA, et al. The effects of salsalate on glycemic control in patients with type 2 diabetes: a randomized trial. *Annals of Internal Medicine* 2010;**152**:346–57.

47. Goldfine AB, Fonseca V, Jablonski KA, et al. Salicylate (salsalate) in patients with type 2 diabetes: a randomized trial. *Annals of Internal Medicine* 2013;**159**:1–12.

48. Larsen CM, Faulenbach M, Vaag A et al. Interleukin-1-receptor antagonist in type 2 diabetes mellitus. *New England Journal of Medicine* 2007;**356**:1517–26.

49. Larsen CM, Faulenbach M, Vaag A, et al. Sustained effects of interleukin-1 receptor antagonist treatment in type 2 diabetes. *Diabetes Care* 2009;**32**:1663–8.

50. Doyle TA, de Groot M, Harris T, et al. Diabetes, depressive symptoms, and inflammation in older adults: results from the Health, Aging, and Body Composition Study. *Journal of Psychosomatic Research* 2013;**75**:419–24.

51. Hayashino Y, Mashitani T, Tsujii S, Ishii H, Diabetes Distress and Care Registry at Tenri Study Group. Elevated levels of hs-CRP are associated with high prevalence of depression in Japanese patients with type 2 diabetes: the Diabetes Distress and Care Registry at Tenri (DDCRT 6). *Diabetes Care* 2014;**37**:2459–65.

52. Laake JP, Stahl D, Amiel SA, et al. The association between depressive symptoms and systemic inflammation in people with type 2 diabetes: findings from the South London Diabetes Study. *Diabetes Care* 2014;**37**:2186–92.

53. **Danese A, Pariante CM, Caspi A**, et al. Childhood maltreatment predicts adult inflammation in a life-course study. *Proceedings of the National Academy of Sciences of the United States of America* 2007;**104**:1319–24.
54. **Moulton CD, Pickup JC, Ismail K.** The link between depression and diabetes: the search for shared mechanisms. *Lancet Diabetes and Endocrinology* 2015;**6**:461–7.
55. **Stringhini S, Batty GD, Bovet P**, et al. Association of lifecourse socioeconomic status with chronic inflammation and type 2 diabetes risk: the Whitehall II prospective cohort study. *PLoS Med* 2013;**10**:e1001479.
56. **Kemp DE, Ismail-Beigi F, Ganocy SJ**, et al. Use of insulin sensitizers for the treatment of major depressive disorder: a pilot study of pioglitazone for major depression accompanied by abdominal obesity. *Journal of Affective Disorders* 2012;**136**:1164–73.
57. **Hu Y, Xing H, Dong X**, et al. Pioglitazone is an effective treatment for patients with post-stroke depression combined with type 2 diabetes mellitus. *Experimental and Therapeutc Medicine* 2015;**10**:1109–14.
58. **Dai Y, Mehta JL, Chen M.** Glucagon-like peptide-1 receptor agonist liraglutide inhibits endothelin-1 in endothelial cell by repressing nuclear factor-kappa B activation. *Cardiovascular Drugs and Therapy* 2013;**27**:371–80.
59. **Makdissi A, Ghanim H, Vora M**, et al. Sitagliptin exerts an antinflammatory action.*Journal of Clinical Endocrinology & Metabolism* 2012;**97**:3333–41.
60. **Moulton CD, Pickup JC, Amiel SA**, et al. Investigating incretin-based therapies as a novel treatment for depression in type 2 diabetes: Findings from the South London Diabetes (SOUL-D) Study. *Primary Care Diabetes* 2016;**10**:156–9.
61. **da Silva Dias IC, Carabelli B, Ishii DK**, et al. Indoleamine-2,3-dioxygenase/kynurenine pathway as a potential pharmacological target to treat depression associated with diabetes. *Molecular Neurobiology* 2016;**53**:6997–7009.

Chapter 6

Hypothalamic–pituitary–adrenal axis

Allan H. Young and Mario F. Juruena

Introduction

The relationship between stress and affective (mood) disorders is a strong example of a field of study that can be best understood from an integrative perspective. During acute stress, adaptive physiological responses occur, including increased adrenocortical hormone secretion, primarily cortisol. Whenever an acute interruption of this balance occurs, illness may result. Particularly interesting are psychological stress (i.e. stress in the mind) interactions with the nervous, endocrine, and immune systems. It is now broadly accepted that psychological stress may change the internal homeostatic state of an individual [1].

During acute stress, adaptive physiological responses occur, which include hyperactivity of the hypothalamic–pituitary–adrenal (HPA) axis. Whenever there is an acute interruption of this balance, illness may result. The social and physical environments have an enormous impact on our physiology and behaviour, and they influence the process of adaptation or 'allostasis'. It is correct to state that at the same time that our experiences change our brain and thoughts, namely, changing our mind, they are also changing our neurobiology [2].

Physiology of the HPA axis

The HPA axis constitutes one of the major endocrine systems that maintains homoeostasis when the organism is challenged or stressed. Activation of the HPA axis is perhaps the most important endocrine component of the stress response [3]. Abnormal activation of the HPA axis, as well as increased circulating levels of cortisol, is one potential explanation for many of the features of depression, and many previous studies have described an impaired HPA negative feedback, leading to hypercortisolaemia, in the most severe forms of depression [4].

Cortisol mediates its action, including feedback regulation of the HPA axis, through two distinct intracellular corticosteroid receptor subtypes in the brain: the type I, high-affinity, mineralocorticoid receptor (MR) and type 2, glucocorticoid receptor (GR) [5]. The type I receptor (MR) has a limited distribution, and it is found in relatively high density in the hippocampus and sensory and motor sites outside the hypothalamus. The expression of type II receptors (GR) is more widespread, and they are found in the hippocampus, the amygdala, the hypothalamus, and the catecholaminergic cell bodies of the brain stem [6]. There is a theory that suggests that a GR defect may mediate the impaired negative feedback thought to cause hypercortisolaemia in depression [7].

Under basal levels of cortisol, negative feedback is mediated mainly through the MR in the hippocampus, whereas under stress and high cortisol concentrations, feedback is mediated by the less sensitive GR in the hippocampus, hypothalamus, and pituitary gland. The balance in these MR- and GR-mediated effects on the stress system is of crucial importance to the set point of the HPA axis activity [5].

It is proposed that the maintenance of corticosteroid homeostasis and the balance in MR-/GR-mediated effects limit vulnerability to stress-related diseases in genetically predisposed individuals. Stress-induced activation of the HPA axis generally involves stimulated release of corticotropin-releasing factor (CRF) from the paraventricular nucleus (PVN) of the hypothalamus into the portal venous circulation, where CRF stimulates the synthesis of proopiomelancortin, the precursor of adrenocorticotropic hormone (ACTH) from anterior pituitary cells. Arginine-vasopressin (AVP) is a potent synergistic factor with CRF in stimulating ACTH secretion [8].

In the hypothalamus, the PVN receives fibres from a number of brain areas, notably the brain stem and limbic system (e.g. amygdala and the septal areas). It is thought that these afferents may be important in HPA responses to behavioural and emotional stimuli and may play a role in corticosteroid feedback. Several peptides are released alongside and interact with CRF at the level of the anterior pituitary and alter the stimulatory action of ACTH secretion [9]. Increases in circulating ACTH stimulate glucocorticoid release from the adrenal cortex (see Fig. 6.1).

The division of the adrenal cortex into separate layers is important since zones produce different steroids [10]. Box 6.1 summarizes the adrenal steroids. Cortisol is produced by the zona fasciculata at the rate of 12–15 mg/m² of body surface area per day. However, more than 90% of the circulating cortisol is bound to corticosteroid-binding globulin (CBG) in humans and rodents. Also, it has been observed that both exogenous glucocorticoid administration and

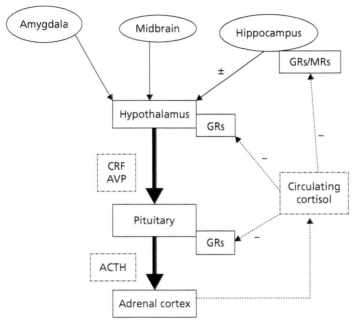

Fig. 6.1 Schematic diagram of hypothalamic–pituitary–adrenal (HPA) axis. It describes regulation and negative feedback (–) of cortisol via glucocorticoid receptors (GRs) and mineralocorticoid receptors (MRs).

endogenous increases in plasma cortisol (e.g., Cushing's syndrome) result in a 30–40% decrease in the plasma CBG concentration. Thus, CBG levels fluctuate according to glucocorticoid concentration [11,12].

Adrenocorticotropic hormone is secreted in irregular bursts throughout the day, and plasma cortisol tends to rise and fall in response to this pulsatile secretion. In humans, the bursts are most frequent in the early morning and least frequent in the evening. The biological clock responsible for the diurnal ACTH rhythm is thought to be located in the suprachiasmatic nuclei of the hypothalamus. Changes in the activity of these neurones increase the release of CRF and AVP by the PVN during usual times of peak activity. Consequently, it is thought that the secretion of CRF and AVP also follows a pulsatile pattern. However, CRF levels in human peripheral plasma are very low and do not exhibit circadian variation, and, therefore, these levels cannot be used reliably to assess hypothalamic CRF release relevant to the HPA axis. An important feature is the intrinsic rhythmicity of the HPA axis with regard not only to the diurnal variation but also to the pulsatility, which is similar to the rhythm found within the reproductive and growth hormone axes [10].

Box 6.1 Adrenal steroids

Three sets of steroids produced by the adrenal cortex

- Aldosterone (mineralocorticoid) from zona glomerulosa
- Cortisol (corticosterone in some rodents; glucocorticoid) from zona fasciculata
- Dehydroepiandrosterone from zona reticularis (primates)

Separate control systems for the three regions

- Glomerulosa: angiotensin II (via renal renin)
- Fasciculata: adrenocorticotropic hormone (pituitary)
- Reticularis: largely unknown

Mineralocorticoids and glucocorticoids both bind to the mineralocorticoid receptor present in target tissues, including the brain

- High expression in several areas, including the hippocampus, anterior hypothalamus

Glucocorticoids also bind to the glucocorticoid receptor expressed much more widely in the brain

Both MR and GR bind as dimmers to a range of palindromic glucocorticoid receptor elements (GREs) following activation by adrenal steroids

Glucocorticoids at least may also interact with membrane bound receptors in the brain

- e.g., GABAA or NMDA receptors
- Recent evidence indicates that the classical steroid receptors themselves may mediate such membrane effects

Binding to GRE activates or suppresses a wide range of downstream genes

A wide variation in cortisol levels is observed among individuals in response to a stressor. This variability is so marked that in any one individual, it is not always possible to distinguish a stress response from a spontaneously occurring pulse. Young and Altemus [13] put forward a totally different hypothesis that acute stressors simply 'advance' a spontaneous cortisol pulse rather than activate cortisol release as an independent variable, thereby acting as a synchronizer or *zeitgeber* for the ultradian cortisol rhythm, whose effectiveness will depend on a number of variables that control the individual's endogenous rhythm. Finally, pulsatility analysis enables us to examine multiple aspects of

Box 6.2 Factors that affect corticosteroid secretion

◆ Corticosteroids are secreted in distinct pulses
  There is a rapid fall in plasma levels after each pulse
  This pulse generator increases its activity in the morning (in humans) or in the evening (in rats)
  The pulse generator is controlled by both genetic and epigenetic factors
  Pulsatile frequency is increased with age
◆ Early-life exposure to adversity (either physical or social) has persistent affects on later HPA axis function
◆ There are sex differences in HPA activity.
◆ Gonadal steroids in adulthood also alter HPA activity

the control of the HPA axis, extending our understanding well beyond mean cortisol levels [13].

Glucocorticoids control their own synthesis and release by completing a negative feedback loop at the level of the anterior pituitary, hypothalamus, and other higher centres, including the mesencephalic reticular formation. The circulating concentration of cortisol is a major influence at both the hypothalamic and pituitary levels (see Box 6.2). The negative feedback mechanisms constitute a rate-sensitive fast feedback system and a delayed feedback system. Fast feedback is proportional to the rate of rising of steroid concentrations and perhaps serves to limit the amplitude of the response. In contrast, delayed feedback is related to the ambient concentration of corticosteroid and is frequently the consequence of repeated or continuous administration of high doses of glucocorticoids. Delayed feedback may persist for days or weeks after the steroid treatment is withdrawn [9–11].

The glucocorticoid receptors

Steroid hormones are small, lipid-soluble ligands that diffuse across cell membranes. Unlike the receptors for peptide hormones, which are located in the cell membrane, the receptors for these ligands are localized in the cytoplasm. In response to ligand binding, steroid hormone receptors translocate to the nucleus, where they regulate the expression of certain genes by binding to specific hormone response elements (HREs) in their regulatory regions. Type I receptors are thought to be involved in controlling the basal expression of CRF and AVP at the nadir of diurnal ACTH secretion and in controlling peak ACTH secretion [14,15]. Type II receptors are considered to be involved in control of stress-induced ACTH secretion. According to the 'nucleocytoplasmic traffic' model of GR action, the GR in its 'inactivated' form resides primarily in the cytoplasm in association with a multimeric complex of chaperone proteins including several heat shock proteins (HSPs). After being bound by steroid, the GR undergoes a conformational change, dissociates from the chaperone protein complex, and translocates from the cytoplasm to the nucleus, where it either binds to glucocorticoid response elements (GREs) on DNA or interacts with other transcription factors. GREs can confer either positive or negative regulation of the genes to which they are linked. Glucocorticoid receptors have a low affinity but high capacity for cortisol and are very responsive to changes in cortisol concentrations [14,15].

Studies on the subcellular localization of the MR have been controversial. In the lack of corticosteroid hormone, MR is present both in the cytoplasm and in the nucleus. However, the presence of corticosteroid hormone induced a rapid nuclear accumulation of the MR. The MR has a high affinity for endogenous glucocorticoids: the *in vitro* dissociation constant/ionization constant (K_d/K_i) is 0.13 nM for cortisol binding to human MR and 0.5 nM for corticosterone binding to mouse MR. In contrast, the GR has a low affinity for endogenous glucocorticoids: the *in vitro* K_d/K_i is 15 nM for cortisol binding to human GR and 5 nM for corticosterone binding to mouse GR. Under basal levels of cortisol, negative feedback is mediated mainly through the MR in the hippocampus, whereas under stress and high cortisol concentrations, the less sensitive GR in the hippocampus, hypothalamus, and pituitary gland come into play. The balance in these MR- and GR-mediated effects on the stress system is of crucial importance to the set point of the HPA axis activity [16]. Spencer et al. [15] and de Kloet et al. [5] have clarified that GR activation is necessary for the HPA feedback regulation when levels of glucocorticoids are high (response to stress, circadian peak) but that MR also plays an important role by modulating GR-dependent regulation.

Brain corticosteroid balance in health and disease

Data on corticosteroid receptor diversity led de Kloet et al. [10] to a working hypothesis that in rodents, 'tonic influences of corticosterone are exerted via hippocampal MRs, while the additional occupancy of GRs with higher levels of corticosterone mediates feedback actions aimed to restore disturbances in homeostasis'. This proposal provides a receptor-based version of Selye's classical 'pendulum hypothesis' on opposing effects of mineralocorticoids and glucocorticoids in host defence. In humans, MRs are thought to be involved in the tonic inhibitory activity within the HPA axis, but GRs appear to 'switch off' cortisol production at times of stress [17]. According to Pace and Spencer [18], MRs may be necessary for glucocorticoid regulation of HPA axis activity during mild stressors but not during stressors that result in a stronger corticosterone response. It is proposed that the maintenance of corticosteroid homeostasis and the balance in MR/GR-mediated effects limit vulnerability to stress-related diseases in genetically predisposed individuals [5].

States associated with hyperactivation

Hyperactivity of the HPA axis in depression is one of the most consistent findings in psychiatry. A significant percentage of patients with major depression have been shown to exhibit increased concentrations of cortisol in plasma, urine, and cerebrospinal fluid (CSF); an exaggerated cortisol response to adrenocorticotropic hormone (ACTH); and an enlargement of both the pituitary and adrenal glands [4]. Adrenal hypertrophy in patients with depression has been demonstrated, and this finding is likely to explain why the cortisol response to CRF is similar in subjects with depression and control subjects because the enlarged adrenal gland is capable of compensating for the blunted ACTH response to CRF commonly observed in patients with depression [16]. Increased pituitary volume in these patients has also been described, and it has also been considered a marker of HPA axis activation. The first episode of a psychosis has also been found to be associated with a larger pituitary volume, and it has been suggested that this is due to activation of the HPA axis; the smaller pituitary volume in subjects with established psychosis could also be the consequence of repeated episodes of HPA axis hyperactivity. In general, HPA axis changes appear to be state-dependent, tending to improve upon resolution of the depressive syndrome. In fact, previous studies have described an impaired HPA negative feedback, leading to hypercortisolaemia [16,17–19].

A spectrum of other conditions may be associated with increased and prolonged activation of the HPA axis, including anorexia nervosa with or without malnutrition, obsessive–compulsive disorder, panic anxiety, chronic active alcoholism, alcohol and narcotic withdrawal, poorly controlled diabetes mellitus, and hyperthyroidism [20]. Another group of states is characterized by hypoactivation of the stress system, rather than sustained activation, in which chronically reduced secretion of CRF may result in pathological hypoarousal and an enhanced HPA negative feedback. Patients with posttraumatic stress disorder, atypical depression, seasonal depression, and chronic fatigue syndrome fall into this category [21,22], see Fig. 6.2.

The dysregulations situate themselves at different levels of the HPA axis, and the experimental findings can be classified under basal hormonal changes, *post mortem* findings, and results from imaging studies and functional tests.

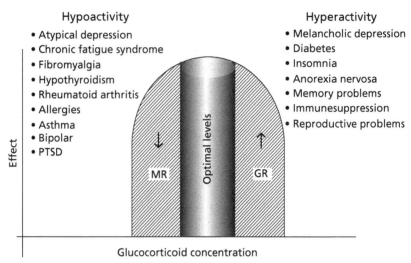

Hypoactivity
- Atypical depression
- Chronic fatigue syndrome
- Fibromyalgia
- Hypothyroidism
- Rheumatoid arthritis
- Allergies
- Asthma
- Bipolar
- PTSD

Hyperactivity
- Melancholic depression
- Diabetes
- Insomnia
- Anorexia nervosa
- Memory problems
- Immunesuppression
- Reproductive problems

Effect

MR   Optimal levels   GR

Glucocorticoid concentration

Fig. 6.2 Effect of glucocorticoid concentration and balance between mineralocorticoid (MR) and Glucocorticoid receptors (GR) and activity of hypothalamic–pituitary–adrenal (HPA) axis, with different impact on psychopathology.

Theories as to the causes of abnormal HPA axis function in depression are that it is related to either (1) increased central drive at the hypothalamic level or (2) downregulation of GRs. Taking the first theory, it has been suggested that hypercortisolism represents a defect at or above the level of the hypothalamus, resulting in the hypersecretion of CRF and AVP [4]. CRF itself has behavioural effects in animals that are similar to those seen in patients with depression including alterations in activity, appetite, and sleep [21]. The second theory suggests that a defect of GRs may also explain the hypercortisolaemia seen in depression, via impaired negative feedback control of the HPA axis by glucocorticoids. Various research groups have suggested that the overactivity of the HPA axis in depression may be due to an abnormality of the GR at the limbic–hippocampal level [7–10]. This abnormality then results in a defect in or resistance to glucocorticoid. In fact, several findings in depression are consistent with an abnormality of the GR. Most notably, patients with depression fail to show most of the physical symptoms of corticosteroid excess, despite the frequent presence of hypercortisolism, suggesting that peripheral GRs may be abnormal or insensitive in depression. Consistent with the fact that GR is more important in the regulation of the HPA axis when endogenous levels of glucocorticoids are high [5] and with the fact that patients with major depression exhibit impaired HPA negative feedback in the context of elevated circulating levels of cortisol [16], a number of studies have described reduced GR function in patients with depression (GR resistance) and have concluded that antidepressants act by reversing these putative GR changes [16,23,24].

Because a wide variety of stressors reliably activate the HPA axis and because glucocorticoids are the end-products of HPA axis activation, these hormones have been most commonly seen as the agents provocateurs, or even in extreme cases as the physical embodiment, of stress-induced pathology [16,23,24]. Indeed, it has been suggested that prolonged overproduction of glucocorticoids, whether as a result of ongoing stress or a genetic predisposition to HPA axis hyperactivity, damages brain structures (especially the hippocampus) essential for HPA axis restraint. Such damage, in turn, has been hypothesized to lead to a feed-forward circuit in which ongoing stressors drive glucocorticoid overproduction indefinitely: the 'glucocorticoid cascade hypothesis'. Because of the capacity of high concentrations of glucocorticoids to disrupt cellular functioning in ways that can lead to a host of ills, this glucocorticoid overproduction is believed to contribute directly to many of the adverse behavioural and physiological sequelae associated with chronic stress [25,26].

Assessing the impaired HPA negative feedback

Functioning of the HPA axis can be assessed under basal as well as under challenged conditions. Basal cortisol mainly reflects adrenal functioning, whereas several challenge paradigms target different levels of the HPA axis [6–11]. Cortisol is secreted with a pulsatory diurnal rhythm, with a peak (average increase of 50%) approximately 30 minutes after awakening and a progressive decline during the day with lowest levels around midnight. Basal cortisol may be assessed in several bodily fluids such as saliva, urine, blood (serum or plasma), and cerebrospinal fluid. Whereas salivary free cortisol and urinary free cortisol consist almost entirely of the (free) biologically active fraction, in blood, less than 10% of the cortisol is free. The major part is bound to cortisol-binding globulin or other proteins and, therefore, biologically inactive. A distinction can be made between psychosocial stress challenges and pharmacological stress challenges. Examples of the psychosocial stress challenges are cognitive stress challenges, challenges using trauma related acoustic stimuli, or trauma scripts. The most often used psychosocial stress challenge is the Trier Social Stress Test (TSST) that combines social-evaluative threat and uncontrollability [27].

The dexamethasone suppression test (DST) was the first and is, to date, the most studied biological marker in research on depressive disorders. In 1968, Bernard Carroll and colleagues [28] showed that patients with depression fail to suppress plasma cortisol to the same extent as controls without depression.

This impaired feedback inhibition by dexamethasone has been demonstrated in patients with depression by a variety of studies, many occurring in the 1970s and the 1980s. However, in the 1990s, several studies found that the sensitivity of the DST in the diagnosis of the DSM-III defined the melancholic subclass of major depression was only approximately 35–45%, although the specificity was higher at approximately 70–89% [29,30]. A meta-analysis to determine the significance of differences in rates of no suppression of cortisol indicated a high probability that a greater rate of cortisol no suppression occurs in psychotic depression (64% versus 41% in patients without psychosis). The DEX/CRH test combines both, the DST and the corticotrophin-releasing hormone (CRH) stimulation test [29,30]. Watson et al. [31] compared the use of the DEX/CRH test and the DST in patients with mood disorders and controls, and suggested that the two tests measure common pathology but that the DEX/CRH test is more specific and hence has better diagnostic utility. Nevertheless, the DEX/CRH test remains limited by the pharmacokinetic profile of dexamethasone and the lack of MR activity.

Prednisolone is a synthetic glucocorticoid that, like dexamethasone, is widely used as an anti-inflammatory and immunosuppressive drug. Prednisolone mimics cortisol in many ways. Like cortisol, it binds to CBG, and its half-life is similar to that of cortisol. However, the most important of these similarities is that prednisolone and cortisol are similar in their abilities to bind and activate the GR and the MR [17,32–34]

HPA axis in depression and implications for diabetes

Once cortisol is released from the adrenal cortex in response to ACTH stimulation, it functions to increase blood glucose levels through its action on glycogen, protein, and lipid metabolism. In the liver, cortisol stimulates gluconeogenesis and, in adipose tissue, activates lipolysis and free fatty acids (FFA) to be released into the circulation. Cortisol also has a permissive effect on glucagon and catecholamine action, thereby contributing to insulin resistance and increased blood glucose levels at the expense of glycogen, protein, and lipid storage [35,36].

There is growing evidence that depression may cause major life-threatening and disabling diseases, such as diabetes mellitus [36]. The metabolic syndrome is a clustering of risk factors associated with a particularly high risk of cardiovascular events and diabetes.

Dysregulation of the HPA axis is typically associated with chronic stress, and some studies have described an association between depression and high cortisol levels, and, in turn, elevated levels of cortisol have been related to metabolic syndrome components such as abdominal obesity and glucose intolerance [35].

There is now evidence that insulin exerts important functions in neural development and synaptic plasticity [37]. These findings have led to the hypothesis that insulin insufficiency may lead to the defects in neurocognition commonly observed in depression. Disrupted control of adrenocorticotropic hormone (ACTH) release from pituitary corticotrophs and direct stimulation of corticotrophin-releasing hormone of the adrenal gland with or without the release of ACTH leads to hyperactivation of the HPA in patients with diabetes. Furthermore, the impairment of glucocorticoid negative feedback sensitivity in patients with diabetes also results in increased activity of the HPA axis: following glucocorticoid administration, these patients exhibit a greater incidence of no suppression of pituitary–adrenal activity compared with non-diabetic individuals [38]. Corticosteroids have been demonstrated to exert a tonic inhibitory control of hippocampal 5-HT1A receptors; this finding is of particular salience given the serotonin deficiency that occurs in depression. Once established, the HPA axis dysregulation and hypercortisolaemia may further contribute to a hyperglycaemic or poorly controlled diabetic state and has been associated with increased chronic complications of diabetes in adult studies [39].

There are two possible mechanisms underlying the association between type 2 diabetes and the onset of depression. First, biochemical changes associated with diabetes could account for the increased risk of depression [40]. For example, hyperglycaemia and hyperinsulinaemia increase the activity of the HPA axis, inducing arousal of the nervous system, which in turn may promote depression [41]. Second, depression in patients with diabetes may be viewed as the result of the burden of the disease. This is supported by the finding that when the burden of diabetes increases, the probability of mood symptoms increases as well [42].

Patients with present type 2 diabetes frequently show alterations of the HPA axis negative feedback [43] suggestive of an impairment of corticosteroid receptor sensitivity. HPA axis disturbance seems to be particularly important for people with diabetes since the degree of cortisol secretion is related to the presence and number of diabetes complications [44].

At baseline, diabetes patients had increased glucocorticoid, but normal mineralocorticoid sensitivity in the presence of hypercortisolaemia. The action of dexamethasone, which exclusively binds to GR, and of prednisolone, which binds to both GR and MR, is respectively a proxy for glucocorticoid and mineralocorticoid sensitivity [17,33]. Such disturbance in the regulation of the HPA axis may contribute to deterioration in diabetes by enhancing the effect of cortisol and its anti-insulin actions, including the inhibition of glucose uptake in adipocytes and fibroblasts, increasing hepatic gluconeogenesis, sensitizing the liver to catecholamines and glucagon, and elevating blood glucose [45].

This review suggests that in diabetes the ability to match the body's response to a stressor involves modulation of corticosteroid receptor sensitivity, an evidence of insufficient corticosteroid signalling. Moreover, insufficient corticosteroid signalling may also increase arousal and thus play a role in stress-related pathology.

Conclusion

Type 2 diabetes is associated with a lack of stress-induced modulation of glucocorticoid and mineralocorticoid sensitivity in the HPA axis. Emphasis on modulating glucocorticoids in stress-related pathology encourages the development of therapeutic strategies to modulate glucocorticoid-signalling pathways.

In conclusion, our review suggests a synergistic relationship between depression, cortisol, and diabetes. Persons with hypercortisolaemic depression, in particular, may be at risk for having the metabolic syndrome, and therefore have an increased risk of developing diabetes.

References

1. **Young AH.** Cortisol in mood disorders. *Stress*. 2004;7:205–8.
2. **Juruena MF** Early-life stress and HPA axis trigger recurrent adulthood depression. *Epilepsy & Behavior* 2014;38:148–59.
3. **Nemeroff CB, Evans DL.** Correlation between the dexamethasone suppression test in depressed patients and clinical response. *American Journal of Psychiatry* 1984;141:247–9.
4. **Gold PW, Goodwin FK, Chrousos GP.** Clinical and biochemical manifestations of depression. Relation to the neurobiology of stress (2). *New England Journal of Medicine* 1988;319:413–20.
5. **de Kloet ER, Vreugdenhil E, Oitzl MS, Joels M.** Brain corticosteroid receptor balance in health and disease. *Endocrine Reviews* 1998;19(3):269–301.
6. **McEwen BS.** Allostasis and allostatic load: implications for neuropsychopharmacology. *Neuropsychopharmacology* 2000;22:108–24.
7. **Modell S, Yassouridis A, Huber J, Holsboer F.** Corticosteroid receptor function is decreased in depressed patients. *Neuroendocrinology* 1997;65:216–22.
8. **Juruena MF, Cleare AJ, Bauer ME, Pariante CM.** Molecular mechanisms of glucocorticoid receptor sensitivity and relevance to affective disorders. *Acta Neuropsychiatrica* 2003;15:354–67.
9. **Juruena MF, Cleare AJ, Pariante CM.** The hypothalamic pituitary adrenal axis, glucocorticoid receptor function and relevance to depression. *Revista Brasileira de Psiquiatria* 2004;26:189–201.

10. Herbert J, Goodyer IM, Grossman AB, et al. Do corticosteroids damage the brain? *Journal of Neuroendocrinology* 2006;**18**:393–411.

11. Chrousos GP. The hypothalamic–pituitary–adrenal axis and immune-mediated inflammation. *New England Journal of Medicine* 1995;**332**:1351–62.

12. Frairia R, Agrimonti F, Fortunati N, et al. Influence of naturally occurring and synthetic glucocorticoids on corticosteroid-binding globulin-steroid interaction in human peripheral plasma. *Annals of the New York Academy of Sciences*1988;**538**:287–303.

13. Young EA, Altemus M. Puberty, ovarian steroids, and stress. *Annals of the New York Academy of Sciences* 2004;**1021**:124–33.

14. Fejes-Toth G, Pearce D, Naray-Fejes-Toth A. Subcellular localization of mineralocorticoid receptors in living cells: effects of receptor agonists and antagonists. *Proceedings of the National Academy of Sciences* 1998;**95**:2973–8.

15. Spencer RL, Kim PJ, Kalman BA, Cole MA. Evidence for mineralocorticoid receptor facilitation of glucocorticoid receptor-dependent regulation of HPA axis activity. *Endocrinology* 1998;**139**:2718–26.

16. de Kloet ER, Joels M, Holsboer F. Stress and the brain: from adaptation to disease. *Nature Reviews Neuroscience* 2005;**6**:463–75.

17. Juruena MF, Pariante CM, Papadopoulos AS, et al. Prednisolone suppression test in depression: prospective study of the role of HPA axis dysfunction in treatment resistance. *British Journal of Psychiatry* 2009;**194**: 342–9.

18. Pace TW, Spencer RL. Disruption of mineralocorticoid receptor function increasescorticosterone responding to a mild, but not moderate, psychological stressor. *American Journal of Physiology. Endocrinology and Metabolism* 2005;**288**:E1082–8.

19. Holsboer F. The corticosteroid receptor hypothesis of depression. *Neuropsychopharmacology* 2000;**23**:477–501.

20. Tsigos C, Chrousos GP. Hypothalamic–pituitary–adrenal axis, neuroendocrine factors and stress. *Journal of Psychosomatic Research* 2002;**53**:865–71.

21. Juruena MF, Cleare AJ. Overlap between atypical depression, seasonal affective disorder and chronic fatigue syndrome. *Revista Brasileira de Psiquiatria* 2007;**29**:20–7.

22. Palma BD, Tiba PA, Ricardo BM, et al. Immune outcomes of sleep disorders: the hypothalamic-pituitary-adrenal axis as a modulatory factor. *Revista Brasileira de Psiquiatria* 2007;**29**(suppl.1):33–8.

23. McQuade R, Young AH. Future therapeutic targets in mood disorders: the glucocorticoid receptor. *British Journal of Psychiatry* 2000;**177**:390–5.

24. Watson S, Gallagher P, Ritchie JC, et al. Hypothalamic–pituitary–adrenal axis function in patients with bipolar disorder. *British Journal of Psychiatry* 2004;**184**:496–502.

25. Sapolsky RM. Glucocorticoids and hippocampal atrophy in neuropsychiatric disorders. *Archives of General Psychiatry* 2000;**57**:925–35.

26. McEwen BS, Seeman T. Protective and damaging effects of mediators of stress. Elaborating and testing the concepts of allostasis and allostatic load. *Annals of the New York Academy of Sciences* 1999:30–47.

27. de Kloet CS, Vermetten E, Geuze E, et al. Assessment of HPA-axis function in posttraumatic stress disorder: pharmacological and non-pharmacological challenge tests, a review. *Journal of Psychiatric Research* 2006;**40**:550–67.

28. **Carroll BJ, Martin FIR, Davies B.** Resistance to suppression by dexamethasone of plasma 11-O.H.C.S. levels in severe depressive illness. *British Medical Journal 1968;***3**:285–7.

29. **Nelson JC, Davis JM.** DST studies in psychotic depression: a meta-analysis. *American Journal of Psychiatry* 1997;**154**:1497–503.

30. **Ribeiro SC, Tandon R, Grunhaus L, Greden JF.** The DST as a predictor of outcome in depression: a meta-analysis. *American Journal of Psychiatry* 1993;**150**:1618–29.

31. **Watson S, Gallagher P, Smith MS,** et al. The dex/CRH test—is it better than the DST? *Psychoneuroendocrinology* 2006;**31**:889–94.

32. **Juruena MF, Cleare AJ, Papadopoulos AS,** et al. Different responses to dexamethasone and prednisolone in the same depressed patients. *Psychopharmacology (Berlin)* 2006;**189**:225–35.

33. **Juruena MF, Pariante CM, Papadopoulos AS,** et al. The role of mineralocorticoid receptor function in treatment-resistant depression. *Journal of Psychopharmacology* 2013;**27**:1169–79.

34. **Pariante CM, Papadopoulos AS, Poon L,** et al. A novel prednisolone suppression test for the hypothalamic–pituitary–adrenal axis. *Biological Psychiatry* 2002;**51**:922–30.

35. **Bjorntorp P, Rosmond, R.** Hypothalamic origin of the metabolic syndrome X. *Annals of the New York Academy of Sciences* 1999;**892**:297–307.

36. **Brown LC, Majumdar SR, Newman, S.C, Johnson JA.** History of depression increases risk of type 2 diabetes in younger adults. *Diabetes Care* 2005;**28**:1063–7.

37. **Huang CC, Lee CC, Hsu KS.** The role of insulin receptor signaling in synaptic plasticity and cognitive function. *Chang Gung Medical Journal* 2010;**33**:115–25

38. **Hudson JI, Hudson MS, Rothschild AJ,** et al. Abnormal results of dexamethasone suppression tests in nondepressed patients with diabetes mellitus. *Archives of General Psychiatry* 1984;**41**:1086–9.

39. **Chiodini I, Adda G, Scillitani A,** et al. Cortisol secretion in patients with type 2 diabetes: relationship with chronic complications. *Diabetes Care* 2007;**30**:83–8.

40. **Talbot F, Nouwen A.** A review of the relationship between depression and diabetes in adults: is there a link? *Diabetes Care* 2000;**23**:1556–62.

41. **Chan O, Inouye K, Riddell MC, Vranic M, Matthews SG.** Diabetes and the hypothalamo-pituitary-adrenal (HPA) axis. *Minerva Endocrinologica* 2003;**28**:87–102.

42. **Musselman DL, Betan E, Larsen H, Phillips LS.** Relationship of depression to diabetes types 1 and 2: epidemiology, biology, and treatment. *Biological Psychiatry* 2003;**54**:317–29.

43. **Bruehl H, Rueger M, Dziobek I,** et al. HPA axis dysregulation and memory impairments in type 2 diabetes. *Journal of Clinical Endocrinology & Metabolism* 2007;**92**:2439–45.

44. **Rohleder N, Wolf JM, Kirschbaum** C. 2003. Glucocorticoid sensitivity in humans-interindividual differences and acute stress effects. *Stress* **6**, 207—222.

45. **Chan O, Inouye K, Akirav E,** et al. Insulin alone increases HPA activity, and diabetes lower speak stress responses. *Endocrinology* 2005;**146**:1382–90.

Chapter 7

Gut–brain axis: Physiology and pathology

Carla Petrella, Giuseppe Nisticò,
and Robert Nisticò

Introduction

Who has never felt tightness or a 'butterfly' feeling in the stomach? Who has never experienced the sensation of missing/increased appetite in the presence of a stressful situation?

While the idea that the brain can alter the intestinal function has long been recognized and accepted, the concept that signals from the gut can have an effect on mood, behaviour, and cognitive function is less common [1]. The reciprocal impact of the gastrointestinal (GI) tract on brain function is well summarized in the concept of the 'gut–brain axis', which provides a bidirectional homeostatic route of communication between the 'little' and the 'big' brain. The gut–brain axis forms a complex two-way relationship. It enables the brain to influence gastrointestinal functions, such as motility, secretion, and mucin production as well as immune functions, including the modulation of cytokine production in the mucosal immune system.

The increasing knowledge of this complex system has highlighted the multiplicity and the varied nature of the different components of the axis. In particular, experimental studies during the past years have shown that the neuronal circuits have a pivotal but not unique role in the interrelation between the gut and the brain. Hormonal and immunological routes, as well as the enteric microbiota, integrate bidirectional information, building a complex network, the dysfunction of which can have pathophysiological consequences.

Anatomy and physiology of the mammalian gut–brain axis: an overview

Neuronal connection involves the central nervous system (CNS), the autonomic nervous system (ANS), and the enteric nervous system (ENS).

Neuronal control

The ENS

The ENS consists of a network of hundreds of millions of neurons and glial cells clustered in small ganglia, which are connected by nerve bundles and organized in two major layers: the myenteric plexus (or *Auerbach's* plexus) and the submucosal plexus (or *Meissner's* plexus). The ENS controls motor functions, changes local blood flow, regulates mucosal transport and secretions, and interacts with the immune and endocrine systems of the gut. It still controls these functions when the intestine is completely separated from the CNS, even if, of course, it is not autonomous [2]. In fact, the ENS (the 'gut's brain') receives modulatory input from the brain and provides information to the brain via ascending neural circuits [3]. Sensory afferent vagal fibres from the GI tract activate the dorsal motor nucleus of the vagus and the nucleus of the solitary tract, transmitting physiological sensations centrally. The dorsal motor nucleus of the vagus and the nucleus of the solitary tract/area postrema form the backbone vagal complex, which integrates the received enteric information, allowing the coordination of various intestinal processes.

The ANS

The vagus nerve is the major pathway for signals originating from the foregut and the proximal colon, whereas parasympathetic nerves innervate the distal colon. The sympathetic system primarily exerts an inhibitory influence on the gut, decreasing intestinal motor function and secretion via the release of neurotransmitters such as noradrenaline. The autonomic input from the gut is connected to the limbic system. Communication between the limbic and autonomic systems provides the neural circuitry underlying the strong link between behaviour and gut function in health (such as stomach 'butterflies') and disease (such as irritable bowel syndrome/IBS).

Humoral control

The humoral components of the gut-brain axis are mainly regulated by the hypothalamic–pituitary–adrenal (HPA) axis and the enteroendocrine system.

The HPA axis

The HPA axis is responsible for stress responses, resulting in the release of cortisol, adrenaline, and noradrenaline. Chronic psychological stress is associated with a perturbation in the HPA axis and related to enhanced abdominal pain and altered intestinal barrier function [4]. Postnatal alterations of the HPA axis because of different emotional events can cause not only pathophysiological modifications of the behaviour and the neuroendocrine system, but also of the homeostasis of the gastrointestinal tract in adults.

The enteroendocrine cells

Enteroendocrine cells (EECs) are specialized cells distributed throughout the gastrointestinal epithelium [5]. Under appropriate stimulation, they are capable of sensing luminal content, modulating homeostatic functions, and producing and releasing a variety of hormones and signalling molecules. Among these, glucagon-like peptide-1 (GLP-1), which regulates postprandial glucose levels, promotes satiety, and has an inhibitory effect on energy intake, is particularly important in the context of diabetes. Another interesting molecule is serotonin (5-HT), with 95% of the total amount being produced in the GI tract. Serotonin is a polyfunctional signalling molecule, playing a major role in promoting intestinal motility through a combination of neuronal and mucosal mechanisms. In the CNS, serotonin plays an important role in regulating mood, sleep, body temperature, sexuality, and appetite.

Secretory products can act locally in the mucosa, reach distant targets through release into the bloodstream or act directly on nerve endings close to the site of release. In this regard, direct or indirect communication of EECs with nerves is a major mechanism underlying EEC function in the gut mucosa through peptide release. Hormones released by EECs act on receptors located on the vagal and spinal neurons and influence neuronal pathways in the bidirectional brain–gut communication. This information sends positive or negative feedback to the CNS, which modulates functions of the GI tract, glucose homeostasis, and satiety.

The gut microbiota

The gastrointestinal tract hosts 10^{14} bacterial cells, distributed unevenly along its entire length. Microbial colonization begins at birth following contact with maternal and environmental bacteria. Different modes of childbirth (natural or caesarean) and feeding (breast-fed or formula-fed) change the composition of the intestinal microbiota [6,7]. Mammary microbiota derives from the enteromammary pathway, through which maternal gut commensal bacteria cross the intestinal barrier to the lymph/blood circulation and reach the mammary gland epithelium. The distribution of the gut microbiota shows spatial and temporal variation in both humans and rodents. During weaning, bacterial colonization further changes until adulthood. Even the adult bacterial ecosystem may vary, influenced by various factors, such as the place where we live [8]. In addition, because of modifications in lifestyle and nutritional behaviour, as well as an increase in infection rates and inflammatory diseases (which need more medication), the microbiota also undergoes significant changes towards old age. The microorganisms have a symbiotic relationship with their host and perform many important health-promoting functions. The gut microbiota play essential roles in protecting against pathogens, metabolizing dietary nutrients and drugs, absorbing and distributing dietary fat, producing vitamins, and enhancing immune responses [9].

Role in intestinal homeostasis

The processes that regulate homeostasis of the GI tract (in terms of motor and secretory functions, permeability, and immune system) ensure proper control of physiological functions. Most aspects of GI physiology are under neural control, particularly the ENS, whose functional maturation is completed within the microenvironment of the postnatal gut, under the influence of gut microbiota and the mucosal immune system.

Germ-free (GF) and antibiotic-treated animals (mice or rats) represent useful tools to investigate the influence of the microbiota in the modulation of physiological and pathological functions. Concerning the ENS, it has been shown that GF mice present a reduced number of enteric neurons that is associated with deficits in gut motility. Reconstitution of GF mice with conventional microbiota normalized the neuronal density and gut physiology [10]. Among the mechanisms responsible for the effects of microbiota on intestinal motility, it has been hypothesized that intestinal microbiota could modulate gut motility through the release of neuroendocrine factors such as gastrin, serotonin, and motilin [11].

The interactions between the host and its microbiota are crucial for the preservation of tissue homeostasis. In homeostasis, the intestinal immune cells maintain a balance between defence against pathogens and tolerance towards luminal antigens. Mucosal innate immune responses are essential for eliciting adaptive immune responses, which may become the major drivers of chronic tissue inflammation. Intestinal epithelial cells are considered highly relevant for the 'education' of the innate immune system. These cells express toll-like receptors (TLRs), pattern recognition receptors (PRRs), and NOD-like receptors (NOD-1/NOD-2), whose activation predisposes to local inflammation [12]. Signals that are released by the microbiota might influence the interactions between neurons of the ENS and intestinal muscularis macrophages to facilitate gastrointestinal motility.

Role in brain homeostasis

The concept that the microbiome plays a role in the physiological homeostasis of the brain is becoming more evident. It is increasingly accepted that the gastro-intestinal microbiota contributes substantially to shaping the development of the CNS. Recent studies have revealed the importance of microbiota in several CNS functions [13]. In this regard, a novel conceptual model of a 'microbiome–gut–brain axis' assigns a key role to the commensal microorganisms, not only in the control of metabolic, immune, and trophic functions of the intestine, but also for the proper functioning of the CNS. The parallel development of the CNS and the microbiota in early life and the bidirectional communication between these organs puts the bacterial components in a position where they may exert substantial influence over the developing brain [14]. Evidence gathered from animals with altered commensal flora indicates that rodent behavioural responses are influenced by the bacterial status of the gut when manipulated by inflammation, infection, or drugs [15].

Microbiome can interact with the brain through the vagal afferent nerves that convey sensory (ENS) information from viscera to the CNS. In particular, vagal activation seems to be necessary for a range of effects of gut microbiome on brain functions [1]. Other possible mechanisms that allow the gut micro-biota to influence the gut–brain axis act via the neurotransmitters they produce (serotonin and GABA) [16], which may well reach systemic circulation and hence potentially have an impact on brain development. In early life, serotonin is considered an essential signalling molecule that regulates the development of many systems throughout the body. The lack of serotonin in the CNS affects the proper wiring of the brain and may predispose to the emergence of neurodevelopmental disorders.

Regulation of energy balance

Regulation of food intake

One main example of gut–brain communication is the control of food intake, whose regulation is crucial for energy homeostasis. Depending on energy metabolism in the host, the gut microbiota undergoes modification in terms of number and bacterial composition. In particular, it has been observed that during regular feeding, the meal induces an exponential growth phase of bacterial populations in the large intestine in a time usually associated with activation of satiety pathways. When the bacterial population size declines in the postprandial state, owing to the natural lysis and elimination of bacteria, the feeling of satiety also declines. This results in a renewed feeling of hunger and the onset of the next meal. Concerning the microbiome composition, an association between the gut microbiota, body mass index, and adiposity has recently been put in evidence. The mechanism through which bacteria could influence satiety is unknown. Bacteria are able to produce/release small proteins, lipids, and sugars, which could interact with the satiety pathways through the gut epithelium in a more or less specific manner. Direct or indirect activation of EECs by bacterial signals triggers release of peptide YY (PYY) and GLP-1, thereby transmitting satiety. Paracrine actions of bacteria-derived molecules on 5-HT producing enterochromaffin cells might activate the ENS, thus regulating intestinal motility and gut barrier permeability, including the access of bacterial signals to the vagal afferents [17].

The possible involvement of the gut bacteria in the regulation of host appetite offers a new integrative homeostatic model that extends our knowledge on the multifaceted mechanisms of satiety.

Regulation of glucose metabolism

The gut–brain axis plays a pivotal role in the maintenance of glucose metabolism. This process is hypothesized to involve cooperative and coordinated interactions between central (brain) and peripheral (pancreatic and intestinal) regulatory systems. After a meal, nutrients in the gastrointestinal tract are absorbed into the circulation. Rising blood glucose levels trigger pancreatic β cells to secrete insulin, which lowers blood glucose levels both by inhibiting hepatic glucose production and by stimulating glucose uptake into insulin-sensitive tissues (primarily muscle and adipose tissue). The intestine and stomach secrete metabolic hormones (grouped under the term of incretins, e.g. GLP-1, ghrelin) that control insulin release and action as well as food intake. In addition, nervous afferents from the gut are able to detect various stimuli, owing to the activation of chemo- and mechanoreceptors, and to transmit these signals to the CNS. The main structures involved in the control of glucose homeostasis are the hypothalamus and brainstem [18]. Specifically, the arcuate nucleus, located in the mediobasal hypothalamus, contains neurons sensitive to both hormones (ghrelin, leptin, GLP-1) and nutrients (glucose, fatty acids). Projections that are responsible for integration of peripheral signals from the gut and able to promote glucose disposal by both insulin-dependent and -independent mechanisms originate from this nucleus.

The role of microbiota in the glucose metabolism is under investigation. Different pilot studies performed in humans have shown that prebiotic treatment increases GLP-1 and PYY, while decreasing ghrelin [19]. Interestingly, recent studies have demonstrated that some specific bacteria (e.g. *Bifidobacterium* spp., *Lactobacillus* spp. or *Akkermansia muciniphila*) contribute to this modulation via direct or indirect mechanism. Altogether, this recent evidence provides new insights both for the understanding of an alternative way to control glucose homeostasis and for the investigation of new therapeutic strategies in metabolic dysfunctions.

Gut–brain axis deregulation

Functional intestinal disorders

Functional gastrointestinal disorders (FGIDs) are the most common GI disorders in the general population. IBS is the most widely recognized FGID accounting for up to 50% of visits to primary care physicians for GI disorders and affecting between 7% and 10% of the world's population [20].

There is general consensus that microbiome–gut–brain axis perturbations play a crucial role in the onset and exacerbation of FGID symptomatology, even though the basic mechanisms are not well established. Clinical studies have observed specific alterations in the composition of the gut microbiota in IBS. On the other hand, it is known that manipulation of the gut microbiome influences the pattern of symptoms in IBS [21]. Certainly, FGIDs result from the reciprocal interaction of altered gut physiology and psychological factors via the gut–brain axis. Of note, psychiatric disorders such as anxiety and depressive illness are common features in patients with FGIDs [22].

Despite advances in this field of research, effective treatment of GI symptoms in IBS still remains a challenge because of the complexity of the pathophysiological mechanisms underlying the communication between the intestinal microbiota, the gut, and the brain.

Role in CNS-related disorders

Autism

Accumulating evidence suggests a role for GI microbiota in neuropsychiatric diseases including autism spectrum disorders (ASDs). Indeed, GI disturbances are frequently observed in children with ASDs and this is possibly linked to an abnormal composition of the gut microbiota [23], manifested by a decrease in bifidobacteria and an increase in lactobacilli and bacteroidetes species. It is difficult to understand whether these alterations are the cause or direct consequence of the condition, or whether they are the result of atypical eating behaviour exhibited by children with ASDs. Notably, changes in the faecal concentrations of the short-chain fatty acids have been found in individuals with ASDs [24], highlighting that the production of specific metabolites might contribute to influence brain activity. Accordingly, administration of short-chain fatty acid propionic acid induces typical autistic-like behaviours in rodents

[25]. Metabolic abnormalities have also been linked to ASD patients, possibly resulting in the change of amino acid levels and consequent inflammation. Alteration in carbohydrate digestion and absorption might also occur in some ASD patients, although it is not clear how this may affect the neurological and behavioural profile.

Although there is increasing knowledge that the gut–brain axis plays a crucial role in ASDs, future studies are mandatory to clarify the possible cause–effect relationship and the underlying mechanisms.

Anxiety and depression

The majority of patients suffering from IBS manifest clinical depression and anxiety [26]. Extensive preclinical research investigated the relationship between microbiota and behaviour relevant to mood and anxiety. In this regard, different strains of GF animals manifested decreased anxiety in specific anxiety-related behavioural paradigms, including the elevated plus maze or light–dark box tests [27]. Notably, the low anxiety profile was still evident following colonization with specific pathogen-free (SPF) intestinal microbiota, highlighting that gut–brain interactions occurring early in life are able to influence brain activity in adulthood. Several possible mechanisms mediating the effect of gut microbiota on brain development and plasticity have been recently highlighted. Among these, neurotrophins (brain-derived neurotrophic factor (BDNF)) and neurotransmitter systems including GABA, glutamate, and serotonin have been implicated [28]. Another experimental research strategy to understand how microbiota modulates brain function is to induce infections through the administration of enteric pathogens to rodents. Accordingly, both *Trichuris muris* and *Citrobacter rodentium* increased anxiety-like behaviour following transplantation. Similarly, oral administration of subclinical doses of *Campylobacter jejuni* led to anxiety-like behaviour. How infection signals to the brain and affects behaviour is puzzling and involves multiple routes of entry. Many of the above-described effects were dependent on vagal activation, even though vagal-independent mechanisms have also been described. Notably, vagus nerve stimulation, which mimics afferent signalling from the gut, has proven beneficial in clinical depression and improves cognition in animals and humans [29].

Another approach consists in exposing animals either to probiotics or to antimicrobial agents. A recent study using functional magnetic resonance imaging reported that a 4-week intake of a fermented milk product by healthy women affected brain activity in regions that control central processing of emotion and sensation. In line with this, *Lactobacillus helveticus* R0052 and *Bifidobacterium longum* administration to human volunteers induced beneficial effects on anxiety- and depression-related behaviour, which was associated with lower urinary free cortisol levels [30]. Furthermore, probiotic consumption alleviated anxiety and stress and exerted antidepressant effects in patients with IBS or major depression [31]. Of note, a low but persistent inflammatory condition has been reported in clinical depression, which may be linked to gut permeability [32]. These clinical evidences were also confirmed in animal studies in which a beneficial impact of probiotic administration on anxiety- and depressive-like behaviour has been demonstrated as being dependent on vagal activation and the modulation of neurotransmitters [33]. Conversely, administration of antibiotics in SPF mice, which induce perturbation of the microbiota and intestinal dysbiosis, increased exploratory behaviour and modulated hippocampal BDNF levels [34]. These effects were independent of vagus nerve activation, suggesting the presence of alternative mechanisms in the dysbiosis-induced animal model.

Role in obesity and diabetes

Obesity is defined as a massive expansion of the adipose tissue. It is typically associated with a wide cluster of metabolic alterations, including glucose homeostasis disorders such as glucose intolerance, insulin resistance, and type 2 diabetes (T2D), which result from a combination of genetic and environmental factors. Low-grade chronic inflammation may contribute to the development of related disorders such as insulin resistance, T2D, and cardiovascular diseases [35]. Deregulation of the gut–brain axis is also recognized in human and animal models of obesity. In particular, a reduced sensitivity to postprandial gut peptides (cholecystokinin, GLP-1), as well as reduced vagal sensitivity to nutrients has been shown extensively in several scientific reports. The involvement of microbiome in obesity was first shown through the use of GF mice, which display reduced adiposity when compared to normal mice and exhibit resistance to diet-induced obesity due, in part, to reduced energy extraction from the diet. High-fat feeding can induce drastic and rapid changes in the gut microbiome. Obese rodents and humans exhibit significantly altered gut microbiota, with changes in composition and/or reductions in diversity. Moreover, several studies in humans have found a causal link between the composition of the gut microbiota and obesity.

Numerous studies have shown that the composition of the gut microbiota is also altered in diabetic patients, although results regarding the species involved are controversial. In view of the importance of intestinal microbiota in the regulation of energy balance and the digestive process, it is not surprising that it could also intervene in glucose tolerance. Concerning the mechanism through which gut microbiota is associated with T2D, different hypotheses are under investigation. Dysbiosis can contribute to the increase of chronic systemic inflammation, a characteristic of T2D, mediated by increased plasma lipopoly-saccharide (LPS). Recent studies suggested that an altered bowel function of the intestinal barrier contributes to the pathogenesis of diabetes. The major effect of impaired barrier functionality is the increase in plasmatic LPS, due to bacterial penetration.

Although further studies are needed to respond to different open questions concerning the role of microbiota in the ethiopathogenesis of such metabolic disorders, present knowledge offers a new potential therapeutic target for the prevention and management of these pathologies.

Conclusions

The gut–brain axis consists of a bidirectional communication system involving anatomic and humoral pathways. Therefore, targeting one system within this unit may influence the entire axis. A classical example is represented by the different microbiota-modifying approaches. Indeed, antibiotics, prebiotics, and probiotics have the potential to ameliorate not only functional gut disorders but also stress-related behavioural disturbances. However, there is currently very limited clinical research on the long-term effects of many of these agents in the human population. Nonetheless, targeting the gut–brain axis is certainly promising for novel pharmacological and nutritional strategies in GI and brain disorders, especially when alterations in both systems coexist.

References

1. **Cryan JF, Dinan TG.** Mind-altering microorganisms: the impact of the gut microbiota on brain and behaviour. *Nature Review Neuroscience* 2012;**13**:701–12.
2. **Bayliss WM, Starling EH.** The movements and innervation of the small intestine. *Journal of Physiology* 1899;**24**:99–143.
3. **Furness JB.** The enteric nervous system and neurogastroenterology. *Nature Reviews Gastroenterology & Hepatology* 2012;**9**:286–94.
4. **Wiley JW, Higgins GA, Athey BD.** Stress and glucocorticoid receptor transcriptional programming in time and space: Implications for the brain-gut axis. *Neurogastroenterology & Motility* 2016;**28**:12–25.
5. **Dockray GJ.** Gastrointestinal hormones and the dialogue between gut and brain. *Journal of Physiology,* 2014;**592**:2927–41.
6. **Dominguez-Bello MG, Costello EK, Contreras M**, et al. Delivery mode shapes the acquisition and structure of the initial microbiota across multiple body habitats in newborns. *Proceedings of the National Academy of Sciences of the USA* 2010;**107**:11971–5.
7. **Wang M, Li M, Wu S**, et al. Fecal microbiota composition of breast-fed infants is correlated with human milk oligosaccharides consumed. *Journal of Pediatric Gastroenterology & Nutrition* 2015;**60**:825–33.

8. **De Filippo C, Cavalieri D, Di Paola, M**, et al. Impact of diet in shaping gut microbiota revealed by a comparative study in children from Europe and rural Africa. *Proceeding of the National Academy of Sciences of the USA* 2010;**107**:14691–6.

9. **Cho I, Blaser MJ.** The human microbiome: at the interface of health and disease. *Nature Review Genetics* 2012;**13**:260–70.

10. **Kashyap PC, Marcobal A, Ursell LK**, et al. Complex interactions among diet, gastrointestinal transit, and gut microbiota in humanized mice. *Gastroenterology* 2013;**144**:967–77.

11. **Husebye E, Hellstrom PM, Sundler F, Chen J, Midtvedt T.** Influence of microbial species on small intestinal myoelectric activity and transit in germ-free rats. *American Journal of Physiology. Gastrointestinal and Liver Physiology* 2001;**280**:G368–80.

12. **Pott J, Hornef M.** Innate immune signalling at the intestinal epithelium in homeostasis and disease. *EMBO Reports* 2012;**13**:684–98.

13. **Diaz Heijtz R, Wang S, Anuar F**, et al. Normal gut microbiota modulates brain development and behavior. *Proceedings of the National Academy of Sciences of the USA* 2011;**108**:3047–52.

14. **Stilling RM, Dinan TG, Cryan JF.** Microbial genes, brain & behaviour—epigenetic regulation of the gut-brain axis. *Genes, Brain and Behaviour* 2014;**13**:69–86.

15. **Gareau MG, Sherman PM, Walker WA.** Probiotics and the gut microbiota in intestinal health and disease. *Nature Reviews Gastroenterology & Hepatology,* 2010;**7**:503–14.

16. **O'Mahony SM, Felice VD, Nally K**, et al. Disturbance of the gut microbiota in early-life selectively affects visceral pain in adulthood without impacting cognitive or anxiety-related behaviors in male rats. *Neuroscience* 2014;**277**:885–901.

17. **Fetissov SO.** Role of the gut microbiota in host appetite control: bacterial growth to animal feeding behaviour. *Nature Reviews Endocrinology* 2017;**13**:11–25.

18. **Horvath TL, Diano S.** The floating blueprint of hypothalamic feeding circuits. *Nature Reviews Neuroscience* 2004;**5**:662–7.

19. **Everard A, Lazarevic V, Derrien M**, et al. Responses of gut microbiota and glucose and lipid metabolism to prebiotics in genetic obese and diet-induced leptin-resistant mice. *Diabetes* 2011;**60**:2775–86.

20. **Spiegel BM.** The burden of IBS: looking at metrics. *Current Gastroenterology Reports* 2009;**11**:265–9.

21. **Kennedy PJ, Cryan JF, Dinan TG, Clarke G.** Irritable bowel syndrome: a microbiome-gut-brain axis disorder? *World Journal of Gastroenterology* 2014;**20**:14105–25.

22. **Van Oudenhove L, Aziz Q.** The role of psychosocial factors and psychiatric disorders in functional dyspepsia. *Nature Reviews Gastroenterology & Hepatology* 2013;**10**:158–67.

23. **de Theije CG, Wu J, da Silva SL**, et al. Pathways underlying the gut-to-brain connection in autism spectrum disorders as future targets for disease management. *European Journal of Pharmacology* 2011;**668**(Suppl. 1):S70–80.

24. **Wang L, Christophersen CT, Sorich MJ**, et al. Elevated fecal short chain fatty acid and ammonia concentrations in children with autism spectrum disorder. *Digestive Diseases and Sciences* 2012;**57**:2096–102

25. **Thomas RH, Meeking MM, Mepham JR**, et al. The enteric bacterial metabolite propionic acid alters brain and plasma phospholipid molecular species: further

development of a rodent model of autism spectrum disorders. *Journal of Neuroinflammation* 2012;**9**:153.

26. **Mikocka-Walus A, Knowles SR, Keefer L, Graff L.** Controversies revisited: a systematic review of the comorbidity of depression and anxiety with inflammatory bowel diseases. *Inflammatory Bowel Disease* 2016;**22**:752–62.

27. **Clarke G, Grenham S, Scully P,** et al. The microbiome-gut-brain axis during early life regulates the hippocampal serotonergic system in a sex-dependent manner. *Molecular Psychiatry* 2013;**18**:666–73.

28. **Yano JM, Yu K, Donaldson GP,** et al. Indigenous bacteria from the gut microbiota regulate host serotonin biosynthesis. *Cell,* 2015;**161**:264–76.

29. **Rush AJ, George MS, Sackeim HA,** et al. Vagus nerve stimulation (VNS) for treatment-resistant depressions: a multicenter study. *Biological Psychiatry* 2000;**47**:276–86.

30. **Messaoudi M, Violle N, Bisson JF,** et al. Beneficial psychological effects of a probiotic formulation (Lactobacillus helveticus R0052 and Bifidobacterium longum R0175) in healthy human volunteers. *Gut Microbes* 2011;**2**:256–61.

31. **Rao S, Srinivasjois R, Patole S.** Prebiotic supplementation in full-term neonates: a systematic review of randomized controlled trials. *Archives of Pediatric & Adolescent Medicine* 2009;**163**:755–64.

32. **Berk M, Williams LJ, Jacka FN,** et al. So depression is an inflammatory disease, but where does the inflammation come from? *BMC Medicine* 2013;**11**:200.

33. **Bravo JA, Forsythe P, Chew MV,** et al. Ingestion of Lactobacillus strain regulates emotional behavior and central GABA receptor expression in a mouse via the vagus nerve. *Proceedings of the National Academy of Sciences of the USA,* 2011;**108**:16050–5.

34. **Bercik P, Park AJ, Sinclair D,** et al. The anxiolytic effect of Bifidobacterium longum NCC3001 involves vagal pathways for gut-brain communication. *Neurogastroenterol Motil,* 2011;**23**:1132–9.

35. **Shoelson SE, Goldfine AB.** Getting away from glucose: fanning the flames of obesity-induced inflammation. *Nature Medicine* 2009;**15**:373–4.

Chapter 8

Diabetes distress

Norbert Hermanns, Marijke A. Bremmer, and Frank J. Snoek

Introduction

Diabetes-related distress or diabetes distress is defined as negative emotions in response to the burden of living with and managing the chronic disease diabetes mellitus. Negative emotions associated with diabetes have received increasing attention in the last two decades, with special interest in the relationship between diabetes and depression, a common psychological comorbidity adversely affecting quality of life, morbidity, and mortality of people with diabetes. Diabetes distress and depression are partially overlapping constructs, but they are not identical, since diabetes distress is a negative emotional reaction to perceived specific stressors associated with diabetes, whereas depression is a negative cognitive–affective state, not necessarily related to a stimulus or to a specific cause.

This chapter will focus on diabetes-related emotional distress. In the first part, a definition of psychological distress will be provided and the relationship between psychological distress and chronic somatic diseases is reviewed. In this context, the prevalence and content of diabetes-related distress will be addressed, as well as its relationship with depression. The second part of this chapter deals with the clinical assessment, diagnosis, and treatment of diabetes-related distress.

Psychological distress

The term 'distress' was first introduced by the Hungarian physiologist Hans Selye to distinguish between stress initiated by negative, unpleasant stressors and positive stress ('eustress') [1]. Psychological distress is conceptualized as a negative impact of stressors on emotions. It is a continuous variable rather than a dichotomous outcome and can vary in response to different stressful situations. It is therefore a 'state' measure rather than a 'trait' measure. The latter is conceptualized as a stable and invariant construct, whereas state measures refer to the situational context in which different emotional states can occur [2]. Ridner has defined psychological distress as 'the unique discomforting, emotional state experienced by an individual in response to a specific stressor or demand that results in harm, either temporary or permanent to the person' [3]. The harm mentioned in this definition refers to negative emotions, such as irritability, fear, nervousness, and sadness, which are burdensome in their own right, associated with lower well-being and social functioning, but are not necessarily pathological [4]. Distress is thus defined as an emotional response toward adverse or unpleasant stressors. This emotional response is not only dependent on the stressor per se, but also from the subjective evaluations and appraisal of coping abilities related to the perceived stressor [5]. Therefore, psychological distress is a function of the magnitude of stressors and a persons' individual ability to cope with these specific stressors.

Psychological distress in chronic diseases

As noted by de Ridder et al. [6], chronic illness challenges patients' habitual coping strategies, with the majority eventually reaching good psychological adjustment but for about 30% the adjustment phase is prolonged or unsuccessful. Psychological distress is prevalent in medical patients and often regarded a normal response to the burden of diagnosis and treatment, discomforting symptoms, and negative social implications. In a large representative study, Nakaya et al. [7] assessed the prevalence of elevated non-specific psychological distress (Kessler 6 scale >13) in a community-dwelling Japanese population, including people with and without self-reported somatic diseases. Overall, the risk for psychological distress was elevated in people with (self-reported) somatic diseases compared to the general population. The risk for psychological distress was increased for hypertension, cancer, myocardial infarction, arthritis, and stroke. Diabetes was associated with an overall risk increase of 30% (Fig. 8.1). Illnesses accompanied by pain or disabilities or with a potential life threatening character were associated with a higher risk of psychological distress than metabolic disorders.

Thus, different somatic diseases with different symptom profiles, treatment requirements, and prognoses are associated with different rates of severe psychological distress. These findings suggest an impact of the magnitude of disease-specific or treatment-specific stressors on the prevalence of psychological distress.

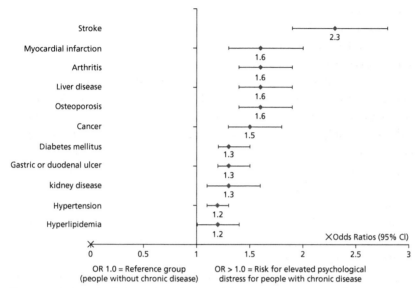

Fig. 8.1 Relative risk of elevated psychological distress in people with different chronic somatic diseases.

Source data from *European Journal of Public Health,* 24, 1, Nakaya N., Kogure M., Saito-Nakaya K. et al., The association between self-reported history of physical diseases and psychological distress in a community-dwelling Japanese population: the Ohsaki Cohort 2006 Study, pp. 45–9, 2014.

Diabetes distress

Diabetes-related distress refers to the negative emotions, for example anger, fears, and worries associated with the burden of living with and managing the chronic disease diabetes mellitus [8]. Diabetes distress has been associated with impaired quality of life [9], reduced diabetes treatment adherence [10], and hyperglycaemia [11–13] and was also found to prospectively predict reduced glycaemic control [11,14].

Diabetes-related distress can be connected to the diagnosis of the disease and its ramifications, the treatment demands, and interactions with the social environment [15,16]. The most prominent emotional diabetes-specific stressor is the uncertainty about developing late complications often associated with feelings of guilt for non-optimal diabetes management. For those on insulin therapy, the risk of hypoglycaemia is a common stressor, sometimes leading to extreme anxiety and avoidance behaviours. Having always to care for the diabetes and dietary issues, thus feeling restricted in the choice of food, are often reported stressors by people with diabetes. Lack of social support is a commonly reported cause of distress in people living with diabetes [15,17–20].

Not only the content but also the level of reported diabetes-related distress can vary across different groups of people with diabetes. Among the differentiating factors are diabetes type, age, treatment regimen, and socio-economic factors. Sources and triggers of diabetes-related distress can differ considerably between groups of people with diabetes. For example, in adolescents with type 1 diabetes, family conflicts are known to be associated with high levels of psychological distress [21]. As mentioned, for insulin-requiring patients, recurrent hypoglycaemia is a driver of high diabetes-related distress and associated with elevated anxiety and depression rates [22,23]. In type 2 diabetes, the transitioning from oral medications to insulin injections is frequently experienced as a stressful event [24,25]. Diabetes-related distress was found to be significantly higher in people with type 2 diabetes treated in secondary diabetes care settings than treated in primary diabetes care settings (4% vs. 19%) [26]. Since level of care is presumably a marker of the severity of diabetes or it's complications, diabetes-related distress can be expected to be more prominent and severe in people with diabetes and other morbidities. Being a member of an ethnic minority is a further correlate of elevated diabetes distress [26,27].

Prevalence of diabetes distress

A recent meta-analysis examined the prevalence of diabetes distress in people with type 2 diabetes living in 17 different countries [28]. Diabetes distress was assessed either by the Problem Areas in Diabetes (PAID) questionnaire or with the Diabetes Distress Scale (DDS). Point prevalence rates were based on 36,998 participants with type 2 diabetes. Overall prevalence of diabetes distress in people with type 2 diabetes was 36% (95% CI 31–41%). Female responders reported significant higher prevalence of diabetes distress than male responders (46% vs. 32%). Also, depression seemed to be a risk factor for diabetes distress with increasing prevalence rates in sub-samples with higher depression rates (see later). A longitudinal study over 18 months showed a somewhat lower proportion of people with type 2 diabetes (29.2%), who reported elevated diabetes-related distress at least at one of three measurement points. In 13% of this group, diabetes distress scores stayed high at least at two measurement points, indicating persistence of diabetes distress [29].

In type 1 diabetes, Fisher et al. [15] observed a prevalence rate of moderate and high diabetes distress of 33.7% and 7.9% respectively. In Germany, Ehrmann et al. [30] observed a point prevalence of diabetes distress of 29.3% in people with type 1 and type 2 diabetes who were in need for diabetes education.

After a 6-month follow-up, persisting diabetes distress was observed in 18.1% of patients and incidence of elevated diabetes distress was 5.3% [30].

Overall, more than one-third of patients with type 2 diabetes are affected by diabetes distress and every eighth person with type 2 diabetes is affected by persistent diabetes distress over an 18-month observational period. In type 1 diabetes every second person reported moderately elevated diabetes distress. Persistently elevated diabetes distress was also higher in type 1 diabetes than in type 2 diabetes. More research is needed especially regarding the prevalence of diabetes distress in type 1 diabetes.

Aetiology of diabetes distress

Besides the objective magnitude of diabetes-related stressors (e.g. treatment complexity, complications) it is the individual perception of these stressors and the appraisal of individual coping abilities that determine the level of diabetes-related distress. The individuals' perception of diabetes-related stressors is influenced by the presence of vulnerability and protective factors [31,32]. A potent vulnerability factor can be pre-existing poor mental health, whereas resilience, social support, and coping abilities are protective factors. Both vulnerability and protective factors are determined by the individual experiences, stressful life events in interaction with a genetic vulnerability, and social factors like the socio-economic status (Fig. 8.2).

This multidimensional aetiology of diabetes-related distress has implications for the clinical management of diabetes distress regarding both assessment and treatment. Besides the reduction of diabetes-related stressors, the modification

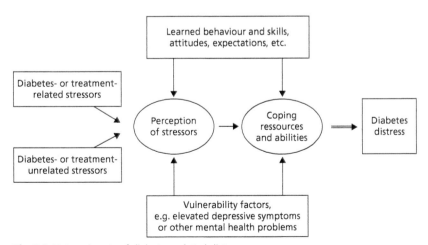

Fig. 8.2 Determinants of diabetes-related distress.

of the perception of stressors in people with diabetes and the enhancement of coping resources including stress management are goals for treatment.

Depression in people with diabetes

Besides elevated diabetes-related distress, depression or elevated depressive symptoms are the most common mental health problems in people with diabetes [29,33–35]. The negative consequences of depression in diabetes have been demonstrated in multiple well-controlled studies. People with diabetes and comorbid depression report a reduced quality of life [36–38], show poorer diabetes self-management [39,40], poorer glycaemic control [12,41], and increased morbidity [42,43], and mortality [44,45].

Depressive symptoms and diabetes-related distress both represent negative emotional experiences and are inter-related, yet the constructs of depression and distress are defined differently. Whereas diabetes distress is defined by its functional relationship to diabetes-specific stressors, depressive symptoms do not require to be related to specific external conditions or events. Differences in diabetes distress and depression may also be explained by factorial analytical findings, which could demonstrate a relative independency of depression and distress symptoms, since depression and distress symptoms could be segregated into two different factors [30,46].

The concept of depression (major depressive disorder in DSM V) is aetiologically neutral [2,47] and defined by a set of symptoms and behaviours [48,49]. The criteria for a full syndromal diagnosis include the presence of at least one out of two core symptoms (depressive mood and/or anhedonia) and at least four out of seven additional symptoms (anergia, diminished concentration, excessive guilt, suicidal thoughts, weight change, insomnia, and psychomotor retardation or agitation) [48,49]. The presence of depressive symptoms or an elevated depression score on a depression questionnaire, without meeting the diagnostic criteria for an episode of major depressive disorder, is often considered as mild or sub-clinical depression.

Epidemiological evidence suggests that a more complicated course of diabetes is associated with an increased depression risk. This would indicate that depression or depressive symptoms might also be partially responsible for the burden of the disease, at least in some people with diabetes.

The overall prevalence of depression is elevated in people with diabetes, but the DESMOND study group found this not to be the case in people with newly diagnosed type 2 diabetes [50]. Likewise, screen-detected people with type 2 diabetes showed relatively low levels of distress and anxiety at the time of diagnosis, with a significant increase during the following 12 months [51].

In line with these observations, depression and depressive symptoms become more prevalent in type 2 diabetes patients who are on oral blood glucose-lowering agents and are progressing to insulin treatment [22]. The occurrence of late complications or the perception of deteriorating health appear to be additional risk factors for depression in people with type 1 and type 2 diabetes [52,53]. The fact that perceived severity of diabetes appears closely associated with depression could be due to the increasing psychological strains associated with a complicated course of diabetes. This fits the 'disablement process' as described by Verbrugge and Jette [54], with increasing adjustment in the face of treatment demands, progressing functional limitations, and loss of social roles adding to the risk of depression. Stigma and social isolation may further add to the burden of living with diabetes and its ramifications, and hamper seeking treatment. The diagnosis of depression does not require the identification of a specific cause. Of course, this does not mean that depressive symptoms are by definition unrelated to the burden of living with diabetes or its treatment.

Depression and diabetes distress

Depression and diabetes distress are inter-related problems in many people with diabetes. Therefore, the association between depression and diabetes distress deserves attention.

There is clear evidence for a strong relationship between depression and diabetes distress. In cross-sectional studies, moderate to high correlations between depression and diabetes distress were observed, with correlation coefficients ranging from 0.50 to 0.60 [11,13,18,55]. Ehrmann et al. [30] showed that elevated depression in people with diabetes and non-elevated diabetes distress longitudinally increased the incident risk for diabetes distress. In people with diabetes and elevated diabetes distress, depression was a barrier for remission to non-elevated diabetes distress. This indicates that depression in diabetes might be a vulnerability factor for diabetes distress, since a negative cognitive-affective state like depression might reduce coping abilities to manage diabetes-related stressors or enhance these stressors [30]. Grouping patients with diabetes according to their level of depression severity (no depression, elevated depressive symptoms and major depressive disorder) yielded highly different mean diabetes distress scores derived from the 20-item PAID scale (Fig. 8.3) [56]. This would suggest that the presence of depressive symptoms or clinical depression is an amplifier for diabetes-related distress. A similar association between elevated depression and diabetes distress was also found in a recent meta-analysis by Perrin et al. [28].

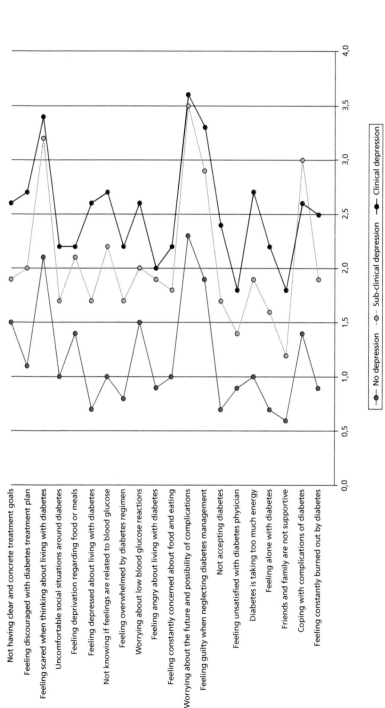

Fig. 8.3 Diabetes distress in people with diabetes and different depression states (no depression *vs.* sub-threshold depression *vs.* clinical depression).

Source data from *Diabetologia*, 49, 3, Hermanns N, Kulzer B, Krichbaum M, et al., How to screen for depression and emotional problems in patients with diabetes: comparison of screening characteristics of depression questionnaires, measurement of diabetes-specific emotional problems and standard clinical assessment, pp. 469–77, 2006.

In summary, depression and diabetes distress are related concepts, but originate from different clinical research traditions. Whereas diabetes distress is defined as a functional negative emotional consequence of diabetes-related stressors, the definition of depression is etiologically neutral. The aetiology of depression is considered multifactorial. Most etiological models for depression are stress–diathesis models in which stressful experiences trigger depression in those who are vulnerable due to biological (chronic diseases, inflammation, genetic) and psychosocial characteristics and circumstances [57]. As a consequence, depressive symptoms may arise due to diabetes-related distress, as illustrated by the often-observed close association between diabetes distress and depressed mood. It is also discussed that depression and diabetes may share a common underlying dimension such as 'emotional distress' [58]. This could explain the responsiveness of depressive symptoms to diabetes distress.

Management of diabetes distress

The clinical management of diabetes-related distress requires assessment and measurement of the distress as well as interventions in people with diabetes and elevated diabetes-related distress.

Assessment of diabetes distress

Dunn and colleagues [59] in Australia were among the first to acknowledge the 'emotional side' of diabetes and developed a measure of emotional adjustment specifically for use in adult patients with diabetes. This self-report scale (ATT39) covered 39 attitude statements describing a person's emotional responses to diabetes, its treatment, its effects on lifestyle, and the future [59]. The ATT39 could be considered the first measure of diabetes-specific distress.

At a later stage, Polonsky and colleagues [17,18,60] in the USA developed two specific psychometric tools to capture diabetes-related distress, the PAID questionnaire and the DDS. Both scales were attested good psychometric qualities [17,18,60] and have been translated into multiple languages, thereby enabling the assessment of diabetes distress in many countries [2,19,43].

The PAID questionnaire is a 20-item self-report measure to capture the emotional burden commonly reported by people living with diabetes, both type 1 and type 2 [17]. The DDS [18] allows for quantification of diabetes-specific emotional distress, defined as the worries, concerns, and fears of individuals struggling with type 1 or type 2 diabetes [12]. The first version of the DDS consisting of 17 items is considered more suited for type 2 diabetes, whereas an enlarged version of the DDS with 28 items was specifically designed for people with type 1 diabetes [15]. The PAID was conceptualized as a one-dimensional measure of distress, but factor analyses identified four inter-related subdomains of distress: disease-related, treatment-related, food related, and social support-related. For the DDS, almost similar domains were extracted for people with type 2 diabetes: emotional burden related to diabetes, physician-related burden, regimen-related burden, and interpersonal distress [18,19]. The DDS type 1 version aims to assess distress specifically for people with type 1 diabetes. It consists of 28 items which built up seven scales: powerlessness, negative social perceptions, physician distress, friend/family distress, hypoglycaemia distress, management distress, and eating distress [15]. The PAID and the DDS have short forms consisting of five [61] and two items respectively [62].

The PAID and the DDS constitute the current standards of measurement of diabetes-related distress. The identification of people with elevated diabetes-related distress is mostly based on elevated scores in the PAID or DDS. An elevated score indicates a higher level of diabetes-related distress. A cut-off-score of 40 in the PAID questionnaire (range 0–100) and a cut-off-score of 3 in the DDS scale (range 1–6) is considered as indicative for elevated diabetes-related distress [50,56,63].

Interventions

A recent meta-analysis examined the impact of different interventions on diabetes distress and glycaemic control [64]. This meta-analysis included 32 studies with 5206 participants in different settings (group vs. individual, use of digital platforms or collaborative care settings) and using 15 different intervention methods. Regarding diabetes distress and glycaemic control, significant effects where observed in the intervention groups compared to the control groups. The effect of the interventions on diabetes distress was small to moderate for distress (standardized mean difference –0.13, 95% CI –0.01 to –0.25) and moderate for glycaemic control (weighted mean difference of glycated haemoglobin (HbA1c) –0.28, 95% CI –0.08 to –0.48) in favour for the intervention groups. Meta-regression analysis failed to demonstrate a significant impact of setting or specific intervention methods on diabetes distress or glycaemic control. Probably because of the high heterogeneity within the different interventions and settings, the results of the meta-analysis indicate that a plethora of different interventions exists, which are efficacious in reducing diabetes-related distress [64]. Albeit formally not significant, different digital platforms, diabetes self-management education, and use of cognitive behavioural approaches showed moderate to large effect size for reducing diabetes distress and appear most promising. However, it may not be the method of delivery that determines effectiveness, but rather the extent to which a given intervention addresses the relationship between one or more diabetes-related stressors and the persons' emotional response. Understanding the underlying causes of diabetes-related distress can help to tailor interventions to the individual's profile. For many people with diabetes the key problem is the emotional burden of living with the day-to-day demands of self-managing diabetes. If treatment-related diabetes distress is prominent, modification of the diabetes treatment regimen may be helpful (e.g. simplification of diabetes treatment, intensification of diabetes insulin treatment to allow more flexibility, modification of glycaemic targets to minimize hypoglycaemic risks). This calls for close collaboration between the diabetes care team and the mental health specialist.

Modern diabetes education programmes are aimed at enhancing self-management abilities for diabetes self-care by enhancing knowledge and skills to cope with the challenges of diabetes and its treatment. These programmes often also address emotional problems in living with diabetes or its treatment. Therefore, it can be expected that modern diabetes education programmes can address negative emotional responses towards diabetes or its treatment. Indeed, diabetes education for people with type 1 diabetes, such as the DAFNE or PRIMAS programmes, reduces diabetes distress by $d = 0.13–0.48$ standard deviations with a median effect size of $d = 0.30$, where d represents the change in diabetes distress expressed as a relative proportion of the standard deviation [65–68]. In MEDIAS 2 ICT, a structured treatment and education programme for people with type 2 diabetes on intensive insulin treatment, the reduction of diabetes distress 6 months after participation in the programme was $d = 0.36$ standard deviations [69].

Psychoeducational programmes for people with diabetes and hypoglycaemia were also able to demonstrate a reduction of diabetes-related distress by $d = 0.23$ standard deviations in the 'HyPOS' programme [70] and a reduction of the relative risk for elevated diabetes distress by 30% in the 'HypoAware' programme [71].

In summary, it can be expected that diabetes education and training programmes augment coping resources to deal with diabetes-related stressors, resulting in a reduction of diabetes-related distress.

Interventions specifically targeting diabetes-related distress like the Reducing Distress and Enhancing Effective Management (REDEEM) programme are focusing on more specific emotional barriers of diabetes management and solutions to overcome or reduce these barriers. In a 1-year follow-up of the REDEEM study, diabetes distress could be reduced between $d = 0.39$ to 0.53 standard deviations, indicating an intermediate effect of such interventions on diabetes distress [72].

In people with diabetes and elevated diabetes distress combined with elevated depressive symptoms, psychotherapeutic interventions based on cognitive behaviour therapy (CBT) have been proven efficacious. Two web-based approaches aiming at a reduction of depressive symptoms as the primary outcome observed a reduction of diabetes-related distress with rather large effect sizes ranging from $d = 0.58$ to $d = 0.44$ standard deviations [73,74]. Face-to-face CBT-based approaches, addressing elevated depressive symptoms by supporting people with diabetes to cope with diabetes-related and diabetes-unrelated stressors also showed a great impact on diabetes distress, with effect sizes in the range $d = 0.66$ to 0.77 standard deviations [75,76]. There is little evidence to date on the mechanisms explaining the impact of depression management on diabetes distress and vice versa. Basic cognitive behavioural techniques, such as cognitive restructuring and behaviour activation, appear to have beneficial effects for patients with depression and/or diabetes distress, but other therapeutic approaches with more focus on acceptance, such as mindfulness, also deserve our attention [77,78]. Evidence to date suggests that patients with high diabetes distress are helped most by programmes addressing the specific stressors of living with diabetes. However, more research is needed to determine whether this holds for all patients, presenting with various combinations of diabetes-specific and generic problems.

Implications for clinical practice

With respect to the clinical management of diabetes distress, distinguishing between patients with and without co-existing depression is important. For patients seriously distressed about their diabetes, but without elevated depressive symptoms, interventions such as the REDEEM project, diabetes self-management programmes, psychoeducation, and supportive counselling are most suitable to improve the patients' problem-solving skills and coping with the daily demands of diabetes self-care.

Patients with diabetes and comorbid depression, but without elevated diabetes distress, might profit most from specialized depression treatment. Although the absence of diabetes distress may suggest there is no psychological link with the somatic comorbidity, effects of diabetes may still play a role on a neuroendocrinological level. A chronic dysregulation of the stress response and cortisol levels as well as a chronic low-grade inflammatory state are shared risk factors in diabetes and depression [79]. Consequently, depression may interfere with sleep habits, eating, and diabetes self-regulation, which may all lead to diminished glycaemic control. Since depression and diabetes interact on several levels, one may presume that, next to standard depression treatment, patients with both diabetes and depression may profit from tailored interventions that target both the body and the brain, separately or in concert. The application of bright light therapy (BLT) might be promising, as BLT might work as an antidepressant and also regulate diurnal variability in sleep, eating, and stress hormones, which are all related to insulin sensitivity [80]. Results on efficacy of BLT are still under way.

People with diabetes with combined depression and diabetes distress constitute the most psychologically vulnerable group. Here, the interaction between mood and diabetes-related issues deserves special attention and patients are likely to benefit most from diabetes-specific depression treatment modalities.

References

1. **Selye H.** *Stress without distress.* Philadelphia, PA: J.B. Lippincott Co, 1974.
2. **Snoek FJ, Bremmer MA, Hermanns N.** Constructs of depression and distress in diabetes: time for an appraisal. *Lancet Diabetes Endocrinol* 2015;**3**:450–60.
3. **Ridner SH.** Psychological distress: concept analysis. *Journal of Advanced Nursing* 2004;**45**:536–45.
4. **Veit CT, Ware JE,** Jr. The structure of psychological distress and well-being in general populations. *J Consult Clin Psychol* 1983;**51**:730–42.
5. **Lazarus RS, Folkman S.** *Stress Appraisal and Coping.* New York: Springer, 1984.
6. **de Ridder D, Geenen R, Kuijer R, van Middendorp H.** Psychological adjustment to chronic disease. *Lancet* 2008;**372**:246–55.
7. **Nakaya N, Kogure M, Saito-Nakaya K,** et al. The association between self-reported history of physical diseases and psychological distress in a community-dwelling Japanese population: the Ohsaki Cohort 2006 Study. *European Journal of Public Health* 2014;**24**:45–9.
8. **Fisher L, Gonzalez JS, Polonsky WH.** The confusing tale of depression and distress in patients with diabetes: a call for greater clarity and precision. *Diabetic Medicine* 2014;**31**:764–72.
9. **Schmitt A, Reimer A, Kulzer B, Haak T, Ehrmann D, Hermanns N.** How to assess diabetes distress: comparison of the Problem Areas in Diabetes Scale (PAID) and the Diabetes Distress Scale (DDS). *Diabetic Medicine* 2016;**33**:835–43.
10. **Schmitt A, Gahr A, Hermanns N, Kulzer B, Huber J, Haak T.** The Diabetes Self-Management Questionnaire (DSMQ): development and evaluation of an instrument to assess diabetes self-care activities associated with glycaemic control. *Health Quality Life Outcomes* 2013;**11**:138.
11. **Fisher L, Glasgow RE, Strycker LA.** The relationship between diabetes distress and clinical depression with glycemic control among patients with type 2 diabetes. *Diabetes Care* 2010;**33**:1034–6.
12. **Schmitt A, Reimer A, Hermanns N,** et al. Assessing diabetes self-management with the Diabetes Self-Management Questionnaire (DSMQ) can help analyse behavioural problems related to reduced glycaemic control. *PLoS One* 2016;**11**:e0150774.
13. **van Bastelaar KM, Pouwer F, Geelhoed-Duijvestijn PH,** et al. Diabetes-specific emotional distress mediates the association between depressive symptoms and glycaemic control in Type 1 and Type 2 diabetes. *Diabetic Medicine* 2010;**27**:798–803.

14. **Fisher L, Mullan JT, Arean P, Glasgow RE, Hessler D, Masharani U.** Diabetes distress but not clinical depression or depressive symptoms is associated with glycemic control in both cross-sectional and longitudinal analyses. *Diabetes Care* 2010;**33**:23–8.

15. **Fisher L, Polonsky WH, Hessler DM,** et al. Understanding the sources of diabetes distress in adults with type 1 diabetes. *Journal of Diabetes Complications* 2015;**29**:572–7.

16. **Peyrot M, Rubin RR, Polonsky WH.** Diabetes distress and its association with clinical outcomes in patients with type 2 diabetes treated with pramlintide as an adjunct to insulin therapy. *Diabetes Technology & Therapeutics* 2008;**10**:461–6.

17. **Polonsky WH, Anderson BJ, Lohrer PA,** et al. Assessment of diabetes-related distress. *Diabetes Care* 1995;**18**:754–60.

18. **Polonsky WH, Fisher L, Earles J,** et al. Assessing psychosocial distress in diabetes: development of the Diabetes Distress Scale. *Diabetes Care* 2005;**28**:626–31.

19. **Snoek FJ, Pouwer F, Welch GW, Polonsky WH.** Diabetes-related emotional distress in Dutch and U.S. diabetic patients: cross-cultural validity of the problem areas in diabetes scale. *Diabetes Care* 2000;**23**:1305–9.

20. **Welch GW, Jacobson AM, Polonsky WH.** The Problem Areas in Diabetes Scale. An evaluation of its clinical utility. *Diabetes Care* 1997;**20**:760–6.

21. **Williams LB, Laffel LM, Hood KK.** Diabetes-specific family conflict and psychological distress in paediatric Type 1 diabetes. *Diabetic Medicine* 2009;**26**:908–14.

22. **Hermanns N, Kulzer B, Krichbaum M, Kubiak T, Haak T.** Affective and anxiety disorders in a German sample of diabetic patients: prevalence, comorbidity and risk factors. *Diabetic Medicine* 2005;**22**:293–300.

23. **Shao W, Ahmad R, Khutoryansky N, Aagren M, Bouchard J.** Evidence supporting an association between hypoglycemic events and depression. *Current Medical Research and Opinion* 2013;**29**:1609–15.

24. **Polonsky WH, Fisher L, Guzman S, Villa-Caballero L, Edelman SV.** Psychological insulin resistance in patients with type 2 diabetes: the scope of the problem. *Diabetes Care* 2005;**28**:2543–5.

25. **Polonsky WH, Hajos TR, Dain MP, Snoek FJ.** Are patients with type 2 diabetes reluctant to start insulin therapy? An examination of the scope and underpinnings of psychological insulin resistance in a large, international population. *Current Medical Research and Opinion* 2011;**27**:1169–74.

26. **Stoop CH, Nefs G, Pop VJ,** et al. Diabetes-specific emotional distress in people with Type 2 diabetes: a comparison between primary and secondary care. *Diabetic Medicine* 2014;**31**:1252–9.

27. **Strandberg RB, Graue M, Wentzel-Larsen T, Peyrot M, Rokne B.** Relationships of diabetes-specific emotional distress, depression, anxiety, and overall well-being with HbA1c in adult persons with type 1 diabetes. *J Psychosom Res* 2014;**77**:174–9.

28. **Perrin NE, Davies MJ, Robertson N,** et al. The prevalence of diabetes-specific emotional distress in people with type 2 diabetes: a systematic review and meta-analysis. *Diabetic Medicine* 2017;**34**:1508–20.

29. **Fisher L, Skaff MM, Mullan JT, Arean P, Glasgow R, Masharani U.** A longitudinal study of affective and anxiety disorders, depressive affect and diabetes distress in adults with Type 2 diabetes. *Diabetic Medicine* 2008;**25**:1096–101.

30. **Ehrmann D, Kulzer B, Haak T, Hermanns N.** Longitudinal relationship of diabetes-related distress and depressive symptoms: analysing incidence and persistence. *Diabetic Medicine.* 2015;**32**:1264–71

31. **Casey P.** Adjustment disorder: new developments. *Current Psychiatry Reports* 2014;**16**:451.

32. **Casey P, Jabbar F, O'Leary E, Doherty AM.** Suicidal behaviours in adjustment disorder and depressive episode. *Journal of Affective Disorders* 2015;**174**:441–6.

33. **Anderson RJ, Freedland KE, Clouse RE, Lustman PJ.** The prevalence of comorbid depression in adults with diabetes: a meta-analysis. *Diabetes Care* 2001;**24**:1069–78.

34. **Kruse J, Schmitz N, Thefeld W.** On the association between diabetes and mental disorders in a community sample: results from the German National Health Interview and Examination Survey. *Diabetes Care* 2003;**26**:1841–6.

35. **Roy T, Lloyd CE.** Epidemiology of depression and diabetes: a systematic review. *Journal of Affective Disorders* 2012;**142**(Suppl.):S8–21.

36. **Egede LE, Grubaugh AL, Ellis C.** The effect of major depression on preventive care and quality of life among adults with diabetes. *General Hospital Psychiatry* 2010;**32**:563–9.

37. **Egede LE, Hernandez-Tejada MA.** Effect of comorbid depression on quality of life in adults with Type 2 diabetes. *Expert Review of Pharmacoeconomics & Outcomes Research* 2013;**13**:83–91.

38. **Goldney RD, Phillips PJ, Fisher LJ, Wilson DH.** Diabetes, depression, and quality of life: a population study. *Diabetes Care* 2004;**27**:1066–70.

39. **Gonzalez JS, Peyrot M, McCarl LA,** et al. Depression and diabetes treatment nonadherence: a meta-analysis. *Diabetes Care* 2008;**31**:2398–403.

40. **Katon W, Russo J, Lin EH,** et al. Diabetes and poor disease control: is comorbid depression associated with poor medication adherence or lack of treatment intensification? *Psychosomatic Medicine* 2009;**71**:965–72.

41. **Lustman PJ, Anderson RJ, Freedland KE, De Groot M, Carney RM, Clouse RE.** Depression and poor glycemic control: a meta-analytic review of the literature. *Diabetes Care* 2000;**23**:934–42.

42. **Black SA, Markides KS, Ray LA.** Depression predicts increased incidence of adverse health outcomes in older Mexican Americans with type 2 diabetes. *Diabetes Care* 2003;**26**:2822–8.

43. **Pouwer F, Skinner TC, Pibernik-Okanovic M,** et al. Serious diabetes-specific emotional problems and depression in a Croatian-Dutch-English survey from the European Depression in Diabetes [EDID] Research Consortium. *Diabetes Research and Clinical Practice* 2005;**70**:166–73.

44. **Katon W, Fan MY, Unutzer J, Taylor J, Pincus H, Schoenbaum M.** Depression and diabetes: a potentially lethal combination. *Journal of General Internal Medicine* 2008;**23**:1571–5.

45. **Zhang X, Norris SL, Gregg EW, Cheng YJ, Beckles G, Kahn HS.** Depressive symptoms and mortality among persons with and without diabetes. *American Journal of Epidemiology* 2005;**161**:652–60.

46. **Schmitt A, Reimer A, Kulzer B, Haak T, Gahr A, Hermanns N.** Assessment of diabetes acceptance can help identify patients with ineffective diabetes self-care and poor diabetes control. *Diabetic Medicine* 2014;**21**;**31**:1446–51.

47. Gonzalez JS, Fisher L, Polonsky WH. Depression in diabetes: have we been missing something important? *Diabetes Care* 2011;**34**:236–9.

48. American Psychiatric Association. *Diagnostic and Statistical Manual of Mental Disorders,* DSM-5, 5th edn. Washington, DC: APA, 2013.

49. World Health Organization. *International Statistical Classification of Diseases and Related Health Problems* 10th Revision (ICD-10) Version for 2008. http://apps whoint/classifications/icd10/browse/2008/en#/V 2008 (accessed October 17 2014).

50. Skinner TC, Carey ME, Cradock S, et al. Depressive symptoms in the first year from diagnosis of Type 2 diabetes: results from the DESMOND trial. *Diabetic Medicine* 2010;**27**:965–7.

51. Thoolen B, de Ridder D, Bensing J, Gorter K, Rutten G. Psychological outcomes of patients with screen-detected type 2 diabetes: the influence of time since diagnosis and treatment intensity. *Diabetes Care* 2006;**29**(:2257–62.

52. Badawi G, Page V, Smith KJ, et al. Self-rated health: a predictor for the three year incidence of major depression in individuals with type II diabetes. *Journal of Affective Disorders* 2013;**145**:100–5.

53. Pouwer F, Beekman AT, Nijpels G, et al. Rates and risks for co-morbid depression in patients with Type 2 diabetes mellitus: results from a community-based study. *Diabetologia* 2003;**46**:892–8.

54. Verbrugge LM, Jette AM. The disablement process. *Social Science & Medicine* 1994;**38**(1):1–14.

55. Fisher L, Skaff MM, Mullan JT, et al. Clinical depression versus distress among patients with type 2 diabetes: not just a question of semantics. *Diabetes Care* 2007;**30**:542–8.

56. Hermanns N, Kulzer B, Krichbaum M, Kubiak T, Haak T. How to screen for depression and emotional problems in patients with diabetes: comparison of screening characteristics of depression questionnaires, measurement of diabetes-specific emotional problems and standard clinical assessment. *Diabetologia* 2006;**49**:469–77.

57. Beck AT. The evolution of the cognitive model of depression and its neurobiological correlates. *American Journal of Psychiatry* 2008;**165**:969–77.

58. Hessler D, Fisher L, Strycker LA, Arean PA, Bowyer V. Causal and bidirectional linkages over time between depression and diabetes regimen distress in adults with type 2 diabetes. *Diabetes Research and Clinical Practice* 2015;**108**:360–6.

59. Dunn SM, Smartt HH, Beeney LJ, Turtle JR. Measurement of emotional adjustment in diabetic patients: validity and reliability of ATT39. *Diabetes Care* 1986;**9**:480–9.

60. Welch G, Weinger K, Anderson B, Polonsky WH. Responsiveness of the Problem Areas In Diabetes (PAID) questionnaire. *Diabetic Medicine* 2003;**20**:69–72.

61. McGuire BE, Morrison TG, Hermanns N, et al. Short-form measures of diabetes-related emotional distress: the Problem Areas in Diabetes Scale (PAID)-5 and PAID-1. *Diabetologia* 2010;**53**:66–9.

62. Fisher L, Glasgow RE, Mullan JT, Skaff MM, Polonsky WH. Development of a brief diabetes distress screening instrument. *Annals of Family Medicine* 2008;**6**:246–52.

63. Fisher L, Hessler DM, Polonsky WH, Mullan J. When is diabetes distress clinically meaningful?: establishing cut points for the Diabetes Distress Scale. *Diabetes Care* 2012;**35**:259–64.

64. **Perrin NE, Bodicoat DH, Davies MJ**, et al. Effectiveness of psycho-eductional interventions for the treatment of diabetes-specific emotional distress and glycaemic control in people with type 2 diabetes: a systematic review and meta-analysis. *Diabetes Care* In press 2017.

65. **DAFNE Study Group**. Training in flexible, intensive insulin management to enable dietary freedom in people with type 1 diabetes: dose adjustment for normal eating (DAFNE) randomised controlled trial. *BMJ* 2002;**325**:746.

66. **Ehrmann D, Bergis-Jurgan N, Haak T, Kulzer B, Hermanns N**. Comparison of the Efficacy of a Diabetes Education Programme for Type 1 Diabetes (PRIMAS) in a randomised controlled trial setting and the effectiveness in a routine care setting: results of a comparative effectiveness study. *PLoS One* 2016;**11**:e0147581.

67. **Hermanns N, Kulzer B, Ehrmann D, Bergis-Jurgan N, Haak T**. The effect of a diabetes education programme (PRIMAS) for people with type 1 diabetes: results of a randomized trial. *Diabetes Research and Clinical Practice* 2013;**102**:149–57.

68. **Hopkins D, Lawrence I, Mansell P**, et al. Improved biomedical and psychological outcomes 1 year after structured education in flexible insulin therapy for people with type 1 diabetes: the U.K. DAFNE experience. *Diabetes Care* 2012;**35**:1638–42.

69. **Hermanns N, Kulzer B, Maier B, Mahr M, Haak T**. The effect of an education programme (MEDIAS 2 ICT) involving intensive insulin treatment for people with type 2 diabetes. *Patient Education and Counseling* 2012;**86**:226–32.

70. **Hermanns N, Kulzer B, Kubiak T, Krichbaum M, Haak T**. The effect of an education programme (HyPOS) to treat hypoglycaemia problems in patients with type 1 diabetes. *Diabetes/Metabolism Research and Reviews* 2007;**23**:528–38.

71. **Rondags SM, de WM, Twisk JW, Snoek FJ**. Effectiveness of HypoAware, a brief partly web-based psychoeducational intervention for adults with type 1 and insulin-treated type 2 diabetes and problematic hypoglycemia: a cluster randomized controlled trial. *Diabetes Care* 2016;**39**:2190–6.

72. **Fisher L, Hessler D, Glasgow RE**, et al. REDEEM: a pragmatic trial to reduce diabetes distress. *Diabetes Care* 2013;**36**:2551–8.

73. **Nobis S, Lehr D, Ebert DD**, et al. Efficacy of a web-based intervention with mobile phone support in treating depressive symptoms in adults with type 1 and type 2 diabetes: a randomized controlled trial. *Diabetes Care* 2015;**38**:776–83.

74. **van Bastelaar KM, Pouwer F, Cuijpers P, Riper H, Snoek FJ**. Web-based depression treatment for type 1 and type 2 diabetic patients: a randomized, controlled trial. *Diabetes Care* 2011;**34**:320–5.

75. **Hermanns N, Schmitt A, Gahr A**, et al. The effect of a Diabetes-Specific Cognitive Behavioral Treatment Program (DIAMOS) for patients with diabetes and subclinical depression: results of a randomized controlled trial. *Diabetes Care* 2015;**38**:551–60.

76. **Petrak F, Herpertz S, Albus C**, et al. cognitive behavioral therapy versus sertraline in patients with depression and poorly controlled diabetes: The Diabetes and Depression (DAD) Study: a randomized controlled multicenter trial. *Diabetes Care* 2015;**38**:767–75.

77. **Tovote KA, Fleer J, Snippe E**, et al. Individual mindfulness-based cognitive therapy andcognitive behavior therapy for treating depressive symptoms in patients with diabetes: results of a randomized controlled trial. *Diabetes Care* 2014;**37**:2427–34.

78. **van Son J, Nyklicek I, Pop VJ, Blonk MC, Erdtsieck RJ, Pouwer F**. Mindfulness-based cognitive therapy for people with diabetes and emotional problems: long-term

follow-up findings from the DiaMind randomized controlled trial. *J Psychosom Res* 2014;77:81–4.

79. **Moulton CD, Pickup JC, Ismail K.** The link between depression and diabetes: the search for shared mechanisms. *Lancet Diabetes Endocrinol* 2015;3:461–71.

80. **Brouwer A, van Raalte DH, Diamant M, Rutters F, van Someren EJ, Snoek FJ,** et al. Light therapy for better mood and insulin sensitivity in patients with major depression and type 2 diabetes: a randomised, double-blind, parallel-arm trial. *BMC Psychiatry* 2015;15:169.

Chapter 9

The association between depression and cognitive impairment in type 2 diabetes

Calum D. Moulton and Clive Ballard

Introduction

There is a worldwide epidemic of dementia, which is expected to increase in prevalence from around 35.6 million in 2010 to approximately 65.7 million by 2030 [1]. However, available treatments for dementia are not disease modifying and produce only modest effects on cognitive decline [2]. It is now established that type 2 diabetes (T2D) increases the risk of incident dementia, even independently of its association with cardiovascular disease (CVD), and around 7% of cases of dementia overall can be attributed to diabetes [3]. The association between diabetes and cognitive impairment is poorly explained by hyperglycaemia alone and is likely to be multifactorial in aetiology.

Depression has emerged as a potential risk factor for cognitive impairment and dementia in T2D. Building on a large evidence base for its association with both T2D and dementia, respectively, there is growing evidence that depression increases the risk of dementia in patients with T2D. If this is the case, depression presents multiple opportunities for treatments to improve cognitive outcomes in T2D.

This chapter will briefly summarize the epidemiology and clinical presentation of cognitive impairment in patients with T2D, before examining key candidate risk factors. The chapter will then scrutinize the evidence to date that has tested depression as a risk factor for cognitive impairment and cognitive decline in patients with T2D. The chapter concludes with suggestions for future multidisciplinary research that could exploit depression as a target for primary and secondary prevention of cognitive decline in patients with T2D.

Clinical presentation of cognitive impairment in T2D

A broad spectrum of cognitive impairment can be observed in people with T2D. This ranges from subtle subjective-only deficits at the mildest end to dementia at the other, with mild cognitive impairment (MCI) falling in between.

Dementia and MCI are clinical diagnoses, made with reference to operationalized criteria [4]. Instead, however, much research into cognitive impairment in T2D has used cognitive tests, some employing self-report measures, such as the Mini-Mental State Examination (MMSE) [5], and others using a more detailed neuropsychological assessment [6]. In the clinic, such tests are supplementary to any clinical diagnosis of MCI or dementia. Indeed, cognitive tests are susceptible to confounding by educational status and concomitant psychopathology such as depression [7].

At the severe end of the spectrum, dementia is generally defined as a progressive deterioration in memory and other cognitive abilities that leads to a significant deterioration in functioning [4]. In addition to a 2.5-fold increased risk of vascular dementia, T2D is associated with a 1.5-fold increased risk of Alzheimer's disease AD [3]. Because AD is far more common overall, T2D leads more commonly to AD than vascular dementia.

Presenting with a less severe phenotype, MCI is used as a term to describe cognitive impairment beyond that expected based on the age and education of the individual but, unlike dementia, is not significant enough to interfere with daily activities [8]. The clinical significance of MCI is debated but it is thought to portend a 10–15% annual conversion rate to dementia [9]. In diabetes, people are 1.5–3 times more likely to progress from MCI to dementia than non-diabetes controls. Moreover, there is some evidence that this progression may be delayed by treatment of vascular risk factors [10]. Diabetes is associated with increased risk of both amnestic- and non-amnestic subtypes of MCI, although the association between non-amnestic MCI and diabetes is weaker when controlled for other vascular risk factors [11].

In addition to MCI and dementia, there is evidence that more subtle cognitive decrements are identifiable in people with T2D, which may be more specifically associated with diabetes. The term *diabetes-associated cognitive decrements* has been developed to describe subtle subjective cognitive deficits that are less severe than MCI. These occur across the lifespan and are thought to progress slowly, if at all [12]. However, the correlates of these subjective decrements remain uncertain and their specificity to diabetes has been questioned [13].

Potential risk factors for cognitive decline in T2D

There has been considerable interest in identifying potentially modifiable factors that may underlie the relationship between T2D and cognitive decline. To date, observational studies have vastly outweighed interventional studies in this area, the latter generally proving unsuccessful. Although considered individually here for ease, isolated modification of risk factors may be one reason for the failure of intervention studies to date. Indeed, 'multiple-hit' studies have shown considerable promise in slowing down cognitive decline in the general population [14].

Glycaemic control

In observational studies, there is mixed evidence to support an association between hyperglycaemia and cognitive decline [15,16]. In by far the largest interventional study to date—the ACCORD-MIND study—intensive glycaemic control was not associated with any difference in cognitive decline after 40 months [17]. However, the study was limited by premature termination because of excess mortality in the intervention group. For hypoglycaemia, there is evidence from well-designed cohort studies and large database studies to support an association between prior episodes and either cognitive impairment or incident dementia in T2D [18,19]. However, the relationship is complicated by a bidirectional effect: dementia significantly increases the risk of subsequent hypoglycaemia, which has important clinical implications when setting glycaemia targets in this population [20].

Cardiovascular risk factors and cardiovascular disease

In cross-sectional studies, hypertension and hyperlipidaemia are both associated with cognitive impairment [21,22]. However, prospective studies examining these risk factors have been far fewer in number with frequent negative findings [23,24]. Furthermore, modification of cardiovascular risk factors in isolation proved ineffective in improving cognitive outcomes in the ACCORD-MIND study [25]. Studies examining the effects of multiple vascular risk factor management in individuals with early-stage T2D and over longer-term follow-up are awaited. In contrast to the mixed findings regarding individual vascular risk factors, the association between cognitive decline and prior CVD, such as stroke, myocardial infarction, or peripheral vascular disease, is far more consistent [18,24]. The reasons for the mismatch between individual vascular risk factors and established CVD are not clear, and it may be that a history of CVD denotes patients at higher overall vascular risk.

Inflammation

In the general population, elevated inflammation is strongly implicated in the pathogenesis of cognitive decline and dementia [26]. Meanwhile, the role of inflammation in the pathogenesis of T2D is established [27]. As such, inflammation has been suggested as a potential risk factor for cognitive decline in patients with T2D. In the Edinburgh Type 2 Diabetes study of 1,066 people aged 60–75 years, elevated concentrations of interleukin-6 were associated with overall cognitive performance on seven tests, even after adjustment for potential confounders [28]. Prospective research is now needed to test whether inflammation is associated with cognitive decline in patients with T2D.

Insulin resistance and defective insulin signalling

There is growing evidence that both insulin resistance and deficiency of insulin may lead to AD. In epidemiological studies, both insulin resistance and central obesity are associated with increased risk of incident dementia, the latter occurring independently of diabetes status [29,30]. Reviewed in detail elsewhere, both insulin resistance and insulin deficiency may lead to AD-like pathology through effects on beta-amyloid, cerebral glucose metabolism, vascular function, and inflammation [31]. Of the small number of intervention studies performed, supplementation of intranasal insulin in patients with early AD has been found to improve declarative memory and attention in the short term [32]. By contrast, clinical trials of insulin sensitizers, such as thiazolidinediones, have not demonstrated consistent benefit in AD patients to date [33].

Depression as a novel risk factor for cognitive decline in T2D

Depression is twice as common in patients with T2D as those in the general population, affecting 10–20% of patients with T2D [34]. As well as predicting premature mortality and increased risk of diabetes complications [35,36], depression has emerged as a potential risk factor for cognitive decline and dementia in T2D. This section firstly outlines key evidence from the general population to support an association between depression and dementia, before critically appraising the major studies to date that have tested this association in patients with T2D.

Evidence from the general population

In prospective cohort studies with 14 and 17 years of follow-up, depression predicted around a twofold increased risk of incident dementia in later life [37,38].

Most studies, however, have focused on late-life depression (age 60 years or older), and such studies face more methodological difficulties in demonstrating a robust prospective association with dementia. For example, the prevalence of depression in patients with established dementia is high [39], and depression and dementia share important features, such as reduced attention and impaired working memory [40]. Moreover, depression can cause poor effort on cognitive testing, leading to a 'depressive pseudodementia' that may be misdiagnosed as MCI or dementia [41]. As such, it is difficult to exclude the possibility that depression is in fact a prodrome or clinical feature of dementia, rather than a risk factor for its subsequent development.

The pathways linking depression and dementia are likely to be multifactorial and multidirectional. There is strong evidence that depression is associated with increased risk of vascular disease [42], although the bidirectional nature of this relationship complicates causality [43]. An elevated inflammatory response is strongly associated with both depression and dementia [44,45], and proinflammatory cytokines have been found to reduce both synaptic plasticity and hippocampal neurogenesis [46]. Depression may lead to activation of the hypothalamic–pituitary–adrenal axis and increased glucocorticoid production, leading subsequently to hippocampal damage and potentially to beta-amyloid accumulation [46,47]. Finally, post-mortem brains of patients with AD with comorbid depression show more pronounced neurofibrillary tangle formation than those from patients who did not have depression [48].

Evidence from studies in type 2 diabetes

Cross-sectional studies

Cross-sectional studies of depression and cognitive function in T2D have produced mixed findings. In an analysis of three mixed ethnicity cohorts ($n = 2,436$), comorbid depression and diabetes significantly increased risk for MCI and AD [49], whereas effects of comorbid diabetes and depression on MCI were inconclusive. This study was strengthened by rigorous cognitive assessment and a consensus definition of depression. In a sample of 225 people with T2D aged 70 or over, those with either dementia or MCI were found to have a 1.8-fold increased risk of concurrent depression, as defined using the Center for Epidemiologic Studies Depression Scale (CES-D) [50]. However, the association with depression was not subjected to any multivariate analysis. In a study of 374 patients all within 6 months of a stroke, comorbidity with either diabetes or depressive symptoms alone (defined using the CES-D) increased the risk of severe cognitive impairment (defined using the Montreal Cognitive Assessment score <20) around twofold. Of note, comorbidity with both depressive symptoms and diabetes approximately tripled the odds of severe cognitive impairment [51].

In a cross-sectional study of 1,790 people with newly diagnosed T2D recruited from primary care in south London, there was no relationship between depression (defined using the Patient Health Questionnaire-9 (PHQ-9)) and cognitive performance on the Telephone Interview for Cognitive Status [44]. Finally, in a cross-sectional analysis of three cohorts with T2D, the 39 participants with comorbid depressive symptoms, as defined using self-report inventories, showed no difference in performance on a range of neuropsychological tests compared to the 327 without depressive symptoms ($p = 0.82$) [52].

Longitudinal studies

Compared with cross-sectional studies, findings from longitudinal studies have been more consistent. In a prospective cohort study of 3,837 primary care patients with diabetes, patients with depression—as defined using the PHQ-9— were more likely to develop dementia (7.9%) than those without depression (4.8%), even after adjustment for potential confounding [53]. However, the study did not exclude any diagnoses of dementia made early in the follow-up period, and diagnoses were based on coding from medical records.

In the Diabetes and Aging Study of 19239 individuals with diabetes, it was found that patients with depression—as defined using the PHQ-8—were twice as likely (2.1% vs. 1.0%) to develop dementia over a 5-year follow-up. This association was robust to potential confounding [54]. The authors attempted to negate the possibility that depression was a dementia prodrome by discounting any diagnoses of dementia made in the first 3 years of follow-up. However, this analysis will not negate this potential limitation completely.

In a Danish national population-based cohort study of 2,454,532 adults, those with comorbid diabetes and depression (95,691) were at increased risk of incident dementia (adjusted hazard ratio 2.17; 95% CI 2.10–2.24). Notably, this risk was greater than the summed risk associated with depression and diabetes individually [55]. In the ACCORD-MIND cohort of 2,977 people at high risk of cardiovascular disease, depression—as defined using the PHQ-9—was associated with greater 40-month decline in performance on a range of neuropsychological tests. These findings remained robust to potential confounding [56].

Finally, in a retrospective study of 2756 Mexican Americans aged 65 or over, those with diabetes or comorbid depression and diabetes had significantly greater cognitive decline over an 11-year period, even after adjusting for confounding. However, depression comorbid with diabetes was not found to increase the effect versus diabetes alone. The study was limited by the measurement of cognition using the MMSE only and the use of self-report diabetes status [57].

Despite the positive findings from these studies, their focus on later life depression means that the methodological limitations discussed in the 'Evidence from the general population' section are not completely negated.

Recommendations for future research

The highest quality observational studies to date have used medical records, which introduces various biases and difficulties establishing causality. Future prospective diabetes cohorts should measure both cognition and depression longitudinally in order to establish that depression is a cause and not a consequence of dementia. Studies of early-life depression would better overcome many of the methodological limitations encountered when testing depression as a risk factor for cognitive decline. Future prospective research should examine the phenotype of depression in more detail in order to test whether different subtypes—whether questionnaire-positive depression, mild depression, or severe depression—are differentially associated with cognitive decline in T2D. This would help to target the patients most likely to benefit from future intervention studies.

A further limitation of database research is the lack of opportunities to define mechanisms by which depression may lead to cognitive decline in T2D. Future cohort studies should be enriched by mechanistic biomarkers, including measures of inflammation, HPA axis function, and endothelial dysfunction, in order to test candidate pathways. There is a need for better understanding of the relative contributions of insulin deficiency and insulin resistance to AD, as well as the degree to which aberrations in central insulin signalling are driven by peripherally or centrally mediated processes. Further *in vitro* research is needed to test the mechanisms by which depression could lead to accumulation of beta-amyloid in diabetes.

In terms of treatment, both observational and interventional studies should test whether treatments for depression in T2D could improve cognitive outcomes. Such studies may test both established antidepressant treatments and novel therapies, such as those acting on the inflammatory response and HPA axis. If depression is indeed a robust risk factor for dementia, the earlier depression is treated, the greater the potential benefit for cognition. For example, whereas treatment of depression in later life could slow down cognitive decline, identification and treatment of high-risk depression patients in earlier life could prevent the onset of dementia altogether.

Conclusion

T2D is an established risk factor for cognitive decline and dementia, yet the reasons for this association are not well understood and poorly explained by glycaemic control alone. There is now good quality observational evidence that depression may be a risk factor for dementia in patients with T2D, although these findings are tempered by the overlap in chronology and clinical presentation between depression and dementia. Longitudinal research across a longer life-course is now needed to test whether depression is a robust risk factor for dementia in T2D, and moreover whether treatment of depression can provide opportunities for secondary and even primary prevention of dementia.

References

1. Prince M, Bryce R, Albanese E, et al. The global prevalence of dementia: a systematic review and metaanalysis. *Alzheimer's Dementia* 2013;**9**:63–75.e2.
2. Scarpini E, Scheltens P, Feldman H. Treatment of Alzheimer's disease: current status and new perspectives. *Lancet Neurology* 2003;**2**:539–47.
3. Cheng G, Huang C, Deng H, Wang H. Diabetes as a risk factor for dementia and mild cognitive impairment: a meta-analysis of longitudinal studies. *Internal Medicine Journal* 2012;**42**:484–91.
4. WHO. *The ICD-10 Classification of Mental and Behavioural Disorders. Clinical Descriptions and Diagnostic Guidelines.* WHO: Geneva, 1992.
5. Bruce DG, Harrington N, Davis WA, Davis TM; Fremantle Diabetes Study. Dementia and its associations in type 2 diabetes mellitus: the Fremantle Diabetes Study. *Diabetes Research and Clinical Practice* 2001;**53**:165–72.
6. Feinkohl I, Aung PP, Keller M, et al. Severe hypoglycemia and cognitive decline in older people with type 2 diabetes: the Edinburgh type 2 diabetes study. *Diabetes Care* 2014;**37**:507–15.
7. Räihä I, Isoaho R, Ojanlatva A, et al. Poor performance in the mini-mental state examination due to causes other than dementia. *Scandinavian Journal of Primary Health Care* 2001;**19**:34–8.
8. Petersen RC, Smith GE, Waring SC, et al. Mild cognitive impairment: clinical characterization and outcome. *Archives of Neurology* 1999;**56**:303–8.
9. Grundman M, Petersen RC, Ferris SH, et al. Mild cognitive impairment can be distinguished from Alzheimer disease and normal aging for clinical trials. *Archives of Neurology* 2004;**61**:59–66.
10. Li J, Wang YJ, Zhang M, et al. Vascular risk factors promote conversion from mild cognitive impairment to Alzheimer disease. *Neurology* 2011;**76**:1485–91.
11. Luchsinger JA, Reitz C, Patel B, et al. Relation of diabetes to mild cognitive impairment. *Archives of Neurology* 2007;**64**:570–5.
12. Koekkoek PS, Kappelle LJ, van den Berg E, et al. Cognitive function in patients with diabetes mellitus: guidance for daily care. *Lancet Neurology* 2015;**14**:329–40.
13. Akbaraly TN, Kivimaki M, Shipley MJ, et al. Metabolic syndrome over 10 years and cognitive functioning in late midlife: the Whitehall II study. *Diabetes Care* 2010;**33**:84–9.

14. **Ngandu T, Lehtisalo J, Solomon A**, et al. A 2 year multidomain intervention of diet, exercise, cognitive training, and vascular risk monitoring versus control to prevent cognitive decline in at-risk elderly people (FINGER): a randomised controlled trial. *Lancet* 2015;**385**:2255–63.

15. **Cukierman-Yaffe T, Gerstein HC, Williamson JD**, et al. Relationship between baseline glycemic control and cognitive function in individuals with type 2 diabetes and other cardiovascular risk factors: the action to control cardiovascular risk in diabetes-memory in diabetes (ACCORD-MIND) trial. *Diabetes Care* 2009;**32**:221–6.

16. **Moulton CD, Stewart R, Amiel SA**, et al. Factors associated with cognitive impairment in patients with newly diagnosed type 2 diabetes: a cross-sectional study. *Aging and Mental Health* 2016;**20**:840–7.

17. **Launer LJ, Miller ME, Williamson JD**, et al. Effects of intensive glucose lowering on brain structure and function in people with type 2 diabetes (ACCORD MIND): a randomised open-label substudy. *Lancet Neurology* 2011;**10**:969–77.

18. **Haroon NN, Austin PC, Shah BR**, et al. Risk of dementia in seniors with newly diagnosed diabetes: a population-based study. *Diabetes Care* 2015;**38**:1868–75.

19. **Lin CH, Sheu WH.** Hypoglycaemic episodes and risk of dementia in diabetes mellitus: 7-year follow-up study. *Journal of Internal Medicine.* 2013;**273**:102–10.

20. **Punthakee Z, Miller ME, Launer LJ**, et al. Poor cognitive function and risk of severe hypoglycemia in type 2 diabetes: post hoc epidemiologic analysis of the ACCORD trial. *Diabetes Care* 2012;**35**:787–93.

21. **Chen G, Cai L, Chen B** et al. Serum level of endogenous secretory receptor for advanced glycation end products and other factors in type 2 diabetic patients with mild cognitive impairment. *Diabetes Care* 2011;**34**:2586–90.

22. **Chen RH, Jiang XZ, Zhao XH**, et al. Risk factors of mild cognitive impairment in middle aged patients with type 2 diabetes: a crosssection study. *Annals of Endocrinology* 2012;**73**:208–12.

23. **Bruce DG, Davis WA, Casey GP**, et al. Predictors of cognitive decline in older individuals with diabetes. *Diabetes Care* 2008;**31**:2103–7.

24. **Bruce DG, Davis WA, Casey GP**, et al. Predictors of cognitive impairment and dementia in older people with diabetes. *Diabetologia* 2008;**51**:241–8a.

25. **Williamson JD, Launer LJ, Bryan RN**, et al. Cognitive function and brain structure in persons with type 2 diabetes mellitus after intensive lowering of blood pressure and lipid levels: a randomized clinical trial. *JAMA Internal Medicine* 2014;**174**:324–33.

26. **Glass CK, Saijo K, Winner B**, et al. Mechanisms underlying inflammation in neurodegeneration. *Cell* 2010;**140**:918–34.

27. **Pickup JC.** Inflammation and activated innate immunity in the pathogenesis of type 2 diabetes. *Diabetes Care* 2004;**27**:813–23.

28. **Marioni RE, Strachan MW, Reynolds RM**, et al. Association between raised inflammatory markers and cognitive decline in elderly people with type 2 diabetes: the Edinburgh Type 2 Diabetes Study. *Diabetes* 2010;**59**:710–13.

29. **Whitmer RA, Gustafson DR, Barrett-Connor E**, et al. Central obesity and increased risk of dementia more than three decades later. *Neurology* 2008,**71**:1057–64.

30. **Yaffe K, Blackwell T, Kanaya AM**, et al. Diabetes, impaired fasting glucose, and development of cognitive impairment in older women. *Neurology* 2004;**63**:658–63.

31. **Craft S, Cholerton B, Baker LD.** Insulin and Alzheimer's disease: untangling the web. *Journal of Alzheimers Disease.* 2013;**33**(Suppl. 1):S263–75.

32. Reger MA, Watson GS, Green PS, et al. Intranasal insulin improves cognition and modulates beta-amyloid in early AD. *Neurology* **2008**:440–8.

33. Harrington C, Sawchak S, Chiang C, et al. Rosiglitazone does not improve cognition or global function when used as adjunctive therapy to AChE inhibitors in mild-to-moderate Alzheimer's disease: two phase 3 studies. *Current Alzheimer Research* 2011,**8**:592–606.

34. Anderson RJ, Freedland KE, Clouse RE, Lustman PJ. The prevalence of comorbid depression in adults with diabetes: a meta analysis. *Diabetes Care* 2001;**24**:1069–78.

35. de Groot M, Anderson R, Freedland KE, Clouse RE, Lustman PJ. Association of depression and diabetes complications: a meta-analysis. *Psychosomatic Medicine* 2001;**63**:619–30.

36. Katon WJ, Rutter C, Simon G, et al. The association of comorbid depression with mortality in patients with type 2 diabetes. *Diabetes Care* 2005;**28**:2668–72.

37. Dal Forno G, Palermo MT, Donohue JE, Karagiozis H, Zonderman AB, Kawas CH. Depressive symptoms, sex, and risk for Alzheimer's disease. *Annals of Neurology* 2005;**57**:381–7.

38. Saczynski JS, Beiser A, Seshadri S, et al. Depressive symptoms and risk of dementia: the Framingham Heart Study. *Neurology* 2010;**75**:35–41.

39. Ballard C, Bannister C, Solis M, et al. The prevalence, associations and symptoms of depression amongst dementia sufferers. *Journal of Affective Disorders*. 1996 **22**;**36**:135–44.

40. Steffens DC, Potter GG. Geriatric depression and cognitive impairment. *Psychological Medicine* 2008;**38**:163–75.

41. Haggerty JJ Jr, Golden RN, Evans DL, Janowsky DS. Differential diagnosis of pseudodementia in the elderly. *Geriatrics* 1988;**43**:61–9.

42. Liebetrau, M., Steen, B, Skoog, I. Depression as a risk factor for the incidence of first-ever stroke in 85-year-olds. *Stroke* 2008;**39**:1960–5.

43. Thomas AJ, Kalaria RN, O'Brien JT. Depression and vascular disease: what is the relationship? *Journal of Affective Disorders* 2004;**79**:81–95.

44. Dowlati Y, Herrmann N, Swardfager W, et al. A meta-analysis of cytokines in major depression. *Biological Psychiatry* 2010;**67**:446–57.

45. Leonard, B. E. Inflammation, depression and dementia: are they connected? *Neurochemistry Research* 2007;**32**:1749–56.

46. Caraci F, Copani A, Nicoletti F, Drago F. Depression and Alzheimer's disease: neurobiological links and common pharmacological targets. *European Journal of Pharmacology* 2010;**626**;64–71.

47. Butters MA, Young JB, Lopez O, et al. Pathways linking late-life depression to persistent cognitive impairment and dementia. *Dialogues in Clinical Neuroscience* 2008;**10**:345–57.

48. Rapp MA, Schnaider-Beeri M, Purohit DP, et al. Increased neurofibrillary tangles in patients with Alzheimer disease with comorbid depression. *American Journal of Geriatric Psychiatry* 2008;**16**:168–74.

49. Johnson LA, Gamboa A, Vintimilla R, et al. Comorbid depression and diabetes as a risk for mild cognitive impairment and Alzheimer's disease in elderly Mexican Americans. *Journal of Alzheimers Disease* 2015;**47**:129–36.

50. **Koekkoek PS, Biessels GJ, Kooistra M,** et al. Undiagnosed cognitive impairment, health status and depressive symptoms in patients with type 2 diabetes. *J Diabetes Complications.* 2015;**29**:1217–22.

52. **Koekkoek PS, Rutten GE, Ruis C,** et al. Mild depressive symptoms do not influence cognitive functioning in patients with type 2 diabetes. *Psychoneuroendocrinology* 2013;**38**:376–86.

53. **Katon WJ, Lin EH, Williams LH,** et al. Comorbid depression is associated with an increased risk of dementia diagnosis in patients with diabetes: a prospective cohort study. *Journal of General Internal Medicine* 2010;**25**:423–9.

51. **Swardfager W, MacIntosh BJ.** Depression, type 2 diabetes, and poststroke cognitive impairment. *Neurorehabilitation and Neural Repair* 2017;**31**:48–55.

54. **Katon W, Lyles CR, Parker MM,** et al. Association of depression with increased risk of dementia in patients with type 2 diabetes: the Diabetes and Aging Study. *Archives of General Psychiatry* 2012;**69**:410–17.

55. **Katon W, Pedersen HS, Ribe AR,** et al. Effect of depression and diabetes mellitus on the risk for dementia: a national population-based cohort study. *JAMA Psychiatry* 2015;**72**:612–9.

56. **Sullivan MD, Katon WJ, Lovato LC,** et al. Association of depression with accelerated cognitive decline among patients with type 2 diabetes in the ACCORD-MIND trial. *JAMA Psychiatry* 2013;**70**:1041–7.

57. **Downer B, Vickers BN, Al Snih S,** et al. Effects of comorbid depression and diabetes mellitus on cognitive decline in older Mexican Americans. *Journal of American Geriatrics Society* 2016;**64**:109–17.

Chapter 10

Treatment of depression in type 2 diabetes

Frank Petrak and Bonnie Röhrig

Introduction

The comorbidity of depression and diabetes is common and impacts medical outcome of patients suffering from both conditions [1,2]. Numerous deteriorating effects of depression were identified in diabetes patients, for example poorer glycaemic control [3,4], increased micro- and macrovascular complications [5], and increased mortality [6,7], among others. Depression also affects psychosocial outcomes in diabetes [8,9]. This has been demonstrated repeatedly for increased diabetes related distress [10], reduced quality of life [8,9], and adherence to diabetes treatment [11,12].

The association between type 2 diabetes and depression is bidirectional and there is increasing evidence for shared biological origins between both conditions. Additionally, the increased vulnerability to depression can be explained by the burden of diabetes and diabetes-related complications among others [1]. Regardless of these well-established facts, there still is an underdiagnosis and undertreatment of depression in people with diabetes [13,14].

This chapter focuses on the treatment of depression in type 2 diabetes patients, starting with treatment goals and an overview of models of healthcare delivery for this specific patient group. A summary of the current state of scientific evidence for the treatment of depression in diabetes patients represents the focus of this chapter, ending with recommendations for clinical practice.

Treatment goals

Considering the adverse interaction between both conditions, it is obvious that depression treatment should focus on medical and psychological outcomes goals simultaneously in people with diabetes [15]. These goals were also highlighted in the only published evidence-based guidelines addressing treatment goals for people with diabetes and comorbid depression. In these guidelines of the German Diabetes Association an equal emphasis is given on psychological and medical targets of depression treatment in diabetes [16].

With regard to the psychological targets, the priority lies in the reduction of symptoms of depression until remission of depression is reached and in the prevention of depression-related suicides. Additional objectives include the improvement of health-related quality of life, the restoration of psychosocial functions, the improvement of coping with and acceptance of diabetes, as well as improvement in healthy lifestyle changes, among others. The most important medical target is to reduce diabetes-related complications and premature mortality. As surrogate marker for subsequent poor prognosis of diabetes, glycated haemoglobin (HbA_{1c}) is currently considered as the primary target variable in most cases. Therefore, the ideal depression treatment in diabetes would be an intervention which simultaneously improves depression symptoms and glycaemic control [15,16].

There is no scientific evidence for the priority of medical or psychological treatment goals for people suffering from depression and diabetes. However, from a clinical perspective it seems favourable to focus first on the rapid improvement or remission of depression. This recommendation is based on the differences in the time course of treatment responses, where response to treatment can be expected within 2–4 weeks for antidepressants and some weeks longer for psychological interventions. By contrast, behaviour changes towards healthier lifestyle or changes regarding diabetes treatment leading to better glycaemic control needs several months until an assessment is meaningful. Most important, improvement of depression may be a prerequisite to good diabetes self-management as people with diabetes may follow their management plan more easily if their mood is improved and they generally feel better first [15].

Healthcare delivery

Models of care for depression in diabetes vary from conventional consultations with psychopharmacological treatment in primary or secondary care, to psychological interventions delivered by different professional groups, to complex interventions such as collaborative care or stepped-care approaches [15,17]. Additionally there is a variety of telemedical and web-based interventions that have received more attention recently [18].

Most psychopharmacological treatments include antidepressants, especially selective serotonin reuptake inhibitors (SSRIs). Psychological interventions include problem-solving techniques, self-management strategies and counselling, cognitive behavioural therapy (CBT), or psychodynamic therapy, among others. Another focus in the treatment of comorbid depression in type 2 diabetes has been on increasing physical activity.

Collaborative care approaches are characterized as team driven, population focused, measurement guided, and evidence-based [19]. In practice this expresses itself in the provision of evidence-based treatment options, interdisciplinary cooperation between healthcare providers, routine monitoring of outcomes and proactive follow-up contacts, self-management training and support for patients, supervision of care managers, and decision support for primary care physicians [17].

On the other hand, stepped-care approaches are characterized by algorithm-based treatment plans allowing individual adaptions to suit the needs and problems of the respective patients. The basic idea of these models is to gradually offer different evidence-based treatments, which generally means the combination of different psychological and psychopharmacological interventions with prespecified cut-offs for the transition to the next step according to treatment response and patient preferences [17].

Recent developments in the treatment of depression in type 2 diabetes are web-based interventions and mobile health applications, focusing on behavioural health coaching and CBT orientated self-management of depression [18].

Evidence from clinical studies

Interventions for the treatment of diabetes and depression have been systematically evaluated within randomized controlled trials (RCTs) since 1998. Existing studies and interventions vary widely in terms of methodology (e.g. comparison condition), settings (e.g. medication, face-to-face intervention, telephone or web-based delivery of treatment, group versus individual treatment), and type of healthcare provider (e.g. primary, secondary or collaborative care). Hence the results of those studies are comparable only to a limited extent.

The following overview of the scientific evidence for the treatment of depression in type 2 diabetes is based on a meta-review published in 2015. This review included all systematic reviews, meta-analyses, and RCTs on any depression intervention for adults with diabetes and depression published until August 2014 [15]. For this chapter we additionally summarize the results of meta-analyses and randomized controlled trials published since the meta-review until September 2016 (see Table 10.1).

Psychological interventions

The 2015 meta-review [15] included 10 RCTs investigating the effects of psychological interventions on depression in diabetes, covering 1,132 patients

Table 10.1 Meta-analyses and RCTs (not included in the meta-analyses) on treatment for depression in diabetes published since the meta-review 2015 of Petrak and colleagues

Reference	Country	Type of intervention	Samples	Number of patients
Psychological interventions				
Uchendu et al. (2016) [22]		Meta-analysis effectiveness of CBT on glycaemic control and psychological outcomes in adults with diabetes	12 RCT	1445
Moncrieft et al. (2016) [23]	USA	RCT Multicomponent life-style interventions on weight, glycaemic control, depressive symptoms	Low income minority patients with T2D	111
Pibernik-Okanovic et al. (2015) [25]	Croatia	RCT Psychoeducation and physical exercises	T2D and subsyndromal depression	179
Hermanns et al. (2015) [24]	Germany	RCT Diabetes-specific CBT	Diabetes and subclinical depression	212
Psychopharmacological interventions				
Kang et al. (2015) [26]	China	RCT paroxetine vs. agomelatine	T2D and Depression	116
Psychopharmacological vs. psychological interventions				
Petrak et al. (2015) [27]	Germany	RCT Diabetes specific CBT vs. sertraline	Diabetes patients with poor glycaemic control and major depression	251
Collaborative and stepped-care interventions				
Stoop et al. (2015) [28]	Netherlands	RCT Stepped care intervention for anxiety and depression	People with diabetes, asthma or COPD in primary care	46
Web-based interventions				
Nobis et al. (2015) [34]	Netherlands	RCT Internet-based guided self-help for depression	Adults with T1D or T2D	260
Pal et al. (2014) [18]		Meta-analysis Computer-based diabetes self-management interventions	16 RCT	3578
Clarke et al. (2016) [30]	Australia	RCT Mobile phone and web-based cognitive behaviour therapy for depressive symptoms	People with diabetes	86

altogether from the USA, China, the Netherlands, and Germany. Most common were the combination of cognitive behavioural therapy (CBT) and diabetes education. It also included other psychological approaches, such as psychodynamic support psychotherapy, mindfulness-based cognitive therapy, psychosocial interventions, and various techniques and strategies (e.g. relaxation techniques, electromyographic feedback, health-education, and self-management). Most of the trials investigating the effects of psychological interventions used usual care as the comparison group. The significant standardized mean differences (SMD) for the primary outcomes ranged from –0.14 to –1.47, which is in agreement with previous research [20,21]. Evidence suggests that psychological interventions also have a positive impact on health-related quality of life, adherence to treatment, and diabetes distress. Results for the improvement of glycemic control ranged from 0.40 to –1.40 and were inconsistent [15].

In addition to the meta-review of 2015 [15], two systematic reviews summarized results for the treatment of depression in type 2 diabetes recently. In accordance with previous results, a meta-analysis reported, that CBT improved depression in people with diabetes in the short, medium, and long-term, but the effect size reduced over time [22]. The influence of CBT on glycaemic control was significant in the short and medium-term but there were no consistent pattern of the effects of CBT on long-term glycaemic control. Similar findings have been observed in a recent study of Moncrieft et al [23], who compared a multicomponent behavioural intervention to usual care. A more recent study compared a short-term diabetes-specific CBT, based on a self-management/empowerment approach, with diabetes education for subclinical depression in people with diabetes. The results indicate that this diabetes-specific programme improved depressive symptoms, diabetes distress, health-related quality of life, and diabetes acceptance. In addition, an improvement of glycaemic control and a decreased risk for a major depression was observed [24]. A Croatian study evaluated the effects of psychoeducation or physical exercises on subsyndromal depression in people with diabetes. Noticeable improvement of depressive symptoms was achieved with no differences between treatment groups and no improvement of glycaemic control was observed in the different interventions [25].

In conclusion, psychological interventions show moderate to good effects in the reduction of depression severity in people with type 2 diabetes and depression. Results concerning glycaemic control, however, are inconsistent and indicate low effectiveness.

Pharmacological interventions

In the 2015 meta-review [15] 12 studies dealt with the evaluation of pharmacological interventions in the treatment of depression in people with diabetes with a total sample of 721 patients primarily evaluating SSRIs (e.g. paroxetine, sertraline, fluoxetine) or tricyclic antidepressants. Most of them were placebo controlled or had an active control group. With a standardized mean difference range from –0.61 to –0.39 antidepressants effectively reduced depression severity compared with placebo. The effectiveness on glycaemic control was also slightly beneficial. Nonetheless, it must be noted that none of the trials reported follow-up data for the long-term effect, so it remains unclear if the reported improvements were stable.

The most recent RCT compared the effectiveness of the antidepressants paroxetine and agomelatine and found an advantage for agomelatine in the long-term follow-up (12 weeks after treatment ending) compared with the short-term follow-up (6 weeks after treatment ending). They also identified a significant improvement of glycaemic control in the agomelatine group [26].

In summary, pharmacological interventions are effective in the treatment of depression in type 2 diabetes. Antidepressants demonstrated the most consistent mild to moderate effect regarding better glycaemic control, but the results are still inconclusive and long-term effects are widely unknown.

Psychopharmacological vs. psychological interventions

A recent multicentre RCT compared a 12-week diabetes-specific behavioural group therapy with sertraline treatment in secondary care settings in patients with poorly controlled diabetes and major depression. Both interventions demonstrated a good short-term (3 months) and long-term effectiveness up to 15 months with a significant advantage for sertraline in the long-term follow-up. Poor glycaemic control remained unchanged in both intervention groups [27].

Collaborative and stepped-care approaches

Five RCTs including only patients with diabetes focused on collaborative and stepped-care approaches and were included in the 2015 meta-review [15]. Post-treatment depression severity and glycaemic control SMDs ranged from 0.00 to –0.54 and –0.13 to –0.68 favouring collaborative care over usual care although these differences did not always reach statistical significance.

Two recent studies confirm these findings. One stepped-care study could find moderate effects for depression in the 6-month follow-up [28] and a study concerning collaborative care could also identify an improvement of depressive symptoms [29].

In summary, collaborative and stepped-care are approaches with a slight to moderate influence on depression and glycaemic control. Owing to the multimodular intervention it remains impossible to identify specific elements (medication or psychological intervention or other variables) responsible for these results.

Web-based interventions and mobile health applications

Mobility and networking have become increasingly integral components of our society. The past few decades have witnessed a definite upsurge in interest in web-based interventions and mobile applications even in healthcare. Considerable efforts have been made in recent years to study and evaluate web-based interventions and mobile applications for the treatment of depression and diabetes. The majority of existing programmes focus on only one disease: diabetes or depression. There have been very few programmes and studies on the comorbidity of both. Existing interventions primarily focus on adherence and self-management. A meta-analysis by Pal et al. [18] investigated the effects of computer-based interventions on self-management in patients with type 2 diabetes. They found small beneficial effects on blood glucose control and no evidence of improvement in depression.

In contrast, a current study on the effectiveness of a mobile phone and web-based cognitive behavioural therapy on depressive symptoms in people with diabetes found persistent improved depressive symptoms [30]. Another study compared the effects of an internet-based guided self help for depression in adults with diabetes with usual care. Sustained effects on depressive symptoms with positive impact on response and remission could be observed [31].

Conclusion of research status

Together these findings have been overwhelmingly interpreted to suggest that different psychological and pharmacological interventions, as well as collaborative and stepped-care approaches show moderately positive effects on depression severity in people with depression and type 2 diabetes. The effectiveness is similar to those in depressive people without diabetes. A small to moderate positive effect on glycaemic control is shown for SSRIs. Some psychological approaches, particularly when combined with diabetes education, also lead to some improvement in glycaemic control, but results are still inconclusive [15].

Most of the studies exhibited methodology limitations (e.g. focus mostly on primary care, most of the studies in the USA), making it difficult to generalize those findings for the treatment of depression in type 2 diabetes in general. For patients in secondary care settings with very poor glycaemic control, neither CBT nor sertraline led to improvement in glycaemic control [27]. In conclusion, despite intense research activities the field has not moved very far when it comes to a convincing 'two-in-one-treatment' with good outcome for depression and diabetes related outcome at the same time.

Future research should challenge the general conclusions of studies that specific interventions are effective for all people with diabetes and depression. This is obviously not the case considering the controversial results for metabolic control and the considerable proportion of non-responders in all trials (as in all depression treatment trials).

It seems to be necessary to focus more on specific characteristics of the patients (e.g. primary vs. secondary care, satisfactory vs. poor glycaemic control, and others). Efforts have to be taken to identify the effective components of complex interventions, appropriate doses, and treatment durations. More active comparison trials are needed to identify the most effective interventions and communication pathways to reach different patient groups. Finally, treatments tailored according to the needs of the specific clinical setting, culture, and country, are of major importance.

Recommendations for clinical practice

The existing standards of healthcare provision vary throughout the world and are mainly influenced by the resources and development statuses. This results in different levels of care ranging from lacks of medical resources and health professionals (limited care), up to evidence-based and cost-effective care (recommended care) right up to the best modern health technologies (comprehensive care) [32]. Most of the few existing evidence-based guidelines for specific treatment for comorbid depression and diabetes are conceptualized for recommended or comprehensive care (e.g. German Diabetes Association, UK National Institute for Health and Care Excellence) [16,33].

There is a lack of scientific evidence for specific treatment recommendations for diabetes-related characteristics such as type of diabetes, level of glycaemic control, or diabetes-related complications (however, these aspects should be taken into consideration in the individual case). Thus, the diabetes management of people with comorbid depression is not any different from those without depression. Diabetes management should follow existing national and international guidelines until new evidence emerges that diabetes-specific depression treatment is associated with better outcomes.

A comprehensive model of stepped care that could be adapted to the level of care in the given setting is recommended here on the basis of recent scientific evidence and the guidelines from the German Diabetes Association. The steps of interventions are defined by severity and persistence of depressive symptoms (which can be grouped to four different categories) [16]. Within the therapy it is necessary to regularly control response and suicidal ideation through all phases and, depending on the severity and development of depression change the step of the intervention. This stepped-care approach should allow a flexible and individual adjustable treatment with the overall goal of complete remission of depression.

Step 1: mild depression (or subthreshold depressive symptoms that cause impairment)

In the case of mild depression a treatment in primary care is possible, a trust-based relationship between patient and physician is essential. The consultation style should be oriented towards problem solving, as well as flexible and supportive to the individual needs of the patients. The most important element in this treatment is information and education about depression, the interaction between diabetes and depression, and its effects on nearly every diabetes and psychosocial outcome. On this basis an individual disease concept should be developed by the patient with the support of the clinician to help identify targets for the intervention (e.g. self-management, poor adherence, dysfunctional thoughts, difficult social interactions, positive activities). This shall help the patients to understand their complex disease pattern and the possibilities to change and to improve it through their own efforts. The course of symptoms should be monitored over 2–4 weeks. If no improvement or even deterioration could be observed, treatment should be escalated to the next step.

Step 2: moderate depression (or persistent mild depression that does not respond to step 1)

A moderate depression indicates a specific antidepressant treatment. The options include antidepressive medications (SSRIs as first choice) and psychological interventions, especially cognitive behavioural approaches. The patient should be fully and thoroughly informed about these options to make an individual and well-considered decision. If treated with antidepressants, this could be realized in primary care and should be monitored carefully to adjust the required dosage or medication. If no improvement with medication, CBT, or even deterioration could be observed, treatment should be escalated to the next step.

Step 3: severe depression (or moderate depression not responding to step 2)

In the case of severe depression a combination of psychotherapy and antidepressant medication (with SSRIs as a first choice drug) is indicated. Depending on severity of depression and individual factors treatment can be delivered as an outpatient or an inpatient treatment. If no improvement or even deterioration could be observed within this treatment step, treatment should be escalated to the next step.

Step 4: very severe depression (or severe depression not responding to step 3)

Very severe depression with a distinct functional impairment requires an inpatient treatment. For this disease severity a complex drug regimen is usually necessary, because psychotherapy is generally insufficient or even not possible in this stage. Psychotherapy can be a treatment option combined with medication after initial response to the treatment.

Conclusions

The comorbidity of type 2 diabetes and depression remains a clinical challenge for patients and healthcare professionals. Patients are confronted with a chronic disease in combination with a high level of suffering, and healthcare professionals in primary care are not always sufficiently trained to identify and treat this comorbid conditions. Thus, further training of healthcare professionals is necessary.

Taken together, the scientific evidence for a variety of treatments for depression in diabetes is somewhat encouraging, demonstrating that depression can be treated with moderate to good results in depressed people with type 2 diabetes. However, the results regarding glycaemic control are less positive, and demonstrate the lack of efficient treatment with convincing effects not only on depression but also on the long-term improvement of glycaemic control, and thus leading to a better prognosis of the diabetes course.

References

1. **Moulton CD, Pickup JC, Ismail K.** The link between depression and diabetes: the search for shared mechanisms. *Lancet Diabetes Endocrinology* 2015;3:461–71.
2. **Snoek FJ, Bremmer MA, Hermanns N.** Constructs of depression and distress in diabetes: time for an appraisal. *Lancet Diabetes Endocrinology* 2015;3:450–60.
3. **Dirmaier J, Watzke B, Koch U,** et al. Diabetes in primary care: prospective associations between depression, nonadherence and glycemic control. *Psychotherapy and Psychosomatics* 2010;79:172–8.

4. Lustman PJ, Anderson RJ, Freedland KE, et al. Depression and poor glycemic control: a meta-analytic review of the literature. *Diabetes Care*. 2000;**23**:934–42.

5. De Groot M, Anderson R, Freedland K, et al. Association of depression and diabetes complications: a meta-analysis. *Psychosomatic Medicine* 2001;**63**:619–30.

6. Egede LE, Nietert PJ, Zheng D. Depression and all-cause and coronary heart disease mortality among adults with and without diabetes. *Diabetes Care* 2005;**28**:1339–45.

7. Richardson LK, Egede LE, Mueller M. Effect of race/ethnicity and persistent recognition of depression on mortality in elderly men with type 2 diabetes and depression. *Diabetes Care* 2008;**31**:880–1.

8. Baumeister H, Hutter N, Bengel J, Härter M. Quality of life in medically ill persons with comorbid mental disorders: a systematic review and meta-analysis. *Psychotherapy and Psychosomatics* 2011;**80**:275–86.

9. Moussavi S, Chatterji S, Verdes E, et al. Depression, chronic diseases, and decrements in health: results from the World Health Surveys. *Lancet* 2007;**370**:851–8.

10. Hermanns N, Kulzer B, Krichbaum M, et al. How to screen for depression and emotional problems in patients with diabetes: comparison of screening characteristics of depression questionnaires, measurement of diabetes-specific emotional problems and standard clinical assessment. *Diabetologia* 2006;**49**:469–77.

11. Gonzalez JS, Peyrot M, McCarl LA, et al. Depression and diabetes treatment nonadherence: a meta-analysis. *Diabetes Care* 2008;**31**:2398–403.

12. Lin EH, Katon W, Von Korff M, et al. Relationship of depression and diabetes self-care, medication adherence, and preventive care. *Diabetes Care* 2004;**27**:2154–60.

13. Katon W, Simon G, Russo J, et al. Quality of depression care in a population-based sample of patients with diabetes and major depression. *Medical Care* 2004;**42**:1222–9.

14. Li C, Ford ES, Zhao G, et al. Prevalence and correlates of undiagnosed depression among U.S. adults with diabetes: the Behavioral Risk Factor Surveillance System, 2006. *Diabetes Research and Clinical Practice* 2009;**83**:268–79.

15. Petrak F, Baumeister H, Skinner TC, Brown A, Holt RI. Depression and diabetes: treatment and health-care delivery. *Lancet Diabetes Endocrinology* 2015;**3**:472–85.

16. Kulzer B, Albus C, Herpertz S, et al. [Pychosocial Aspects of Diabetes Mellitus (Part 1) S2-Guideline Psychosocial Aspects of Diabetes—Long Version] S2-Leitlinie Psychosoziales und Diabetes—Langfassung. *Diabetologie* 2013;**8**:198–242.

17. Baumeister H, Hutter N. Collaborative care for depression in medically ill patients. *Current Opinions in Psychiatry* 2012;**25**:405–14.

18. Pal K, Eastwood SV, Michie S, et al. Computer-based interventions to improve self-management in adults with type 2 diabetes: a systematic review and meta-analysis. *Diabetes Care* 2014;**37**:1759–66.

19. APA. *Dissemination of integrated care within adult primary care settings. The Collaborative Care Model.* Lake St. Louis, MO: APA, 2016.

20. Penckofer S, Doyle T, Byrn M, Lustman PJ. State of the science: depression and Type 2 Diabetes. *Western Journal of Nursing Research* 2014;**36**:1158–82.

21. van der Feltz-Cornelis CM, Nuyen J, Stoop C, et al. Effect of interventions for major depressive disorder and significant depressive symptoms in patients with diabetes mellitus: a systematic review and meta-analysis. *General Hospital Psychiatry* 2010;**32**:380–95.

22. **Uchendu C, Blake H.** Effectiveness of cognitive-behavioural therapy on glycaemic control and psychological outcomes in adults with diabetes mellitus: a systematic review and meta-analysis of randomized controlled trials. *Diabetic Medicine* 2017;**34**:328–39.

23. **Moncrieft AE, Llabre MM, McCalla JR,** et al. Effects of a multicomponent life-style intervention on weight, glycemic control, depressive symptoms, and renal function in low-income, minority patients with type 2 diabetes: results of the community approach to lifestyle modification for diabetes randomized controlled trial. P*sychosomatic Medicine* 2016;**78**:851–60.

24. **Hermanns N, Schmitt A, Gahr A,** et al. The effect of a Diabetes-Specific Cognitive Behavioral Treatment Program (DIAMOS) for patients with diabetes and subclinical depression: results of a randomized controlled trial. *Diabetes Care* 2015;**38**:551–60.

25. **Pibernik-Okanovic M, Hermanns N, Ajdukovic D,** et al. Does treatment of subsyndromal depression improve depression-related and diabetes-related outcomes? A randomised controlled comparison of psychoeducation, physical exercise and enhanced treatment as usual. *Trials* 2015;**16**:305.

26. **Kang R, He Y, Yan Y,** et al. Comparison of paroxetine and agomelatine in depressed type 2 diabetes mellitus patients: a double-blind, randomized, clinical trial. *Neuropsychiatric Disease Treatment* 2015;**11**:1307–11.

27. **Petrak F, Herpertz S, Albus C,** et al. Cognitive Behavioral therapy versus sertraline in patients with depression and poorly controlled diabetes: the Diabetes and Depression (DAD) study: a randomized controlled multicenter trial. *Diabetes Care* 2015;**38**:767–75.

28. **Stoop CH, Nefs G, Pommer AM,** et al. Effectiveness of a stepped care intervention for anxiety and depression in people with diabetes, asthma or COPD in primary care: A randomized controlled trial. *Journal of Affective Disorders* 2015;**184**:269–76.

29. **Hay JW, Katon WJ, Ell K,** et al. Cost-effectiveness analysis of collaborative care management of major depression among low-income, predominantly Hispanics with diabetes. *Value Health* 2012;**15**:249–54.

30. **Clarke J, Proudfoot J, Ma H.** Mobile phone and web-based cognitive behavior therapy for depressive symptoms and mental health comorbidities in people living with diabetes: results of a feasibility study. *JMIR Mental Health* 2016;**3**:e23.

31. **Ebert DD, Nobis S, Lehr D,** et al. The 6-month effectiveness of Internet-based guided self-help for depression in adults with Type 1 and 2 diabetes mellitus. *Diabetic Medicine* 2017;**34**:99–107.

32. **IDF Clinical Guidelines Task Force.** Global Guidelines for Type 2 Diabetes 2012. http://www.idf.org/sites/default/files/IDF-Guideline-for-Type-2-Diabetes.pdf.

33. **Petrak F, Herpertz S, Albus C,** et al. Psychosocial factors and diabetes mellitus: evidence-based treatment guidelines. *Current Diabetes Review* 2005;**1**:255–70.

34. **Nobis S, Lehr D, Ebert DD,** et al. Efficacy of a web-based intervention with mobile phone support in treating depressive symptoms in adults with type 1 and type 2 diabetes: a randomized controlled trial. *Diabetes Care* 2015;**38**:776–83.

Chapter 11

Psychotropic drugs and metabolic risk

Andreas Barthel and Michael Bauer

Introduction

The persistent shift to overweight (as defined with a BMI of 25–29.9 kg/m^2) and obesity (as defined with a BMI $\geq$30 kg/m^2) is one of the biggest challenges to the health systems of our modern societies with a global dimension. According to the WHO [1], the proportion of obese subjects has doubled worldwide since 1980 and in 2014 more than 1.9 billion adults were overweight or obese.

It is well established that an increasing degree of obesity is correlated with a number of specific comorbidities and an increased mortality [2,3]. These comorbidities include in particular metabolic diseases like type 2 diabetes mellitus, dyslipidaemia, and arterial hypertension—summarized as the metabolic syndrome—that are typically associated with cardiovascular complications such as atherosclerosis, myocardial infarction or stroke, retinopathy, and nephropathy with disabling or even deadly consequences [4].Obviously, the current endemic increase in the overweight and obese proportion in our population is based on lifestyle changes with increasing physical inactivity in combination with other social, environmental, and nutritional factors reflected by an increased consumption of refined and energy-rich food [1,5]. Rare causes include hormonal diseases such as hypothyroidism or endogenous hypercortisolism as well as disorders affecting the regulation of food intake and fuel metabolism by the central nervous system such as craniopharyngeoma.

In patients with mental disorders such as schizophrenia and depression the rate of obesity and related disorders as well as the mortality from obesity-related disorders—predominantly cardiovascular disorders (CVD)—is significantly increased compared to with general population [6–8]. On the other hand, obesity itself is frequently associated with symptoms of anxiety or depression [5] and both obesity and depression share common pathophysiological aspects [9]. Further, psychopharmacological treatment of psychiatric disorders with antidepressants, antipsychotics, and mood stabilizing or anxiolytic drugs (summarized as 'psychotropics') is frequently associated with considerable weight gain—reported numbers range up to more than 30 kg in some individuals [7,10–13]. Therefore, we have a vicious circle relating psychiatric disorders with weight gain and obesity on one hand and a therapeutic dilemma complicating this situation on the other hand.

Psychotropic drugs, weight gain, and the metabolic consequences

Weight gain and the underlying changes in body composition related to treatment with psychotropic drugs are commonly attributed to an increased abdominal fat content, although also water retention resulting in oedema has been described for some drugs such as mirtazapine [14–16]. Generally, stimulating effects on orexigenic systems with increased appetite, food craving, and an increased calorie intake are regarded as the major effect for most psychotropics [17,18]. However, the effects on fuel metabolism with a reduced metabolic rate have also been discussed for some classes of psychotropics (tricyclic antidepressants, selective serotonin reuptake inhibitors (SSRIs), and monoamine-oxidase (MAO) inhibitors) [12,19].

Although the precise mechanisms causing these changes are still largely unclear, some basal understanding of the regulation of food intake and energy expenditure exists, allowing the pharmacological actions of psychotropic drugs to be linked with weight gain and consecutive metabolic consequences. Genetic studies—mainly performed in animal models—have provided ample evidence that the signals of nutrient-related hormones regulating fuel metabolism such as insulin or the fat-cell derived hormone leptin are integrated in the central nervous system by hypothalamic structures within the arcuate nucleus. These neuronal structures are related to appetite control, food intake, and the regulation of peripheral fuel metabolism and express regulatory peptides such as NPY/AgRP or αMSH (POMC) [20]. Since NPY/AgRP are known to have orexigenic/anabolic effects on the organism that are opposed by αMSH (POMC), this system comprises not only a sensitive physiological structure in the regulation of metabolism and body composition but also a vulnerable target for exogenous factors. The activity of these neurons is known to be modulated by serotonergic ($5\text{-}HT_{2c}$), histaminergic (H1), and dopaminergic (D2) transmitter systems and most of these receptors typically have a high binding affinity to specific antipsychotic drugs [21]. In addition, many antidepressants exert specific effects on serotonin metabolism in the brain. Further, it has been discussed that the levels of hormones related to food uptake behaviour and the regulation of metabolism such as leptin and ghrelin as well as the signalling mechanisms related to these regulatory peptides may be affected by some antipsychotic drugs [22,23]. Other peripheral effects have also been discussed in this context. Thus, we have a number of potential mechanisms linking the pharmacological action of many psychotropics to the observed weight changes.

The metabolic effects of psychotropics show great interindividual variations. Therefore it is interesting to note that the clinical effectiveness of many antipsychotics is affected by pharmacogenetic polymorphisms. Based on this, it is conceivable that genetic factors may also play a relevant role in psychotropic drug-induced weight gain as well as the development of metabolic adverse effects and studies addressing this question have been performed in particular with antipsychotic drugs [24,25]. It is interesting to note that single nucleotide polymorphisms (SNPs) with potential relevance in this context have been identified mainly in structures functionally related to energy intake and expenditure. For example, among others, these include SNPs located in the promoter regions of the 5-HT$_{2c}$ receptor gene (*HTR2C*) and the leptin gene (*LEP*) and in the genes encoding for the leptin receptor (LEPR) and the melanocortin 4 receptor (MC4-R). A comprehensive overview on current studies relating SNPs to antipsychotic-induced weight gain and the metabolic syndrome is provided by MacNeil and Müller [26]. However, the current evidence of the genetic associations of many of those SNPs has been discussed controversial and raised questions on their clinical relevance. Further, since the pathophysiological sequence of weight gain, insulin resistance, development of the metabolic syndrome, and disease-related endpoints typically occurs over several years, more time for large-scale clinical studies is needed to answer these questions.

Generally, genome-wide association studies (GWAS) have revealed a number of SNPs related to the risk for the development of obesity or type 2 diabetes [27,28]. However, it is estimated that these polymorphisms account for only 10% of the genetically determined risk to develop type 2 diabetes. With regard to the prevention of obesity and type 2 diabetes, it has been discussed whether genetic variants may be associated with different responses to specific measures of prevention such as physical activity or nutritional programmes and results derived from the retrospective analysis of large prevention studies apparently support this hypothesis. So far, the identified polymorphisms associated with the strongest susceptibility for the development of type 2 diabetes are located within the *TCF7L2* gene that encodes for the transcription factor Tcf-4. Interestingly, variants of this gene are also associated with insulin secretion from pancreatic β-cells and the response to treatment with sulphonyl urea and are therefore of potential pharmacogenetic relevance [29].

Taken together, it is clear that we still only know a few isolated pieces of the big puzzle and at this point more robust data are required to develop pharmacogenetics as a valid diagnostic tool to identify patients with psychiatric disorders at risk for metabolic side effects from psychotropic drug treatment.

Antidepressants

Antidepressants are first-line medications for the treatment of acute and chronic major depressive disorders, and anxiety disorders [30,31]. Although antidepressive drugs are known to increase the concentration of specific neurotransmitters such as serotonin and/or norepinephrine and others in central nervous structures by inhibiting the reuptake after release into the synaptic cleft, both the exact pathophysiology and the precise mechanism of action of antidepressants are still largely based on hypotheses. For example, a latent hypercortisolism as a result of an impaired stress response has been assumed in depressive subjects making them per se vulnerable to metabolic aberrations [9]. Further, the clinical effects of antidepressant drugs on mood occur with a delay of some weeks, whereas the effects on neurotransmission appear within minutes to hours. Considering this fragmentary picture on one side and the fact that some antidepressants have profound metabolic side effects whereas others have none, it is conceivable to assume secondary—still unknown—effects responsible for the clinically well-documented effects of certain antidepressants on body weight.

While almost all tricyclic antidepressants are associated with weight gain (particularly in the first months after initiating treatment, frequently dose dependent), the effects of selective reuptake inhibitors may differ more individually with reported weight gain and weight loss for the same compound in different patients. Table 11.1 reviews the evidence for metabolic side effects of antidepressants based on the current literature and summaries of product characteristics (SmPCs). The relative abundance of the side effects noted in the SmPCs is categorized according to standard definitions: very frequent, $\geq 1/10$; frequent, $\geq 1/100$ and $<1/10$; occasionally, $\geq 1/1.000$ and $<1/100$); rare, $<1/1.000$.

A comprehensible review and summary of the current discussion on antidepressant-induced weight changes is provided by Lee et al. [32].

Antipsychotics

Antipsychotics are first-line medications for the treatment of schizophrenia, other psychotic disorders, and delirium, and also commonly for sedating and improving insomnia. Antipsychotics belong to the prototypic class of drugs typically related to weight gain and metabolic side effects [11]. In contrast to

Table 11.1 Metabolic effects of antidepressants

Drug	Class	Weight gain/ metabolic effect	Comment
Tricyclic antidepressants and other non-selective reuptake inhibitors			
Amitriptyline	TCA	+++	
Trimipramine	TCA	N/A	Weight gain reported, frequency not quantified
Doxepine	TCA	N/A	Weight gain reported, frequency not quantified
Clomipramine	TCA	++	
Opipramole	TCA	+	
Selective reuptake inhibitors			
Citalopram	SSRI	++	Weight loss (+)
Sertraline	SSRI	+	Weight loss (+)
Fluoxetine	SSRI	–	Rather weight loss (++)
Escitalopram	SSRI	++	Weight loss (+)
Paroxetine	SSRI	++	
Venlafaxine	SRI	+	Weight loss (+) Increase in serum cholesterol (++)
Duloxetine	SRI	+	Weight loss (++)
Bupropion	SRI	–	Weight loss (+)
Miscellaneous			
Mirtazapine	NaSSA	+++	Peripheral oedema (++)
Tranylcypromine	MAOI	++	Also weight loss (++)
Moclobemide	MAOI	–	

– not reported, –/+ rare, + occasionally, ++ frequent, +++ very frequent, N/A not available; SSRI selective serotonin reuptake inhibitor; SRI other selective reuptake inhibitor; NaSSA noradrenergic and specific serotonergic antidepressant; MAOI monoamine oxidase inhibitor

Source data from Neurology, 35, Gahr M., Connemann B.J., Cabanis M. et al, Metabolic side effects of psychotropic drugs, pp. 559–569, 2016 [53].

first-generation antipsychotics (FGAs), the so-called second-generation antipsychotics (SGAs) have little or no extrapyramidal side effects but are commonly associated with the risk of pronounced weight gain. Mechanistically, the shift of the spectrum of adverse effects from dyskinesia in FGAs to metabolic risks in SGAs is thought to be related to the differences in the receptor binding properties with less D2- and additional hypothalamic H1-receptor antagonism in SGAs than FGAs [33].

The metabolic effects of antipsychotic drugs are of significant clinical relevance since an increased cardiovascular mortality and an increased smoking-related mortality has been documented in patients with schizophrenia [34]. Based on this underlying constellation the need to control for metabolic risk factors particular in these subjects needs to be emphasized. Actually, SGAs such as clozapine and olanzapine are regarded as the psychotropic drugs with the highest risk for metabolic side effects but it should be noted that this assessment may be biased at least in part because these two SGAs have been studied more extensively than other antipsychotics in the context of metabolic side effects. Data from a large current meta-analysis reveal that over prolonged exposure, almost all antipsychotics are associated with weight gain [10]. Therefore, from the metabolic point of view, antipsychotic drug treatment requires thorough monitoring in general.

Table 11.2 reviews the evidence for metabolic side effects of antipsychotics based on the current literature and SmPCs.

Mood stabilizers

This class of drugs is commonly used for the treatment of affective disorders including bipolar disorder [35,36]. In addition to lithium, mood stabilizers include drugs that are also commonly applied in the therapy of epileptic seizures. Antiepileptic drugs are heterogeneous with regard to their effects on weight and metabolism with individual responses for the same compound in different patients. While treatment with valproate and carbamazepine is frequently associated with weight gain, weight loss is commonly associated with the use of topiramate. Based on this finding, prescription of topiramate has been suggested to oppose psychotropic drug-induced weight gain [37].

Based on the current literature and SmPCs, Table 11.3 summarizes the evidence for metabolic side effects of mood stabilizers.

Anxiolytic drugs

Typical drugs of this class include benzodiazepines, although other drugs are also used for the treatment of panic disorders and anxiety. The effects of benzodiazepines on metabolism are limited. Table 11.4 summarizes the evidence for metabolic side effects of anxiolytics based on the current literature and SmPCs.

Table 11.2 Metabolic effects of antipsychotic drugs

Drug	Weight gain/ metabolic effect	Comment
First-generation antipsychotic drugs with low antipsychotic potency		
Promethazine	N/A	Dose-dependent weight gain reported, frequency not quantified
Pipamperone	–	
Melperone	–/+	
Chlorprothixene	+++	increased appetite (++)
First-generation antipsychotic drugs with high antipsychotic potency		
Haloperidol	++	Also weight loss (++)
Perazine	+	
Flupentixole	++	Increased appetite (++)
Fluphenazine	N/A	Weight gain reported, frequency not quantified
Second-generation antipsychotic drugs ('atypical antipsychotics')		
Olanzapine	+++	Hyperglycaemia (++) and hyperlipoproteinaemia (++) reported
Clozapine	++	Impaired glucose tolerance/diabetes mellitus (-/+) reported
Risperidone	++	Increased appetite (++), hyperglycaemia (+), diabetes mellitus (+) and hyperlipoproteinaemia (+) reported
Quetiapine	+++	Increased appetite (++),hyperglycaemia (++), diabetes mellitus (+) and hyperlipoproteinaemia (+++) reported

–not reported, –/+ rare, + occasionally, ++ frequent, +++ very frequent, N/A. not available

Source data from Neurology, 35, Gahr M., Connemann B.J., Cabanis M. et al, Metabolic side effects of psychotropic drugs, pp. 559–569, 2016 [53].

Controlling the metabolic risks in patients with psychiatric disorders

The American Diabetes Association (ADA) together with the American Psychiatric Association (APA), the American Association of Clinical Endocrinologists (AACE), and the North American Association for the Study of Obesity (NAASO) have organized a consensus conference in order to develop clinical guidelines for the identification, evaluation, and treatment of metabolic risks and complications associated with antipsychotic drugs [38].

Table 11.3 Metabolic effects of mood stabilizers

Drug	Weight gain/ metabolic effect	Comment
Anticonvulsants		
Valproate	++	Increased appetite (++); but also weight loss (++) and loss of appetite (++) reported
Carbamazepine	++	Weight gain may be due to water retention
Topiramate	++*	*Based on calculated data; weight loss is clinically predominant (+++)
Lamotrigine	–	
Miscellaneous		
Lithium	++	Dose-dependent weight gain, particularly over the first 2 years of treatment

– not reported, -/+ rare, + occasionally, ++ frequent, +++ very frequent, N/A. not available

Source data from Neurology, 35, Gahr M., Connemann B.J., Cabanis M. et al, Metabolic side effects of psychotropic drugs, pp. 559–569, 2016 [53].

Table 11.4 Metabolic effects of anxiolytic drugs

Drug	Weight gain/ metabolic effect	Comment
Benzodiazepines		
Lorazepam	–	
Diazepam	–	
Bromazepam	–	
Oxazepam	–	Both increased appetite (+) and decreased appetite (+) reported
Miscellaneous		
Pregabaline	++	Increased appetite (++); also weight loss (+) reported; used for the treatment of diabetic neuropathic pain

– not reported, -/+ rare, + occasionally, ++ frequent, +++ very frequent, N/A not available.

Source data from Neurology, 35, Gahr M., Connemann BJ, Cabanis M. et al, Metabolic side effects of psychotropic drugs, pp. 559–569, 2016 [53].

One major question addressed in the resulting joint statement concerned the metabolic screening and the management of weight gain, dyslipidaemia, and type 2 diabetes in patients with psychiatric disorders and a monitoring protocol for patients treated with SGAs was presented. Based on simple anamnestic and clinical data, an initial screening for metabolic risks at baseline and regular clinical follow-up visits are recommended (summarized in Table 11.5). Since increases in weight frequently occur during the first weeks after starting treatment with antipsychotics, weight should initially be monitored monthly during the first 12 weeks and then quarterly, blood pressure, and fasting plasma glucose after 3 months and then annually. However, it is recommended that the frequency of the follow-up assessments should be based on the individual patient's clinical status and course.

Although screening is a simple, but important tool to control metabolic side effects in psychiatric patients requiring only little effort and resources, it should be noted that the frequency and quality of screening for the metabolic syndrome in people prescribed psychotropics is still very limited and requires further improvement [39,40].

In addition to clinical monitoring, psychotropic drug selection is an important point and has to consider the individual patient's metabolic risk. For example, in patients with pre-existing obesity it is essential to be aware of the high weight-gaining potential of SGAs such as clozapine and olanzapine. Therefore, if these drugs are clearly indicated from the psychiatric point of view, limitation to the lowest effective dose may be helpful to control for adverse metabolic effects. To reduce the metabolic risk, switching to another class of psychotropic drugs may also be taken into account [41]. In addition to dietary modifications, persistent physical activity has been well documented to help controlling

Table 11.5 Monitoring metabolic risks in patients treated with psychotropic drugs

Recommended assessment	Recommended frequency
Personal/family history of metabolic syndrome or cardiovascular disease	At baseline, then annually
Weight/height/BMI	At baseline, then monthly during the first 12 weeks, and then quarterly
Waist circumference	At baseline, then annually
Blood pressure	At baseline, after 12 weeks, then annually
Fasting plasma glucose and lipids	At baseline, after 12 weeks, then annually

Source data from Diabetes Care, 27, American Diabetes Association; American Psychiatric Association; American Association of Clinical Endocrinologists; North American Association for the Study of Obesity, Consensus Development Conference on Antipsychotic Drugs and Obesity and Diabetes, pp. 596–601.

weight in patients with mental illness and to improve glucose and lipid metabolism [34,42–45]. Therefore, because of the significantly increased cardiovascular risks, lifestyle interventions based on diet and exercise are essential for the prevention and treatment of metabolic complications in patients with serious mental disorders [46].

Since psychotropic drug-induced weight gain can reach an intriguing extent in individual cases, pharmacological approaches to attenuate this side effect have been discussed intensely. Most data to support this concept have been derived from studies addressing the effects of the antidiabetic drug metformin on the metabolic effects of clozapine and olanzapine. Weight loss is commonly associated with the use of metformin and there is evidence that metformin may not only attenuate psychotropic drug-induced weight gain but also improve metabolic parameters such as dyslipidaemia and insulin resistance [47–50]. In addition, metformin has been found to have preventive effects on the development of type 2 diabetes and, based on this, there are recommendations by the ADA for an early use of metformin in subjects at a metabolically high risk [51,52].

Other drugs with reported effectiveness to reverse psychotropic drug-induced weight gain include some central anorectic stimulants (fenfluramine, sibutramine), the noradrenaline reuptake inhibitor reboxetine (used as an antidepressant), and the antiepileptic drug topiramate [37]. However, compared with metformin, the data on the mentioned compounds in this context are sparse and they all have more and potentially severe side effects. In addition, fenfluramine and sibutramine are no longer approved due to drug safety reasons.

In summary, pharmacological approaches to reverse metabolic side effects of psychotropics should be considered only in individual patients at high metabolic risk due to pre-existing obesity or with an ominous weight gain under psychotropic drug treatment, when other measures such as diet, exercise, and behavioural modifications have failed. Based on the current data, metformin appears to be the drug of choice in this context. However, it should be emphasized that the use of metformin (and other drugs mentioned) is off-label as an attenuate treatment to control weight.

References

1. **WHO.** Obesity and overweight. (2016). http://www.who.int/mediacentre/factsheets/fs311/en/ (accessed 7 February 2018).
2. **Berrington de Gonzalez A, Hartge P, Cerhan JR**, et al. Body-mass index and mortality among 1.46 million white adults. *New England Journal of Medicine* 2010;**363**:2211–19.
3. **WHO.** Physical status: the use and interpretation of anthropometry. Report of a WHO Expert Committee. WHO Technical Report Series 854. Geneva: World Health

Organization. (1995) http://www.who.int/childgrowth/publications/physical_status/en/ (accessed 7 February 2018).

4. **Hanefeld M, Pistrosch F, Bornstein SR, Birkenfeld AL.** The metabolic vascular syndrome—guide to an individualized treatment. *Reviews in Endocrine and Metabolic Disorders* 2016;**17**:5–17.

5. **WHO.** Obesity: preventing and managing the global epidemic. Report of a WHO Consultation. WHO Technical Report Series 894. Geneva: World Health Organization. (2000) http://www.who.int/nutrition/publications/obesity/WHO_TRS_894/en/index. html(accessed 7 February 2018).

6. **Allison DB, Newcomer JW, Dunn AL,** et al. Obesity among those with mental disorders: a National Institute of Mental Health meeting report. *American Journal of Preventative Medicine* 2009; **36**:341–50.

7. **Newcomer JW.** Metabolic considerations in the use of antipsychotic medications: a review of recent evidence. *Journal of Clinical Psychiatry* 2007;**68**(Suppl. 1):20–7.

8. **Vancampfort D, Stubbs B, Mitchell AJ,** et al. Risk of metabolic syndrome and its components in people with schizophrenia and related psychotic disorders, bipolar disorder and major depressive disorder: a systematic review and meta-analysis. *World Psychiatry* 2015;**14**:339–47.

9. **Bornstein SR, Schuppenies A, Wong ML, Licinio J.** Approaching the shared biology of obesity and depression: the stress axis as the locus of gene-environment interactions. *Molecular Psychiatry* 2006;**11**:892–902.

10. **Bak M, Fransen A, Janssen J,** et al. Almost all antipsychotics result in weight gain: a meta-analysis. *PLoS One* 2014;**24**:e94112.

11. **Domecq JP, Prutsky G, Leppin A,** et al. Clinical review: drugs commonly associated with weight change: a systematic review and meta-analysis. *Journal of Clinical Endocrinology & Metabolism* 2015;**100**:363–70.

12. **Jensen GL.** Drug-induced hyperphagia: what can we learn from psychiatric medications? *J Parenteral and Enteral Nutrition* 2008;**32**:578–81.

13. **Nihalani N, Schwartz TL, Siddiqui UA, Megna JL.** Weight gain, obesity, and psychotropic prescribing. *Journal of Obesity* 2011;**2011**:893629.

14. **Correia J, Ravasco P.** Weight changes in Portuguese patients with depression: which factors are involved? *Nutrition Journal* 2014; **13**:117.

15. **Kutscher EC, Lund BC, Hartman BA.** Peripheral edema associated with mirtazapine. *Annals of Pharmacotherapy* 2001;**35**:1494–5.

16. **Laimer M, Kramer-Reinstadler K, Rauchenzauner M,** et al. Effect of mirtazapine treatment on body composition and metabolism. *Journal of Clinical Psychiatry*. 2006;**67**:421–4.

17. **Jensen-Otsu E, Austin GL.** antidepressant use is associated with increased energy intake and similar levels of physical activity. *Nutrients* 2015;**7**:9662–71.

18. **Zimmermann U, Kraus T, Himmerich H,** et al. Epidemiology, implications and mechanisms underlying drug-induced weight gain in psychiatric patients. *Journal of Psychiatric Research* 2003;**37**:193–220.

19. **Gothelf D, Falk B, Singer P,** et al. Weight gain associated with increased food intake and low habitual activity levels in male adolescent schizophrenic inpatients treated with olanzapine. *American Journal of Psychiatry* 2002;**159**:1055–7.

20. **Schwartz MW, Porte D Jr.** Diabetes, obesity, and the brain. *Science* 2005;**307**:375–9.

21. **Balt SL, Galloway GP, Baggott MJ,** et al. Mechanisms and genetics of antipsychotic-associated weight gain. *Clinical Pharmacology & Therapeutics* 2011;**90**:179–83.

22. **Jin H, Meyer JM, Mudaliar S, Jeste DV.** Impact of atypical antipsychotic therapy on leptin, ghrelin, and adiponectin. S*chizophrenia Research* 2008;**100**:70–85.

23. **Monteleone P, Fabrazzo M, Tortorella A,** et al. Pronounced early increase in circulating leptin predicts a lower weight gain during clozapine treatment. *Journal of Clinical Psychopharmacology* 2002;**22**:424–6.

24. **Lett TA, Wallace TJ, Chowdhury NI,** et al. Pharmacogenetics of antipsychotic-induced weight gain: review and clinical implications. *Molecular Psychiatry* 2012;**17**:242–66.

25. **Reynolds GP.** Pharmacogenetic aspects of antipsychotic drug-induced weight gain—a critical review. *Clinical Psychopharmacology Neuroscience* 2012;**10**:71–77.

26. **MacNeil RR, Müller DJ.** Genetics of common antipsychotic-induced adverse effects. *Molecular Neuropsychiatry* 2016;**2**:61–78.

27. **Dupuis J, Langenberg C, Prokopenko I,** et al. New genetic loci implicated in fasting glucose homeostasis and their impact on type 2 diabetes risk. *Nature Genetics* 2010;**42**:105–16

28. **Speliotes EK, Willer CJ, Berndt SI,** et al. Association analyses of 249,796 individuals reveal 18 new loci associated with body mass index. *Nature Genetics* 2010;**42**:937–48.

29. **Pearson ER.** Pharmacogenetics in diabetes. *Current Diabetes Reports* 2009;**9**:172–81

30. **Bauer M, Pfennig A, Severus E,** et al; **World Federation of Societies of Biological Psychiatry.** Task Force on Unipolar Depressive Disorders. World Federation of Societies of Biological Psychiatry (WFSBP) guidelines for biological treatment of unipolar depressive disorders, part 1: update 2013 on the acute and continuation treatment of unipolar depressive disorders. *World Journal of Biological Psychiatry* 2013;**14**:334–85.

31. **Bauer M, Severus E, Köhler S,** et al; **Wfsbp.** Task Force on Treatment Guidelines for Unipolar Depressive Disorders. World Federation of Societies of Biological Psychiatry (WFSBP) guidelines for biological treatment of unipolar depressive disorders. part 2: maintenance treatment of major depressive disorder-update 2015. *World Journal of Biological Psychiatry* 2015;**16**:76–95

32. **Lee SH, Paz-Filho G, Mastronardi C,** et al. Is increased antidepressant exposure a contributory factor to the obesity pandemic? *Translational Psychiatry* 2016;**6**:e759.

33. **He M, Deng C, Huang XF.** The role of hypothalamic H1 receptor antagonism in antipsychotic-induced weight gain. *CNS Drugs* 2013;**27**:423–34.

34. **Brown S, Inskip H, Barraclough B.** Causes of the excess mortality of schizophrenia. *British Journal of Psychiatry* 2000;**177**:212–7.

35. **Kemp DE.** Managing the side effects associated with commonly used treatments for bipolar depression. *Journal of Affective Disorders* 2014;**169** (Suppl. 1):S34–44.

36. **Ketter TA, Miller S, Dell'Osso B,** et al. Balancing benefits and harms of treatments for acute bipolar depression. *Journal of Affective Disorders* 2014;**169**(Suppl. 1):S24–33.

37. **Maayan L, Vakhrusheva J, Correll CU.** Effectiveness of medications used to attenuate antipsychotic-related weight gain and metabolic abnormalities: a systematic review and meta-analysis. *Neuropsychopharmacology* 2010;**35**:1520–30.

38. **American Diabetes Association; American Psychiatric Association; American Association of Clinical Endocrinologists; North American Association for the Study**

of Obesity. Consensus development conference on antipsychotic drugs and obesity and diabetes. *Diabetes Care* 2004;**27**:596–601.

39. **Barnes TR, Bhatti SF, Adroer R, Paton C.** Screening for the metabolic side effects of antipsychotic medication: findings of a 6-year quality improvement programme in the UK. *BMJ Open* 2015;**5**:e007633.

40. **Morrato EH, Newcomer JW, Kamat S**, et al. Metabolic screening after the American Diabetes Association's consensus statement on antipsychotic drugs and diabetes. *Diabetes Care* 2009;**32**:1037–42.

41. **Stroup TS, McEvoy JP, Ring KD**, et al. A randomized trial examining the effectiveness of switching from olanzapine, quetiapine, or risperidone to aripiprazole to reduce metabolic risk: comparison of antipsychotics for metabolic problems (CAMP). *American Journal of Psychiatry* 2011;**168**:947–56.

42. **Bartels SJ, Pratt SI, Aschbrenner KA**, et al. Pragmatic replication trial of health promotion coaching for obesity in serious mental illness and maintenance of outcomes. *American Journal of Psychiatry* 2015;**172**:344–52.

43. **Daumit GL, Dickerson FB, Wang NY** et al. A behavioral weight-loss intervention in persons with serious mental illness. *New England Journal of Medicine* 2013;**368**:1594–602.

44. **Ganguli R.** Behavioral therapy for weight loss in patients with schizophrenia. *Journal of Clinical Psychiatry* 2007;**68**(Suppl. 4):19–25.

45. **Green CA, Yarborough BJ, Leo MC**, et al. The STRIDE weight loss and lifestyle intervention for individuals taking antipsychotic medications: a randomized trial. *American Journal of Psychiatry* 2015;**172**:71–81.

46. **Naslund JA, Aschbrenner KA, Pratt SI, Bartels SJ.** Comparison of people with serious mental illness and general population samples enrolled in lifestyle interventions for weight loss. *Schizophrenia Research* 2015;**169**:486–8.

47. **Baptista T, Rangel N, Fernández V**, et al. Metformin as an adjunctive treatment to control body weight and metabolic dysfunction during olanzapine administration: a multicentric, double-blind, placebo-controlled trial. *Schizophrenia Research* 2007;**93**:99–108.

48. **Jarskog LF, Hamer RM, Catellier DJ**, et al. Metformin for weight loss and metabolic control in overweight outpatients with schizophrenia and schizoaffective disorder. *American Journal of Psychiatry* 2013;**170**:1032–40.

49. **Wu RR, Zhao JP, Guo XF**, et al. Metformin addition attenuates olanzapine-induced weight gain in drug-naive first-episode schizophrenia patients: a double-blind, placebo-controlled study. *American Journal of Psychiatry* 2008;**165**:352–8.

50. **Wu RR, Zhang FY, Gao KM**, et al. Metformin treatment of antipsychotic-induced dyslipidemia: an analysis of two randomized, placebo-controlled trials. *Molecular Psychiatry* 2016;**21**:1537–44.

51. **DeFronzo RA, Abdul-Ghani M.** Type 2 diabetes can be prevented with early pharmacological intervention. *Diabetes Care* 2011;**34**(Suppl. 2):202–209.

52. **Hanefeld M** and **Schaper F.** Drug therapy for the prevention of type 2 diabetes—is there a medical rationale? *British Journal of Diabetes & Vascular Disease* 2011;**11**:168–74.

53. **Gahr M, Connemann BJ, Cabanis M, Denoix N.** Metabolische Nebenwirkungen von Psychopharmaka. *Nervenheilkunde* 2016;**35**:559–69.

Chapter 12

Metabolic surgery and depression

Lidia Castagneto Gissey, James R. Casella Mariolo, Geltrude Mingrone, and Francesco Rubino

Introduction

Environmental and societal changes including a decrease in physical activity, increased consumption of energy-dense foods, a lack of supportive policies in health, agriculture, distribution, and the food industry, and an inadequacy of education in such fields have ultimately led to overweight and obesity. Classified as a chronic, non-communicable disease, obesity is defined as a body mass index (BMI) $\geq$30 kg/m^2. In 1991 the National Institute of Health (NIH) further subdivided this nosological entity by adding a class of 'morbid obesity' intended as a BMI $\geq$35 kg/m^2 with weight-related comorbidities or a BMI $\geq$40 kg/m^2 alone. This subtly progressive condition has most certainly turned into a serious, large-scale health threat, increasing its incidence exponentially and affecting an approximate 13% of the global population [1]. Morbid obesity is associated with augmented rates of morbidity and overall mortality, owing to weight-related complications such as type 2 diabetes mellitus (T2DM), dyslipidaemia, hypertension, cardiovascular disease, joint disease, and sleep apnoea.

Among conditions of psychological pertinence, depression is one of those with the highest prevalence, afflicting an estimated 350 million individuals worldwide [2]. Mental health disorders, specifically depression and binge eating, are more common in patients undergoing bariatric surgery than in the general population [3]. Stigmatization and consequential discrimination of morbidly obese subjects has been hypothesized to trigger or even exacerbate a pre-existing or underlying depressive disorder [4,5]. Consistent with this hypothesis, a significant weight loss has been shown to substantially reduce severity of depression [6].

Bariatric and metabolic surgery

Bariatric and metabolic surgery has established itself over the past several years as an effective treatment not only for morbid obesity but also for its associated comorbidities, above all else T2DM [7–10]. Mounting evidence has proven that bariatric surgery generates substantial improvement in glycaemic control and insulin resistance long before significant body weight reduction has been achieved. Resolution of other obesity-related conditions (i.e. dyslipidaemia, hypertension, hyperuricaemia, sleep apnoea) has also been demonstrated, leading to an abatement of the associated cardiovascular risk [7,9–11]. Bariatric surgery includes various procedures ranging from the mainly 'restrictive' operations (e.g. adjustable gastric banding (AGB), sleeve gastrectomy (SG)) to the predominantly 'malabsorptive' ones (e.g. Roux-en-Y gastric bypass (RYGB), bilio-pancreatic diversion without (BPD) or with duodenal switch (BPD-DS)). Even though bariatric procedures may consist of a principally restrictive or malabsorptive component, all of the widely executed and established operations produce a variable but significant spectrum of metabolic effects in addition to the weight reduction. The aforementioned effects, deriving from manipulation and rearrangement of the gastrointestinal tract involved in bariatric procedures, have allowed it to acquire the denomination of 'metabolic surgery' [12,13].

Non-surgical therapeutic approaches in the management of morbid obesity and its comorbid factors must be taken into consideration and attempted before proceeding to bariatric surgery. Weight loss regimens comprise behavioural and lifestyle alterations, caloric restriction, physical activity, and pharmacologic agents. The treatment of weight-related disturbances such as T2DM, hypertension, and dyslipidaemia includes conventional medical therapy (oral hypoglycaemic agents, incretin mimetics and insulin, hypolipidaemic agents, antihypertensive agents) given as drug monotherapies or drug combinations, in addition to benefits resulting from weight loss.

Nonetheless, an ample body of scientific literature has confirmed the largely superior long-term effects of bariatric/metabolic surgery than conventional medical approaches in terms of weight loss maintenance and improvement or complete remission of comorbid conditions [9,14–17].

Effects of bariatric/metabolic surgery

Bariatric surgery results in significantly greater weight loss than non-surgical interventions. Although variability in terms of the percentage of excess weight loss (%EWL) and BMI change (ΔBMI) among surgical procedures has been documented, all bariatric operations, regardless of the type, generate superior outcomes than conventional treatment. Amidst the most commonly performed bariatric procedures, RYGB and SG produce similar results with regard to weight loss, BPD-DS generates the greatest weight reduction, and all of the aforementioned operations have better improvement in body weight than AGB [18–20].

Substantial improvement of obesity-attributable comorbidities has also been extensively described in literature. T2DM is the weight-related condition most widely investigated after metabolic surgery. Remission of T2DM with normalization of fasting blood glucose and glycated haemoglobin levels has been shown to be highest in morbidly obese, diabetic patients undergoing BPD-DS with remission rates as high as 99.2%, trailed by RYGB (74.4%), SG (61.3%), and AGB (33%) [21]. Hypertension and dyslipidaemia resolution percentages have been reported to be 74% and 68% respectively, while sleep apnoea resolves in 90% of patients [18].

Safety and cost-effectiveness of bariatric/metabolic surgery

Bariatric/metabolic surgery carries an acceptable safety profile, with morbidity and mortality rates superimposable to those of other widespread and established surgical procedures [21,22]. Super-obese patients very often present with augmented cardiovascular and anaesthesiological risk, consequently increasing the operative risk as well. Thanks to the development of laparoscopic surgery and the standardization of surgical techniques, bariatric surgery has improved its safety, reducing complications and mortality rates [19,21,22].

Surgical intervention has also demonstrated to be cost-effective in terms of reducing or even preventing macro- and microvascular complications associated with obesity-related conditions, therefore decreasing its overall health costs in the long term [23].

Prevalence of depression in the general population

Depression is generally defined as a mental state characterized by feelings of sadness, loneliness, despair, low self-esteem, and self-reproach.

The prevalence of depression in the general population is fairly high as it has been reported to range between 7% and 21% [24]. Depression is associated with a poor quality of life and increased mortality [25]. However, the prevalence of depression is often misreported or under-rated and in general it is estimated to be higher than factual figures suggest, since many patients suffering from depression are not correctly diagnosed by general practitioners [26]. In addition, only a limited number of cases require drug treatment [27].

The Center for Epidemiologic Studies Depression Scale is a valuable instrument for depression diagnosis in epidemiological studies [28]. In fact, compared with diagnostic interviews, physicians underestimate the severity of depression in 40% of the cases or give another psychiatric diagnosis in 33% [29].

A sign of the increased dimension of the problem in the USA is the rise in prescriptions of antidepressants from 8% to 14% from 1996 to 2005, with a third to a half of prescriptions specifically for psychiatric conditions [30].

Association between diabetes and depression

The first indication for the association between depression and diabetes dates back to 1684, long before the diagnosis of diabetes mellitus was known as a clinical entity [31]. In fact, it was only in 1776 that Dobson detected a sweet-tasting substance similar in appearance to sugar in the dried urine of diabetic individuals. In 1797, Rollo showed that after eating starchy foods, the sugar content in the urine of patients was increased [32].

Recently, it was proposed that it is the necessity to pursue glycaemic control that stresses diabetic patients, leading them to depression [33]. However, depression was found to be associated to diabetes before the possibility to check blood glucose levels or urine glucose excretion, and before any valid treatment for this disease was available, suggesting that this association derives from different factors [34].

The prevalence of depression in type 1 and type 2 diabetes exceeds that in the general population, with more than 25% of diabetic patients suffering from comorbid depression [35–37]. A meta-analysis looking at the association between depression and diabetes has shown that depression is associated with hyperglycaemia and it explains about 3% of the variance in glycated haemoglobin [38]. An adequate treatment of depressive disorders could potentially increase the number of diabetic patients with good glycaemic control from 41% to 58% [39].

A meta-analysis on 39 studies, involving 20,218 subjects, demonstrated that diabetes doubles the odds of developing depression [40]. Moreover, the likelihood of becoming affected by depression was significantly higher in diabetic women (OR = 1.8) than in diabetic men [40].

Association between morbid obesity and depression

Mood disorders are a frequent comorbidity of morbid obesity. The rate of lifetime mood disorders ranges between 22.4% and 45% [41,42] and the rate of current mood disorders between 11% and 33% [42,43]. A positive association between BMI and suicide risk has also been observed [44].

A recent meta-analysis shows that obese people have a 55% increased risk of developing depression over time and, conversely, depressed individuals have a 58% risk of becoming obese [6]. It is commonly hypothesized that obesity, with its associated health conditions and mobility restrictions, can lead to deterioration of the psychological well-being and secondary depression, eating disorders, distorted body image, and low self-esteem.

Socio-economic status is also associated with depression [45]. According to a recent meta-analysis, individuals with a low socio-economic status have a higher odds ratio (OR = 1.81) of being depressed, with a dose–response relation observed for both education and income [46]. In addition, there is a sexual dimorphism, with a greater depression rate among women than men [47].

Effects of bariatric/metabolic surgery on depression

The effect of bariatric surgery on mood disorders is uncertain. Some studies suggest that bariatric surgery is associated with improvements in depressive disorders [6,45–47]. However, other studies indicate that the number of suicides has increased. A large retrospective cohort study examined the long-term mortality among 9,949 patients who had undergone Roux-en-Y gastric bypass versus 9,628 severely obese controls and found a 50% increase in suicides in the surgery group without, however, a statistical significance [48]. Tindle et al. [49] observed an overall suicide rate of 6.6 per 10,000 among patients who underwent bariatric surgery, compared with 2.4% in sex-matched subjects in the general American population. Thirty per cent of the suicides occurred within the first 2 years and almost 70% occurred within 3 years after surgery. Nevertheless, this study did not take into account the effect of obesity on depression and suicide or that of baseline depressive symptomatology.

A systematic review and meta-analysis of the literature revealed a suicide rate of 4.1/10,000 person-years (95% CI 3.2–5.1/10,000 person-years) after bariatric surgery, which was significantly higher than the general population [50]. In a recent study, the adjusted hazard ratio for attempted suicide after gastric bypass was about three times higher than in the general non-obese population [51].

In a case–control study comparing lifestyle modification to bariatric surgery in 85 morbidly obese patients 1 year after the operation, similar beneficial effects on symptoms of depression and quality of life were obtained in both groups, suggesting that even small weight loss can be as effective as bariatric surgery [52].

Indeed, there is unanimous consent that weight loss after bariatric surgery improves the physical component of quality of life; however, this improvement often does not affect the mental aspect of depression, and anxiety [53]. Improvement of physical health and higher satisfaction with daily life represents a common outcome of weight loss surgery, nonetheless, social relationships or sexual performance do often not improve [54].

In addition, a retrospective population-based cohort study including 11,115 Swedish patients reported that alcohol abuse was doubled after gastric bypass. This is particularly worrisome in view of the more rapid absorption of alcohol linked to the fast gastric emptying [55].

A major drawback of the studies on depression and/or suicide and bariatric surgery is that they do not compare patients with the same baseline psychiatric disorders as, in fact, mild to severe depressive symptoms are observed in most candidates for bariatric surgery.

Guidelines

The practice guidelines for the treatment of patients affected by major depressive disorder issued by the American Psychiatric Association [56] states that:

> A careful and ongoing evaluation of suicide risk is necessary for all patients with major depressive disorder [I]. Such an assessment includes specific inquiry about suicidal thoughts, intent, plans, means, and behaviours; identification of specific psychiatric symptoms or general medical conditions that may increase the likelihood of acting on suicidal ideas [I].

However, there is no specific reference to depression in the guidelines or in the recommendations for bariatric/metabolic surgery as an absolute or relative contraindication to surgery.

In 1991, the National Institutes of Health consensus statement for metabolic surgery recommended that patients should be 'selected carefully after evaluation by a multidisciplinary team with medical, surgical, psychiatric, and nutritional expertise' [57].

The NICE guidelines [58] address the problem to assess 'any psychological problems' and to 'carry out a comprehensive preoperative assessment of any psychological or clinical factors that may affect adherence to postoperative care requirements (such as changes to diet) before performing surgery' and recommend providing 'psychological support before and after surgery'. In addition, NICE states that multidisciplinary evaluation is vital to providing best patient care and in current NHS arrangements, the follow-up team may include bariatric physicians, dieticians, practitioner psychologists or psychiatrists, specialised nursing staff, physiotherapists or exercise specialists, and surgeons.

The most recent recommendations for the gastrointestinal surgical treatment of obesity in diabetic patients have been issued during the 2nd Diabetes Surgery Summit (DSS-II), convened in collaboration with six leading international diabetes organizations: the American Diabetes Association, International Diabetes Federation, Chinese Diabetes Society, Diabetes India, European Association for the Study of Diabetes, and Diabetes UK. The DSS-II [39] recommends that 'Patients' eligibility for metabolic surgery should be assessed by a multidisciplinary team including surgeon(s), internist(s) or diabetologist(s)/endocrinologist(s), and dietician(s) with specific expertise in diabetes care. Also, depending on individual circumstances, other relevant specialists could be consulted to evaluate the patient'.

The American Society for Metabolic and Bariatric Surgery (ASMBS) in its consensus statement [59] states that 'Mental status is a difficult area in which to define standards for patient selection. Selected screening for severe depression, untreated or undertreated mental illnesses associated with psychoses, active substance abuse, bulimia nervosa, and socially disruptive personality disorders may help avoid adverse postoperative outcomes. History of compliance with non-operative therapy may be beneficial in assessing the risk-to-benefit ratio of bariatric surgery'. However, major depression does not represent a contraindication to gastro-intestinal surgery.

The only guidelines that contraindicate bariatric/metabolic surgery in subjects with depression are the 'Interdisciplinary European Guidelines on Metabolic and Bariatric Surgery' issued by an expert panel derived from IFSO-EC (International Federation for the Surgery of Obesity—European Chapter) and EASO (European Association for the Study of Obesity) [60]. These guidelines state that 'Non-stabilized psychotic disorders, severe depression, personality and eating disorders, unless specifically advised by a psychiatrist experienced in obesity' represent a contraindication to surgery. In addition, they affirm that:

> Pre-operative psychological evaluation should always include assessment of psychopathology such as personality examination as well as assessment of his/her expectation/motivation, diet history, lifestyle (i.e. nutritional behaviour, physical activity habits, life conditions), social support network. Pre-operative evaluation enables identification of interventions that can enhance long-term compliance and weight maintenance (i.e., crisis intervention, psychological support, psychotherapy, etc.). The goal is to enhance patients' motivation and ability to comply with nutritional, behavioural and psycho-social changes before and after bariatric surgery. Pre-operative examination leverages psychological support in case of patient's psychological disorder relapse post-operatively (depression, anxiety, etc.). Pre-operative evaluation should detect potential psychological contraindications to surgery, such as severe eating disorders and others highlighted in 'Contraindications Specific for Bariatric Surgery' [61].

Antidepressant therapy and weight gain

Treatment with antidepressants is often accompanied by weight gain, in particular when tricyclic antidepressants and the atypical neuroleptics clozapine and olanzapine are used [5]. Any of these drugs act on several neurotransmitter systems such as the serotonergic, dopaminergic, and histaminergic systems with subsequent central effects on appetite and satiation regulation [38].

However, psychotropic drugs leading to weight gain, such as clozapine and olanzapine, activate the tumour necrosis factor (TNF)-α system and stimulate leptin secretion from the adipose tissue [62–64]. Leptin reduces appetite and food intake; however, this effect can be reduced or even abolished by psychotropic drugs, which may induce a state of leptin resistance/suppression. In addition, by stimulating the secretion of cytokines, these drugs can impair TNF-α receptor sensitivity that may lead to a lack of body weight control and, as a result, to an increase in caloric intake [65–69].

References

1. **WHO**. Obesity. Fact Sheet 311, Updated June 2016. http://www.who.int/mediacentre/factsheets/fs311/en/ (accessed 8 February 2018).

2. **WHO**. Depression. Fact Sheet 369, Updated April 2016. http://www.who.int/mediacentre/factsheets/fs369/en/ (accessed 8 February 2018).

3. **Dawes AJ, Maggard-Gibbons M, Maher AR**, et al. Mental health conditions among patients seeking and undergoing bariatric surgery: a meta-analysis. *Journal of the American Medical Association* 2016;**315**:150–63.

4. **Dixon JB, Dixon ME, O'Brien PE**. Depression in association with severe obesity: changes with weight loss. *Archives of Internal Medicine* 2003;**163**:2058–65.

5. **Rand CS, Macgregor AM**. Morbidly obese patients' perceptions of social discrimination before and after surgery for obesity. *Southern Medical Journal* 1990;**83**:1390–5.

6. **Hayden MJ, Dixon JB, Dixon ME, Shea TL, O'Brien PE**. Characterization of the improvement in depressive symptoms following bariatric surgery. *Obesity Surgery* 2011;**21**:328–35.

7. **Ikramuddin S, Korner J, Lee WJ**, et al. Roux-en-Y gastric bypass vs intensive medical management for the control of type 2 diabetes, hypertension, and hyperlipidemia: the Diabetes Surgery Study randomized clinical trial. *Journal of the American Medical Association* 2013;**309**:2240–9.

8. **Mingrone G, Panunzi S, De Gaetano A**, et al. Bariatric-metabolic surgery versus conventional medical treatment in obese patients with type 2 diabetes: 5 year follow-up of an open-label, single-centre, randomised controlled trial. *Lancet* 2015;**386**:964–73.

9. **Schauer PR, Bhatt DL, Kirwan JP** et al. STAMPEDE Investigators. Bariatric surgery versus intensive medical therapy for diabetes—3-year outcomes. *New England Journal of Medicine* 2014;**370**:2002–13.

10. **Sjöström L, Lindroos AK, Peltonen M,** et al. Swedish Obese Subjects Study Scientific Group. Lifestyle, diabetes, and cardiovascular risk factors 10 years after bariatric surgery. *New England Journal of Medicine* 2004;**351**:2683–93.

11. **Sjöström L, Peltonen M, Jacobson P,** et al. Bariatric surgery and long-term cardiovascular events. *Journal of the American Medical Association* 2012;**307**:56–65.

12. **Buchwald H, Avidor Y, Braunwald E,** et al. Bariatric surgery: a systematic review and meta-analysis. *Journal of the American Medical Association* 2004;**292**:1724–37.

13. **Rubino F, Shukla A, Pomp A,** et al. Bariatric, metabolic, and diabetes surgery: what's in a name? *Annals of Surgery* 2014;**259**:117–224.

14. **Kashyap SR, Bhatt DL, Schauer PR; STAMPEDE Investigators.** Bariatric surgery vs. advanced practice medical management in the treatment of type 2 diabetes mellitus: rationale and design of the Surgical Therapy And Medications Potentially Eradicate Diabetes Efficiently trial (STAMPEDE). *Diabetes Obesity and Metabolism* 2010;**12**:452–4.

15. **Mingrone G, Panunzi S, De Gaetano A** et al. Bariatric surgery versus conventional medical therapy for type 2 diabetes. *New England Journal of Medicine* 2012;**366**:1577–85.

16. **Vest AR, Heneghan HM, Agarwal S,** et al. Bariatric surgery and cardiovascular outcomes: a systematic review. *Heart* 2012;**98**:1763–77.

17. **Wing RR.** Long-term effects of a lifestyle intervention on weight and cardiovascular risk factors in individuals with type 2 diabetes mellitus: four-year results of the Look AHEAD trial. *Archives of Internal Medicine* 2010;**170**:1566–75.

18. **Chang SH, Stoll CR, Song J,** et al. The effectiveness and risks of bariatric surgery: an updated systematic review and meta-analysis, 2003-2012. *JAMA Surgery* 2014;**149**:275–87.

19. **Colquitt JL, Pickett K, Loveman E, Frampton GK.** Surgery for weight loss in adults. *Cochrane Database of Systematic Reviews* 2014;**8**:CD003641.

20. **Picot J, Jones J, Colquitt JL,** et al. The clinical effectiveness and cost-effectiveness of bariatric (weight loss) surgery for obesity: a systematic review and economic evaluation. *Health Technology Assessment* 2009;**13**:1–190.

21. **Flum DR, Belle SH, King WC,** et al. Perioperative safety in the longitudinal assessment of bariatric surgery. Longitudinal Assessment of Bariatric Surgery (LABS) Consortium, *New England Journal of Medicine* 2009;**361**:445–54.

22. **Yu J, Zhou X, Li L** et al. The long-term effects of bariatric surgery for type 2 diabetes: systematic review and meta-analysis of randomized and non-randomized evidence. *Obesity Surgery* 2015;**25**:143–58.

23. **Buchwald H, Estok R, Fahrbach K,** et al. Trends in mortality in bariatric surgery: a systematic review and meta-analysis. *Surgery* 2007;**142**:621–32.

24. **Hoerger TJ, Zhang P, Segel JE,** et al. Cost-effectiveness of bariatric surgery for severely obese adults with diabetes. *Diabetes Care* 2010;**33**:1933–9.

25. **Bromet E, Andrade LH, Hwang I,** et al. Cross-national epidemiology of DSM-IV major depressive episode. *BMC Medicine* 2011;**9**:90.

26. **Spijker J, Graaf R, Bijl RV,** et al. Functional disability and depression in the general population. Results from the Netherlands Mental Health Survey and Incidence Study (NEMESIS). *Acta Psychiatrica Scandinavica* 2004;**110**:208–14.

27. **Mitchell AJ, Vaze A, Rao S.** Clinical diagnosis of depression in primary care: a meta-analysis. *Lancet* 2009;**374**:609–19.

28. **Demyttenaere K, Bruffaerts R, Posada-Villa J,** et al. WHO World Mental Health Survey Consortium. Prevalence, severity, and unmet need for treatment of mental disorders in the World Health Organization World Mental Health Surveys. *Journal of the American Medical Association* 2004;**291**:2581–90.

29. **Radloff L.** The CES-D Scale: A self-report depression scale for research in the general population. *Applied Psychological Measurement* 1977;**1**:385–401.

30. **Tiemens BG, von Korff M, Lin EHB.** Diagnosis of depression by primary care physicians versus a structured diagnostic interview: understanding discordance. *General Hospital Psychiatry* 1999;**21**:87–96.

31. **Olfson M, Marcus SC.** National patterns in antidepressant medication treatment. *Archives of General Psychiatry* 2009;**66**:848–56.

32. **Willis T.** Diabetes: A Medical Odyssey. New York: Tuckahoe, 1971.

33. **Karamanou M, Protogerou A, Tsoucalas G,** et al. Milestones in the history of diabetes mellitus: the main contributors. *World Journal of Diabetes* 2016;**7**:1–7.

34. **Lustman PJ, Anderson RJ, Freedland KE,** et al. Depression and poor glycemic control: a meta-analytic review of the literature. *Diabetes Care* 2000;**23**:934–942.

35. **Lustman PJ, Clouse RE.** Depression in diabetes: the chicken or the egg? *Psychosomatic Medicine* 2007;**69**:297–9.

36. **Eaton WW, Mengel M, Mengel L, Larson D, Campbell R, Montague RB.** Psychosocial and psychopathologic influences on management and control of insulin-dependent diabetes. *International Journal of Psychiatry in Medicine* 1992;**22**:105–117.

37. **Gavard JA, Lustman PJ, Clouse RE.** Prevalence of depression in adults with diabetes: an epidemiological evaluation. *Diabetes Care* 1993;**16**:1167–78.

38. **Murrell SA, Himmelfarb S, Wright K.** Prevalence of depression and its correlates in older adults. *American Journal of Epidemiology* 1983;**117**:173–85.

39. **Wells KB, Stuart A, Hays RD,** et al. The functioning and well-being of depressed patients: results from the medical outcomes study. *Journal of the American Medical Association* 1989;**262**:914–19.

40. **Pijl H, Meinders E.** Bodyweight change as an adverse effect of drug treatment: Mechanisms and management. *Drug Safety* 1996;**14**:329–42.

41. **Rosenthal R, Rubin DB.** A simple, general purpose display of magnitude of experimental effect. *Journal of Educational Psychology* 1982;**74**:166–9.

42. **Anderson RJ, Freedland KE, Clouse RE, Lustman PJ.** The prevalence of comorbid depression in adults with diabetes: a meta-analysis. *Diabetes Care* 2001;**24**:1069–78.

43. **Kalarchian MA, Marcus MD, Levine MD,** et al. Psychiatric disorders among bariatric surgery candidates: relationship to obesity and functional health status. *American Journal of Psychiatry* 2007;**164**:328–34.

44. **Rosenberger PH, Henderson KE, Grilo CM.** Psychiatric disorder comorbidity and association with eating disorders in bariatric surgery patients: a cross-sectional study using structured interview-based diagnosis. *Journal of Clinical Psychiatry* 2006;**67**:1080–5.

45. **de Zwaan M, Enderle J, Wagner S** et al. Anxiety and depression in bariatric surgery patients: a prospective, follow-up study using structured clinical interviews. *Journal of Affective Disorders* 2011;**133**:61–8.

46. Heneghan HM, Heinberg L, Windover A, et al. Weighing the evidence for an association between obesity and suicide risk. *Surgery for Obesity and Related Diseases* 2012;8:98–107.

47. Rutledge T, Braden AL, Woods G, et al. Five-year changes in psychiatric treatment status and weight-related comorbidities following bariatric surgery in a veteran population. *Obesity Surgery* 2012;**22**:1734–11.

48. Lier HO, Biringer E, Hove O, Stubhaug B, Tangen T. Quality of life among patients undergoing bariatric surgery: associations with mental health-A 1 year follow-up study of bariatric surgery patients. *Health and Quality of Life Outcomes* 2011;**26:9**:79.

49. Mitchell JE, King WC, Chen JY, et al. Course of depressive symptoms and treatment in the longitudinal assessment of bariatric surgery (LABS-2) study. *Obesity* 2014;**22**:1799–806.

50. Adams TD, Gress RE, Smith SC, et al. Long-term mortality after gastric bypass surgery. *New England Journal of Medicine* 2007;**357**:753–61.

51. Tindle HA, Omalu B, Courcoulas A, et al. Risk of suicide after long-term follow-up from bariatric surgery. *American Journal of Medicine* 2010;**123**:1036–42.

52. Peterhänsel C, Petroff D, Klinitzke G, et al. Risk of completed suicide after bariatric surgery: a systematic review. *Obesity Reviews* 2013;**14**:369–82.

53. Backman O, Stockeld D, Rasmussen F, Näslund E, Marsk R. Alcohol and substance abuse, depression and suicide attempts after Roux-en-Y gastric bypass surgery. *British Journal of Surgery* 2016;**103**:1336–42.

54. Pagoto S, Bodenlos JS, Kantor L, et al. Association of major depression and binge eating disorder with weight loss in a clinical setting. *Obesity* 2007;**15**:2557–9.

55. Booth H, Khan O, Prevost AT, Reddy M, Charlton J, Gulliford MC; King's Bariatric Surgery Study Group. Impact of bariatric surgery on clinical depression. Interrupted time series study with matched controls. *Journal of Affective Disorders* 2015;**174**:644–9.

56. Vangoitsenhoven R, Frederiks P, Gijbels B, et al. Long-term effects of gastric bypass surgery on psychosocial well-being and eating behaviour: not all that glitters is gold. *Acta Clinica Belgica* 2016;**3**:1–8.

57. Ostlund MP, Backman O, Marsk R, et al. Increased admission for alcohol dependence after gastric bypass surgery compared with restrictive bariatric surgery. *JAMA Surgery* 2013;**148**:374–7.

58. American Psychiatric Association. Practice guideline for the treatment of patients with major depressive disorder (revision). *American Journal of Psychiatry* 2000;**157**:1–45.

59. Hubbard VS, Hall WH. Gastrointestinal surgery for severe obesity. *Obesity Surgery* 1991;**1**:257–65.

60. Stegenga H, Haines A, Jones K, Wilding J; Guideline Development Group. Identification, assessment, and management of overweight and obesity: summary of updated NICE guidance. *British Medical Journal* 2014;**349**:g6608.

61. Reprinted by permission from Springer: *Obesity Surgery*, 24, Fried M, Yumuk V, Oppert JM, et al. International Federation for Surgery of Obesity and Metabolic Disorders-European Chapter (IFSO-EC); European Association for the Study of Obesity (EASO); European Association for the Study of Obesity Obesity Management Task Force (EASO OMTF). Interdisciplinary European guidelines on metabolic and bariatric surgery, 2014, pp. 42–55.

62. **Buchwald H.** Consensus Conference Statement Bariatric surgery for morbid obesity: Health implications for patients, health professionals, and third-party payers. *Surgery for Obesity and Related Diseases* 2005;**1**:371–81.

63. **Fried M, Yumuk V, Oppert JM**, et al. International Federation for Surgery of Obesity and Metabolic Disorders-European Chapter (IFSO-EC); European Association for the Study of Obesity (EASO); European Association for the Study of Obesity Obesity Management Task Force (EASO OMTF). Interdisciplinary European guidelines on metabolic and bariatric surgery. *Obesity Surgery* 2014;**24**:42–55.

64. **Brömel T, Blum WF, Ziegler A**, et al. Serum leptin levels increase rapidly after initiation of clozapine treatment. *Molecular Psychiatry* 1998;**3**:76–80.

65. **Kraus T, Haack M, Schuld A**, et al. Body weight and leptin plasma levels during treatment with antipsychotic drugs. *American Journal of Psychiatry* 1999;**156**:312–14.

66. **Pollmächer T, Hinze-Selch D, Mullington J.** Effects of clozapine on cytokines and soluble cytokine receptors. *Journal of Clinical Psychopharmacology* 1996;**16**:403–9.

67. **Argiles JM, Lopez-Soriano J, Busquets S, Lopez-Soriano FJ.** Journey from cachexia to obesity by TNF. *FASEB Journal* 1997;**11**:743–51.

68. **Berken GH, Weinstein DO, Stern WC.** Weight gain: a side-effect of tricyclic antidepressants. *Journal of Affective Disorders* 1984;**7**:133–8.

69. **Rubino F, Nathan DM, Eckel RH**, et al. Delegates of the 2nd Diabetes Surgery Summit. Metabolic Surgery in the Treatment Algorithm for Type 2 Diabetes: a joint statement by international diabetes organizations. *Diabetes Care* 2016;**39**:861–7.

Chapter 13

Novel pharmacological targets

Calum D. Moulton

Introduction

Depression is a common comorbidity in patients with type 2 diabetes (T2D) and is associated with a twofold increased risk of complications and premature mortality [1–3]. The link is bidirectional: diabetes increases the risk of incident depression by around 20%, whereas depression increases the risk of incident diabetes by up to 60% [4,5]. However, the mechanisms linking depression and T2D are incompletely understood and poorly explained by psychological and behavioural factors alone [2,3,6]. Moreover, current treatments for depression in T2D do not consistently improve biomedical outcomes. Novel treatment strategies are therefore warranted.

There is growing evidence that depression and T2D may in fact be linked by shared biological mechanisms. Such mechanisms may include elevated systemic inflammation, dysfunction of the hypothalamic–pituitary–adrenal (HPA) axis, elevated insulin resistance, vitamin D deficiency, and sleep disturbance, which may in turn interact with one another. All of these pathways present opportunities for pharmacological modification through the repositioning of readily available treatments. If effective, the modification of these pathways provides the opportunity to improve depression and diabetes simultaneously and to improve biomedical outcomes.

After summarizing the limitations of current pharmacotherapy for depression in T2D, this review will scrutinize the evidence for novel pharmacological targets, emphasizing intervention studies where possible. The study will summarize the evidence to make recommendations for future research.

Limitations of current antidepressant treatments in T2D

Standard treatment for depression includes antidepressant medications or psychological therapy such as cognitive behavioural therapy. There is good evidence that antidepressant medications lead to significant short-term and longer term improvements in depression in patients with T2D [7,8]. Likewise, cognitive behavioural therapy has been used to treat depression in T2D, producing positive effects on depressive symptoms, albeit not always sustained [9].

In a purely psycho-behavioural model of depression in T2D, depression would lead to worsening diabetes self-care and increased risk of diabetes complications over time. In such a model, successful treatment of depression would be expected to translate into improvements in both glycaemic control and biomedical outcomes. Frequently, however, this is not the case. For example, in the Pathways study of 329 people with comorbid diabetes and major depression and/or dysthymia, isolated treatment of depression did not improve glycaemic control [10]. In the related field of cardiovascular disease (CVD), standard pharmacological and psychological treatment of depression has not been found to reduce recurrent cardiovascular events or mortality [11,12].

In recent years, a hypothesis has emerged that could explain the limitations of current therapy. Rather than being separate conditions with separate disease mechanisms, depression and T2D may both be driven by shared mechanisms [6]. The failure of standard therapies to improve outcomes could represent nonmodification of these underlying mechanisms. This hypothesis is attractive in that it provides the potential for disease-modifying treatments that could improve longer term outcomes. Major candidate novel pathways will be studied in turn.

Novel pharmacological targets

Inflammation

In the general population, meta-analyses have found higher circulating concentrations of cytokines, including tumour necrosis factor (TNF)-α and interleukin (IL) 6, than in non-depressed controls [13,14]. Prospectively, elevated cytokines are associated with incident depressive symptoms, suggesting a causal role [15]. Of intervention studies to date, a small meta-analysis reported that adjunctive therapy with the non-steroidal anti-inflammatory drug (NSAID) celecoxib reduced depressive symptoms compared with controls [16]. In a placebo-controlled trial, the TNF antagonist infliximab did not improve depressive symptoms after 12 weeks compared with placebo [17]. However, in the subset ($n = 21$) with high baseline C-reactive protein (CRP) concentrations, the remission rate was greater in the infliximab group. An important caveat is that this was a treatment-resistant sample, whose external validity is limited. To date, a lack of high-quality clinical trials of anti-inflammatory agents in depression have been performed.

By comparison, elevated inflammation is robustly implicated in the pathogenesis of T2D. In meta-analyses, elevated concentrations of IL-1β, IL-6, and CRP are consistently predictive of T2D onset [18]. In well-designed randomized controlled trials (RCTs), both biological agents, such as the IL-1 receptor antagonist, and broad-spectrum anti-inflammatory agents, such as NSAIDs, have produced sustained improvements in glycaemic control [19,20]. Inflammation is likewise a strong predictor of cardiovascular complications in patients with T2D [21], suggesting that reduction in inflammation could reduce long-term morbidity and mortality in addition to glycaemic control.

If predictive of both depression and T2D, inflammation is a plausible candidate as a shared mechanism for both conditions. Of the observational research to date, two large, well-designed T2D cohorts have reported higher concentrations of circulating inflammatory markers in patients with depression than in non-depressed controls, even after adjusting for pro-inflammatory confounders [22,23]. However, prospective epidemiological findings have not yet been reported, meaning causality cannot yet be inferred.

Intervention studies targeting inflammation in comorbid depression and T2D have been scarce. In a placebo-controlled, double-blind study of 30 patients with T2D, levels of fatigue were found to improve in patients receiving IL-1β antagonism compared with placebo [24]. In a secondary analysis of the South London Diabetes cohort of 1,735 people with newly diagnosed T2D, we compared treatment with incretin-based therapies—a class that includes dipeptidyl peptidase (DPP) IV inhibitors and glucagon-like peptide (GLP) 1 receptor agonists—against other hypoglycaemic agents for 1-year change in depressive symptoms [25]. We found a greater improvement in depressive symptoms in the incretin group, which correlated with reduction in CRP but not glycated Haemoglobin (HbA1c), suggesting that reduction in inflammation may mediate this effect. There are, however, other possible mechanisms. In a cross-sectional study of 1,335 Chinese adults, increased DPP-IV activity was independently associated with increased depressive symptoms, elevated IL-6 and CRP, as well as negatively with neuropeptide-Y (NPY), even after adjustment for potential confounders [26]. Normally degraded by endogenous DPP-IV, NPY is a neuropeptide expressed both in the central nervous system and in peripheral circulation that has antidepressive and anxiolytic properties in animal models [26,27]. As such, the potential antidepressive effects of DPP-IV inhibitors could result from reduction in pro-inflammatory cytokines, an increase in NPY availability, or a combination of both.

In summary, there is promising observational evidence to support inflammation as a novel pharmacological target for depression in T2D. Well-designed prospective epidemiological studies and intervention studies of anti-inflammatory therapies are now needed in patients with comorbid depression and T2D.

Hypothalamic–pituitary–adrenal axis

The HPA axis has an important role in controlling physiological reactions to stress, leading to pulsatile alterations in endogenous glucocorticoids. However, there is mounting evidence that chronic dysregulation of the HPA axis can have deleterious consequences. Chronic stress with associated hypercortisolaemia may contribute to metabolic syndrome, insulin resistance, and T2D [28]. Likewise, there is evidence that HPA axis dysregulation is associated both with depression and with resistance to antidepressants [29]. Clinical hypercortisolism (Cushing's syndrome) leads to T2D in one-third of patients and depression in up to 80% of patients [30,31]. Blunting of the normal diurnal cortisol curve is a shared feature of depression, incident diabetes, and higher HbA1c in established diabetes [29,30].

Despite its plausibility, few studies have tested subclinical hypercortisolism as a shared mechanism for depression and T2D. In a cross-sectional study of 61 patients with T2D, comorbid major depression was associated with elevated CRP levels and 24-hour urinary free cortisol [32]. In a dexamethasone/corticotrophin-releasing hormone test of 15 patients with depression and 17 controls, plasma cortisol concentrations and peak cortisol values correlated with homoeostatic model assessment insulin resistance (HOMA-R) in patients with depression but not in controls [33].

Of potential treatments, a 2008 Cochrane review scrutinized previous trials of antiglucocorticoid treatments for depression, including metyrapone, spironolactone, and mifepristone. The authors reported an overall improvement in depressive symptoms in five trials of non-psychotic depression [34]. However, a subsequent study of 165 patients receiving metyrapone or placebo—much larger than the proof-of-concept studies cited by the Cochrane review—found no effect on depressive symptoms [35]. Moreover, the external validity of many HPA-modifying studies is limited, as most have targeted hospitalized or treatment-refractory patients [34]. Recent studies using fludrocortisone and spironolactone—both including outpatients—did not find overall benefit on depressive symptoms [36,37]. Even fewer studies have attempted to modify the HPA axis in patients with comorbid depression and T2D. In an open-label study of 17 patients with T2D, candesartan, an angiotensin receptor antagonist, led to reduced cortisol compared with baseline, which was paralleled by improvement in depressive symptoms [38]. However, this trial was limited by its small sample and open-label design.

Overall, dysregulation of the HPA axis shows strong biological plausibility as a shared mechanism for depression and T2D. However, in patients with both depression and T2D, there is little epidemiological- or intervention research to support this currently. Well-powered epidemiological studies measuring HPA function in comorbid depression and T2D are awaited, and the likely benefit of HPA-modifying treatments may be higher in patients with more severe depression and/or established hypercortisolaemia.

Insulin resistance

The case for biological links between depression and T2D would be strengthened by a positive association between depression and insulin resistance. A meta-analysis of 21 studies reported a small but statistically significant cross-sectional association between depression and insulin resistance [39]. One of the few prospective studies to date reported that depression was associated with high HOMA-IR and incident diabetes in middle-aged women, mediated mostly through central adiposity [40].

Intervention studies modifying insulin resistance to treat depression have been few in number. In a 6-week metformin-controlled study of 50 patients with polycystic ovarian syndrome and major depressive disorder, pioglitazone produced significant improvement in depressive symptoms. However, this occurred independently of changes in insulin sensitivity, suggesting other mechanisms may mediate this effect [41]. In a 12-week, open-label study of 23 patients with depression, pioglitazone produced significant improvement in depressive symptoms, paralleled by reductions in inflammation and insulin resistance. The study was limited by its small sample size and an open-label study design with no placebo control [42]. In a placebo-controlled double-blind RCT of 37 patients with non-remitting depression, pioglitazone was associated with improved depressive symptoms in correlation with improvement in glucose metabolism, but only in patients with elevated insulin resistance at baseline [43].

In summary, more prospective epidemiological studies are needed to define the temporal relationship between depression, insulin resistance, and T2D onset. The independence of insulin resistance from both peripheral inflammation and adiposity needs to be more clearly established to support a causal relationship with depression. Future intervention studies should test whether treatment of depression in patients with insulin resistance can delay or even prevent progression to T2D.

Vitamin D

Vitamin D is a promising biomarker of both depression and T2D. For T2D, a 2013 meta-analysis of 21 prospective studies ($n = 76,220$) reported an inverse association between circulating vitamin D levels and incidence of T2D [44]. As possible mechanisms, vitamin D signalling can lead to stimulation of insulin release, and vitamin D may have anti-inflammatory effects that reduce insulin resistance [45]. The latter is supported by studies showing an association between low vitamin D markers and increased CRP [46]. In CVD research, a study of 7,358 patients with previous CVD found that low vitamin D levels were associated with increased risk of incident depression, even after adjustment for confounders [47]. In depression, meanwhile, a 2013 meta-analysis found a negative association between vitamin D levels and depression incidence [48]. However, a subsequent meta-analysis of seven trials of vitamin D supplementation for depression found no overall effect, although efficacy was seen in the two studies that recruited patients with clinical depression [49].

Studies of vitamin D as a biomarker of depression in patients with T2D have been few. In a subsample of 351 participants from the Hoorn study, there was no significant association between baseline vitamin D levels and glucose metabolism and incident diabetes over a 1-year follow-up [50]. There was, however, a trend towards an inverse association of vitamin D with prospective changes in glycaemic control. A 2016 study of 2,786 Chinese patients with T2D found a significant negative association between serum levels of vitamin D and depression [51].

To date, one intervention study has tested vitamin D supplementation for its effect on depression and insulin resistance. Over 8 weeks, this randomized, double-blind trial of 40 patients reported significant improvement in depressive symptoms, insulin secretion, and insulin resistance markers with vitamin D compared with placebo [52]. Further prospective epidemiological studies and intervention studies in patients with depression and comorbid T2D are awaited.

Sleep and circadian rhythms

Disrupted sleep, altered circadian rhythms, and extremes of sleep duration are features of depression, insulin resistance, and T2D [53–55]. Longitudinally, there is accumulating evidence that sleep disturbance is predictive of both depression and diabetes, and specific alterations of sleep architecture have been found to predict both depression and T2D separately [55]. At a cellular level, clock genes are associated with regulation of the circadian rhythm, whose expression is controlled by environmental cues such as light–dark cycles [56]. Recently, evidence has emerged that clock gene expression is associated with the incidence of T2D [57] and with fasting glucose concentrations [58]. Patients with depression, meanwhile, show changes in the expression of various clock genes, which may persist even following standard antidepressant treatment

[59], although prospective findings are limited. Some authors have suggested that the rapid antidepressant actions of low-dose ketamine and sleep deprivation therapy might be due to resetting of abnormal clock genes and subsequent restoration of circadian rhythms [60]. Studies testing clock gene expression in relation to incident depression and T2D together are now warranted.

Summary and future directions

Based on the available evidence, inflammation and vitamin D are likely to provide the strongest novel pharmacological targets to treat depression and T2D at present. However, further prospective observational research is needed to imply stronger shared causality with depression and T2D. Furthermore, biomarkers that are practical for epidemiological studies, such as HOMA-IR and peripheral cytokine concentrations, may be imprecise markers of central and peripheral biological processes. Therefore, strong basic science research is needed to delineate more precisely how candidate biological pathways can cause both depression and T2D. In parallel, intervention studies are needed to track the temporal relationship—ideally over multiple time points—between changes in biological mediators and changes in depressive symptoms. Importantly, future intervention studies should not focus primarily on patients with severe or resistant depression, as this departs from the majority of patients with depression and T2D.

Careful consideration should be given to the nature of future interventions and their potential risks and benefits. Vitamin D has the advantages that the intervention is clearly defined and unlikely to produce serious side-effects. For inflammation, however, it is not known whether to target defined biological pathways, such as IL-1 inhibition, or to use more 'broad-based' anti-inflammatory agents, such as NSAIDs, and neither is without risk. For example, cyclo-oxygenase-2 inhibitors such as celecoxib are associated with increased thrombosis risk, posing particular problems in diabetes patients. Biological cytokine-blocking therapies—generally administered via injection—can have serious side-effects because of their immune-suppressive properties [61]. As such, repurposing of established diabetes therapies with anti-inflammatory effects, such as incretin-based therapies, could be safer and better tolerated.

Although this review has considered candidate biological pathways in isolation, most of the candidate biological pathways are known to interact with one-another. For example, there are established bidirectional relationships between the HPA axis and innate inflammatory response; between insulin resistance and innate inflammation; between inflammation and sleep disturbance; between vitamin D deficiency and inflammation and so forth. This makes it difficult to define the most appropriate target for interventions. A promising approach in this regard could be 'multiple-hit' interventions. DPP-IV inhibitors, for example, have positive effects on NPY and on inflammation. However, careful monitoring of candidate biological pathways against changes in depressive symptoms is needed to maximize the mechanistic value of this approach.

Conclusion

There is mounting evidence that biological mechanisms have a causative role in depression and T2D. In recent years, observational evidence and tentative interventional evidence have suggested that such mechanisms, in particular inflammation and vitamin D deficiency, may link the two conditions. Longitudinal observational studies and carefully designed intervention studies are now needed to test causality and the modifiability of novel mechanisms. Unlike current antidepressant treatments, targeting shared biological pathways has the potential to improve depression and diabetes together, as well as reducing longer term morbidity and mortality in the growing population with comorbid depression and T2D.

References

1. **Anderson RJ, Freedland KE, Clouse RE, Lustman PJ.** The prevalence of comorbid depression in adults with diabetes: a meta analysis. *Diabetes Care* 2001;**24**:1069–78.
2. **de Groot M, Anderson R, Freedland KE, Clouse RE, Lustman PJ.** Association of depression and diabetes complications: a meta-analysis. *Psychosomatic Medicine* 2001;**63**:619–30.
3. **Katon WJ, Rutter C, Simon G,** et al. The association of comorbid depression with mortality in patients with type 2 diabetes. *Diabetes Care* 2005;**28**:2668–72.
4. **Mezuk B, Eaton WW, Albrecht S, Golden SH.** Depression and type 2 diabetes over the lifespan: a meta-analysis. *Diabetes Care* 2008;**31**:2383–90.
5. **Nouwen A, Winkley K, Twisk J,** et al; **European Depression in Diabetes (EDID) Research Consortium.** Type 2 diabetes mellitus as a risk factor for the onset of depression: a systematic review and meta-analysis. *Diabetologia* 2010;**53**:2480–6.
6. **Moulton CD, Pickup JC, Ismail K.** The link between depression and diabetes: the search for shared mechanisms. *Lancet Diabetes Endocrinol* 2015;**3**:461–71.
7. **Echeverry D, Duran P, Bonds C, Lee M, Davidson MB.** Effect of pharmacological treatment of depression on A1C and quality of life in low-income Hispanics and African Americans with diabetes: a randomized, double-blind, placebo-controlled trial. *Diabetes Care* 2009;**32**:2156–60.
8. **Lustman PJ, Clouse RE, Nix BD,** et al. Sertraline for prevention of depression recurrence in diabetes mellitus: a randomized, double-blind, placebo-controlled trial. *Archives of General Psychiatry* 2006;**63**:521–9.
9. **Safren SA, Gonzalez JS, Wexler DJ,** et al. A randomized controlled trial of cognitive behavioral therapy for adherence and depression (CBT-AD) in patients with uncontrolled type 2 diabetes. *Diabetes Care* 2014;**37**:625–33.

10. **Katon WJ, Von Korff M, Lin EH**, et al. The Pathways Study: a randomized trial of collaborative care in patients with diabetes and depression. *Archives of General Psychiatry* 2004;**61**:1042–9.

11. **Berkman LF, Blumenthal J, Burg M**, et al. Effects of treating depression and low perceived social support on clinical events after myocardial infarction: the Enhancing Recovery in Coronary Heart Disease Patients (ENRICHD) Randomized Trial. *Journal of the American Medical Association* 2003;**289**:3106–16.

12. **Glassman AH, O'Connor CM, Califf RM**, et al. Sertraline treatment of major depression in patients with acute MI or unstable angina. *Journal of the American Medical Association* 2002;**288**(6):701–9.

13. **Dowlati Y, Herrmann N, Swardfager W**, et al. A meta-analysis of cytokines in major depression. *Biological Psychiatry* 2010;**67**:446–57.

14. **Liu Y, Ho RC, Mak A.** Interleukin (IL)-6, tumour necrosis factor alpha (TNF-α) and soluble interleukin-2 receptors (sIL-2R) are elevated in patients with major depressive disorder: a meta-analysis and meta-regression. *Journal of Affective Disorders* 2012;**139**:230–9.

15. **Pasco JA, Nicholson GC, Williams LJ**, et al. Association of high-sensitivity C-reactive protein with *de novo* major depression. *British Journal of Psychiatry* 2010;**197**:372–7.

16. **Na KS, Lee KJ, Lee JS, Cho YS, Jung HY.** Efficacy of adjunctive celecoxib treatment for patients with major depressive disorder: a meta-analysis. *Progress in Neuro-Psychopharmacology & Biological Psychiatry* 2014;**48**:79–85.

17. **Raison CL, Rutherford RE, Woolwine BJ**, et al. A randomized controlled trial of the tumor necrosis factor antagonist infliximab for treatment-resistant depression: the role of baseline inflammatory biomarkers. *JAMA Psychiatry* 2013;**70**:31–41

18. **Wang X, Bao W, Liu J**, et al. Inflammatory markers and risk of type 2 diabetes: a systematic review and meta-analysis. *Diabetes Care* 2013;**36**:166–75.

19. **Goldfine AB, Fonseca V, Jablonski KA**, et al. Salicylate (salsalate) in patients with type 2 diabetes: a randomized trial. *Annals of Internal Medicine* 2013;**159**:1–12

20. **Larsen CM, Faulenbach M, Vaag A**, et al. Sustained effects of interleukin-1 receptor antagonist treatment in type 2 diabetes. *Diabetes Care* 2009;**32**:1663–8.

21. **Pickup JC, Mattock MB.** Activation of the innate immune system as a predictor of cardiovascular mortality in type 2 diabetes mellitus. *Diabetic Medicine* 2003;**20**:723–6.

22. **Hayashino Y, Mashitani T, Tsujii S**, et al. Elevated levels of hs-CRP are associated with high prevalence of depression in Japanese patients with type 2 diabetes: the Diabetes Distress and Care Registry at Tenri (DDCRT 6). *Diabetes Care* 2014;**37**:2459–65.

23. **Laake JP, Stahl D, Amiel SA**, et al. The association between depressive symptoms and systemic inflammation in people with type 2 diabetes: findings from the South London Diabetes Study. *Diabetes Care* 2014;**37**:2186–92.

24. **Cavelti-Weder C, Furrer R, Keller C**, et al. Inhibition of IL-1beta improves fatigue in type 2 diabetes. *Diabetes Care* 2011;**34**:e158.

25. **Moulton CD, Pickup JC, Amiel SA, Winkley K, Ismail K.** Investigating incretin-based therapies as a novel treatment for depression in type 2 diabetes: Findings from the South London Diabetes (SOUL-D) Study. *Prim Care Diabetes* 2016;**10**:156–9.

26. **Zheng T, Liu Y, Qin S**, et al. Increased dipeptidyl peptidase-4 activity is associated with high prevalence of depression in middle-aged and older adults: a cross-sectional study. *Journal of Clinical Psychiatry* 2016;**77**:e1248–55.

27. **Canneva F, Golub Y, Distler J,** et al. DPP4-deficient congenic rats display blunted stress, improved fear extinction and increased central NPY. *Psychoneuroendocrinology* 2015;**53**:195–206.

28. **Chrousos GP.** The role of stress and the hypothalamic-pituitary-adrenal axis in the pathogenesis of the metabolic syndrome: neuroendocrine and target tissue-related causes. *International Journal of Obesity and Related Metabolic Disorders* 2000;**24**(Suppl. 2):S50–5.

29. **Stetler, C, Miller GE.** Depression and hypothalamic–pituitary–adrenal activation: a quantitative summary of four decades of research. *Psychosomatic Medicine* 2011;**73**:114–26.

30. **Hackett RA, Kivimaki M, Kumar I, Steptoe A.** Diurnal cortisol patterns, future diabetes, and impaired glucose metabolism in the Whitehall II cohort study. *Journal of Clinical Endocrinology & Metabolism* 2016;**101**:619–25.89.

31. **Pivonello, R, Isidori AM, de Martino MC,** et al. Complications of Cushing's syndrome: state of the art. *Lancet Diabetes Endocrinology* 2016;**4**:611–629.

32. **Alvarez A, Faccioli J, Guinzbourg M.** Endocrine and inflammatory profiles in type 2 diabetic patients with and without major depressive disorder. *BMC Research Notes* 2013;**6**:61.

33. **Yokoyama K, Yamada T, Mitani H.** Relationship between hypothalamic-pituitary-adrenal axis dysregulation and insulin resistance in elderly patients with depression. *Psychiatry Research* 2015;**226**:494–8.

34. **Gallagher P, Malik N, Newham J,** et al. Antiglucocorticoid treatments for mood disorders. *Cochrane Database of Systematic Reviews* 2008;**23**(1):CD005168.

35. **Ferrier IN, Anderson IM, Barnes J,** et al. Randomised controlled trial of Antiglucocorticoid augmentation (metyrapone) of antiDepressants in Depression (ADD Study). Efficacy and Mechanism Evaluation. Southampton: NIHR Journals Library, 2015.

36. **Hinkelmann K, Hellmann-Regen J, Wingenfeld K,** et al. Mineralocorticoid receptor function in depressed patients and healthy individuals. *Progress in Neuro-psychopharmacology & Biological Psychiatry* 2016;**71**:183–8

37. **Otte C, Hinkelmann K, Moritz S,** et al. Modulation of the mineralocorticoid receptor as add-on treatment in depression: a randomized, double-blind, placebo-controlled proof-of-concept study. *Journal of Psychiatric Research* 2010;**44**:339–46.

38. **Pavlatou MG, Mastorakos G, Lekakis I,** et al. Chronic administration of an angiotensin II receptor antagonist resets the hypothalamic-pituitary-adrenal (HPA) axis and improves the affect of patients with diabetes mellitus type 2: preliminary results. *Stress* 2008;**11**:62–72

39. **Kan C, Silva N, Golden SH,** et al. A systematic review and metaanalysis of the association between depression and insulin resistance. *Diabetes Care* 2013;**36**:480–89.

40. **Everson-Rose SA, Meyer PM, Powell LH,** et al. Depressive symptoms, insulin resistance, and risk of diabetes in women at midlife. *Diabetes Care* 2004;**27**: 2856–62.

41. **Kashani L, Omidvar T, Farazmand B,** et al. Does pioglitazone improve depression through insulin-sensitization? Results of a randomized double-blind metformin-controlled trial in patients with polycystic ovarian syndrome and comorbid depression. *Psychoneuroendocrinology* 2013;**38**:767–76

42. **Kemp DE, Schinagle M, Gao K**, et al. PPAR-γ agonism as a modulator of mood: proof-of-concept for pioglitazone in bipolar depression. *CNS Drugs* 2014;**28**:571–81

43. **Lin KW, Wroolie TE, Robakis T, Rasgon NL.** Adjuvant pioglitazone for unremitted depression: Clinical correlates of treatment response. *Psychiatry Res*earch 2015;**230**:846–52.

44. **Song Y, Wang L, Pittas AG**, et al. Blood 25-hydroxy vitamin D levels and incident type 2 diabetes: a meta-analysis of prospective studies. *Diabetes Care* 2013;**36**:1422–8.

45. **Alvarez JA, Ashraf A.** Role of vitamin d in insulin secretion and insulin sensitivity for glucose homeostasis. *International Journal of Endocrinology* 2010:351385.

46. **Amer M, Qayyum R.** Relation between serum 25-hydroxyvitamin D and C-reactive protein in asymptomatic adults (from the continuous National Health and Nutrition Examination Survey 2001 to 2006). *American Journal of Cardiology.* 2012;**109**:226–30.

47. **May HT, Bair TL, Lappé DL**, et al. Association of vitamin D levels with incident depression among a general cardiovascular population. *American Heart Journal* 2010;**159**:1037–43.

48. **Ju SY, Lee YJ, Jeong SN.** Serum 25-hydroxyvitamin D levels and the risk of depression: a systematic review and meta-analysis. *Journal of Nutritional Health and Aging* 2013;**17**:447–55.

49. **Shaffer JA, Edmondson D, Wasson LT**, et al. Vitamin D supplementation for depressive symptoms: a systematic review and meta-analysis of randomized controlled trials. *Psychosomatic Medicine* 2014;**76**:190–6.

50. **Pilz S, van den Hurk K, Nijpels G**, et al. Vitamin D status, incident diabetes and prospective changes in glucose metabolism in older subjects: the Hoorn study. *Nutrition, Metabolism & Cardiovascular Diseases* 2012;**22**:883–9.

51. **Wang Y, Yang H, Meng P, Han Y.** Association between low serum 25-hydroxyvitamin D and depression in a large sample of Chinese patients with type 2 diabetes mellitus. *Journal of Affective Disorders* 2017;**224**:56–60.

52. **Sepehrmanesh Z, Kolahdooz F, Abedi F**, et al. Vitamin D supplementation affects the Beck Depression Inventory, insulin resistance, and biomarkers of oxidative stress in patients with major depressive disorder: a randomized, controlled clinical trial. *Journal of Nutrition* 2016;**146**:243–8.

53. **Courtet P, Olié E.** Circadian dimension and severity of depression. *European Neuropsychopharmacology* 2012;**22**(Suppl. 3):S476–S481

54. **Hall MH, Muldoon MF, Jennings JR**, et al. Self-reported sleep duration is associated with the metabolic syndrome in midlife adults. *Sleep* 2008;**31**:635–43

55. **Kudlow PA, Cha DS, Lam RW, McIntyre RS.** Sleep architecture variation: a mediator of metabolic disturbance in individuals with major depressive disorder. *Sleep Medicine* 2013;**14**:943–49.

56. **Karthikeyan R, Marimuthu G, Spence DW**, et al. Should we listen to our clock to prevent type 2 diabetes mellitus? *Diabetes Research and Clinical Practice* 2014;**106**:182–90

57. **Corella D, Asensio EM, Coltell O**, et al. CLOCK gene variation is associated with incidence of type-2 diabetes and cardiovascular diseases in type-2 diabetic subjects: dietary modulation in the PREDIMED randomized trial. *Cardiovascular Diabetology* 2016;**15**:4.

58. **Stamenkovic JA, Olsson AH, Nagorny** CL, et al. Regulation of core clock genes in human islets. *Metabolism* 2012;**61**:978–85.

59. Li SX, Liu LJ, Xu LZ, et al. Diurnal alterations in circadian genes and peptides in major depressive disorder before and after escitalopram treatment. *Psychoneuroendocrinology* 2013;**38**:2789–99.

60. **Bunney** BG, Li JZ, **Walsh** DM, et al. Circadian dysregulation of clock genes: clues to rapid treatments in major depressive disorder. *Molecular Psychiatry* 2015;**20**:48–55.

61. British National Formulary, 67th ed. London, UK: Pharmaceutical Press, 2013.

Chapter 14

Novel technologies: What does gastric electrical stimulation offer to the patient with type 2 diabetes and depression?

Harold E. Lebovitz and Shlomo Ben-Haim

Introduction

The combination of diabetes mellitus and depression has been clinically recognized for many years, but it has been only possible to focus on this comorbidity more recently as tools to precisely diagnose depression and to define diabetes control and complications became available. The comorbidity of diabetes mellitus and clinically relevant depression poses a number of important clinical questions [1–3]. Does preceding clinical depression increase the incidence of diabetes mellitus? To what extent does pre-existing diabetes mellitus contribute to the development of depression? Does concomitant depression decrease the effectiveness of diabetes management and increase the rate of microvascular and macrovascular complications? Does concomitant diabetes mellitus worsen the results of depression treatments? The responses to these questions are critical if we are to provide the highest quality care to the population with these comorbid conditions or to those who are at risk of developing them.

A 13-year follow-up of the Epidemiologic Catchment Area Program survey from East Baltimore yielded a cumulative incidence of diabetes mellitus of 5.2% among 1,715 individuals at risk. In logistic models, major depressive disorder (MDD) predicted the onset of diabetes with an estimated relative risk (RR) of 2.23 compared with those without MDD [4]. Subsequently, meta-analyses of large populations which had identified those with incident depression at baseline and followed the entire cohort for periods of 4–8.3 years reported the RR for developing new-onset diabetes to range from 1.22 to 2.31 [5–8].

Several meta-analyses suggested that individuals with diabetes mellitus have an increased risk of developing depression [9–12]. Anderson et al. [10] analysed data from 42 studies and determined that depression was increased twofold in patients with diabetes mellitus compared with those without diabetes. Depression was significantly higher in women with diabetes than men (28% versus 18%). A recent meta-analysis of 16 studies involving 497,223 patients followed for a mean of 5.8 years identified 42,633 incident cases of diabetes mellitus [11]. Higher rates of depression were found in patients with diabetes mellitus than in non-diabetic individuals (1.6 versus 1.4% per year, adjusted RR 1.25, $p < 0.001$).

Patients with diabetes and depression have a significant increase in non-adherence to all aspects of their diabetes management including overall care, appointment keeping, following dietary and physical activity programmes, taking medications as prescribed, and performing glucose monitoring as required [13–17]. In a review of 27 studies examining adherence to oral medications alone or with insulin in patients with type 2 diabetes, 21 of 27 studies showed adherence rates of 38.5–80% [15]. Depression, the tasks of managing diabetes, and costs were among the major factors responsible for non-adherence. Lustman et al. [16] analysed the results of 24 studies and found that depression was associated with a significant increase in hyperglycaemia as measured by glycated haemoglobin (HbA1c) levels.

Depression in patients with diabetes is associated with an increase in diabetic complications and an increase in all-cause mortality [18–22]. Egede et al. [20] evaluated 10,025 patients from the NHANES dataset who were alive and interviewed them in 1982 for diabetes and depression status. Subjects were divided into four groups: (1) no diabetes and no depression (reference group); (2) depression with no diabetes; (3) diabetes with no depression; (4) diabetes and depression. After an 8-year follow-up co-existent diabetes and depression increased all-cause mortality (HR = 2.50) significantly more than depression alone (HR = 1.20) or diabetes alone (HR = 1.88). Similar results were found for coronary heart disease mortality (HR for comorbid diabetes and depression = 2.43). An analysis of 10 studies with 42,363 participants of whom 5,325 had diabetes mellitus and depression and 37,038 only diabetes showed a HR for all-cause mortality of 1.5 for those with diabetes and depression [21]. An analysis of the electronic medical records from the VA healthcare system identified a cohort free of cardiovascular disease in 1999 and 2000 [22]. They were divided into four groups: no diabetes mellitus and no depression ($n = 214,749$); depression alone ($n = 77,568$); type 2 diabetes alone ($n = 12,697$); comorbid type 2 diabetes and depression ($n = 11,659$). A 7-year follow-up for the occurrence of myocardial infarction showed an incidence of 2.6% in those with neither diabetes nor depression, 3.5% in those with depression, 5.9% in those with type 2 diabetes, and 7.4% in those with both depression and diabetes. After adjusting for covariates, patients with either depression alone or type 2 diabetes alone had a 30% increased risk for myocardial infarction. Those with both depression and diabetes had an 82% increased risk for myocardial infarction (HR 1.82).

Contemporary issues

Major unresolved issues in managing patients with comorbid diabetes mellitus and depression focus on developing strategies which can effectively treat each condition. Of great importance are the observations that the treatment of each condition also improves the other condition. Short-term treatment of major depressive disorder (MDD) with antidepressants in patients with diabetes provide a response in 60% and a full remission in 46%, but such a response is short lived as one-third of patients with a successful response will have a relapse or recurrence within 1 year and less than 10% remain depression free for 5 years [23]. Diabetes control in patients with concomitant depression is poor with most patients having HbA1c > 8.0%. Effective treatment of the depression has been reported to improve HbA1c in some (8.3% to 7.7%; 10.5% to 9.5%) [24,25], but not all studies [26,27]. Diabetes management factors which significantly increase depressive symptoms and contribute to the increased non-adherence to both diabetes and depression management are insulin therapy, hypoglycaemia, and finger sticks for blood glucose measurements.

Gastric modulation therapy: an interventional strategy to treat overweight and obese individuals with type 2 diabetes

A new interventional therapy, non-stimulatory gastric electrical stimulation (GES) under development for the treatment of overweight and obese patients with type 2 diabetes has several unique characteristics which might make it a reasonable treatment for patients with comorbid diabetes and depression [28,29]. The DIAMOND device (Fig. 14.1) has been described in detail previously [29]. Three pairs of electrodes are implanted under laparoscopic conditions into the fundal, anterior, and posterior antral regions of the stomach. The electrodes are attached to a pulse generator (IPG) which is placed in a pocket created by the surgeon in the abdominal subcutaneous fat. In DIAMOND II, a charging coil is attached to the IPG. The characteristics of the non-stimulatory electric pulse is set by an external programmer. The device automatically detects food ingestion by a change in impedance of the fundal electrodes as the fundus dilates and by a decrease in electrical slow wave activity detected by the antral electrodes. When the food detection signals are received by the IPG, it sends electric pulses to the antral electrodes timed to arrive during the refractory

DIAMONDII-System Components

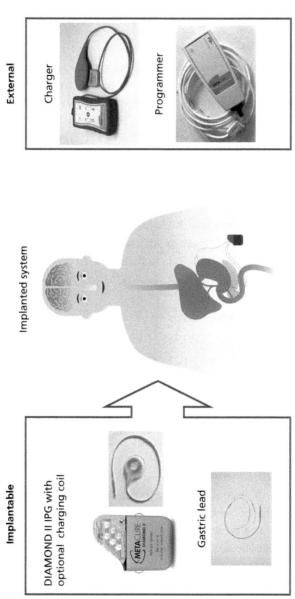

Implantable

Implanted system

External

DIAMOND II IPG with
optional charging coil

Charger

Gastric lead

Programmer

Fig. 14.1 Components of the DIAMOND II gastric electrical stimulatory device. A pair of electrodes is implanted into the fundus and anterior and posterior antral regions of the stomach as shown in the figure. The electrodes are attached to the impulse generator which is imbedded in a pocket in the abdominal fat created by the surgeon. The impulse generator is charged weekly by external current from the charger which is placed over the charging coil which is attached to the IPG. The characteristics of the electric impulse generated is set by the programmer. The DIAMOND device is an experimental device being developed for the treatment of overweight and obese patients with type 2 diabetes not adequately controlled on oral antidiabetic agents and is not currently approved for clinical use.

period of the intrinsic electrical signal. Such a pulse does not change the rate of antral contraction, but does increase the force of contraction and increases the neural signals transmitted from the antrum to the hindbrain. The battery in the IPG is recharged weekly by placing the charger which is connected to an external electric source over the charging coil of the IPG. Gastric contractility modulation (GCM) is delivered for 75 minutes (15 minutes on, alternating with 15 minutes off) starting at meal detection. The electrical impulses are delivered to the antral electrodes synchronized to the local intrinsic gastric slow wave. Electrical pulses use a biphasic symmetric waveform having a phase duration of 6 ms, a repetition rate of 83 Hz, a pulse duration of 1,200 ms and an amplitude of 5–10 mA depending on the patient's tolerability.

Clinical results of gastric electrical stimulation

Over 150 patients with type 2 diabetes inadequately controlled (HbA1c >7.0% and <10.5%) with oral antihyperglycaemic agents have been or are being treated with the DIAMOND device for periods ranging from 1 to 5 years. Table 14.1 presents results from one study in which patients were followed longitudinally for as long as 24 months [28]. A more detailed analysis of 50 patients from that study who had complete weight data over 12 months and glycaemic control data (HbA1c) over 1–2 years are shown in Table 14.2.

The patients had a mean age of 52.5 years and were equally divided between males and females. The baseline HbA1c was 8.3% and body weight was 107 kg. The mean decrease in HbA1c was 0.8% and the mean decrease in body weight was –4.3 kg or 4.2% of the baseline body weight. As has been shown in previous publications, the decrease in HbA1c is a linear function of the baseline HbA1c before the initiation of DIAMOND therapy [28,29]. The higher the baseline HbA1c the greater is the decrease (baseline mean 8.7%, decrease –1.13%) and

Table 14.1 Effect of DIAMOND treatment on glycaemic control in overweight and obese patients with type 2 diabetes inadequately controlled on oral antihyperglycaemic agents: longitudinal data in 61 patients over 2 years

	Baseline	6 months	12 months	18 months	24 months
Number	61	60	47	28	23
Mean	8.32	7.40	7.48	7.28	7.44
SD	0.81	1.01	1.06	0.95	1.27
SEM	0.10	0.13	0.15	0.17	0.26
p		0.0000002	0.0000002	0.0000006	0.0001

Table 14.2 Effect of DIAMOND treatment on glycaemic control and weight loss in 50 overweight or obese patients with type 2 diabetes inadequately controlled on oral antihyperglycaemic agents (metformin alone or combined with sulfonylureas and/or thiazolidinediones)

	Total population	Normal triglycerides (≤1.7 mmol/L)	High triglycerides (>1.7 mmol/L)
Number	50	32	18
Age (years)	52.5	53.0	51.6
Gender (M/F)	24/26	17/15	7/11
Baseline weight (kg)	107.1 ± 3.5	103.0 ± 4.2	112.1 ± 6.2
Weight loss at 1 year (kg)	−4.3 ± 1.0*	−4.7 ± 1.1*	−3.5 ±0.9**
Weight loss at 1 year (%)	−4.2 ± 0.8		
Baseline HbA1c (%)	8.33 ± 0.12	8.38 ± 0.16	8.24 ± 0.20
Decrease in HbA1c (%) at last value between 12 and 24 months	−0.81 ± 0.17*	−1.08 ± 0.20*	−0.34 ± 0.195
Mean Triglyceride over 1 year (mmol/L)	1.77 ± 0.15	1.31 ± 0.05	2.59 ± 0.32

$*p < 0.001$; $**p < 0.002$.

the lower the baseline the less is the decrease (mean baseline HbA1c 7.5%, decrease 0.11%). The response in individual patients is also a function of the fasting plasma triglyceride levels and is documented in Table 14.2. A comparison of the relationship between baseline HbA1c and change in HbA1c in this set of normal and high triglyceride groups was analysed using analysis of covariance (ANCOVA). The analysis showed a statistically significant interaction between the variables: triglyceride group ($p = 0.02$), baseline HbA1c ($p = 0.001$) and decrease in HbA1c at 12 months of DIAMOND treatment [28]. Their interaction was statistically significant ($p < 0.01$). Baseline HbA1c, the triglyceride group, and their interaction accounts for 40% of the variability of the HbA1c decrease [28].

DIAMOND treatment causes a modest weight loss in addition to its glycaemic improvement. This weight loss is due to a decrease in body fat and a reduction in waist circumference, which is a surrogate for visceral fat mass (Table 14.3)

Table 14.3 Effect of DIAMOND treatment for 12 months on metabolic parameters in eight obese Chinese patients with poorly controlled type 2 diabetes

	Baseline	**6 months**	**12 months**
Age (years)	43.9 ± 3.7		
Gender (M/F)	5/3		
Body Mass Index (kg/m²)	29.1 ± 0.7	27.9 ± 1.2*	28.3 ± 1.2*
Body weight (kg_)	80.4 ± 4.0	76.3 ± 4.7*	77.2 ± 4.7*
Body fat (%)	33.5 ± 2.4	28.6 ± 1.0*	30.7 ± 2.9*
Waist circumference (cm)	98.9 ± 0.8	94.3 ± 1.6*	95.0 ± 1.9*
HbA1c (%)	9.1 ± 0.3	7.5 ± 0.3*	8.2 ± 0.5*
Fasting plasma glucose (mmol/L)	10.8 ± 0.9	7.2 ± 0.6*	8.4 ± 0.8*
Systolic blood pressure (mm Hg)	129.0 ± 2.9		124.5 ± 3.8*
Diastolic blood pressure (mm Hg)	78.8 ± 1.5		77.0 ± 1.3
Total cholesterol (mmol/L)	5.0 ± 0.3	4.7 ± 0.3	4.8 ± 0.3

* $p < 0.05$ for paired differences from baseline.

[30]. The decrease in body weight is somewhat greater in patients with normal triglyceride levels than high triglyceride levels but the difference did not achieve statistical significance. However the percentage of patients achieving weight loss of 10 kg or greater was statistically significantly higher (Fisher's exact test) in the normal triglyceride population (7 of 15) than in the high triglyceride population (0 of 16) [28]. Diamond treatment reduces systolic but not diastolic blood pressure (Table 14.3) [30].

An important feature of DIAMOND treatment is that it modifies eating behaviour and increases satiety, resulting in a mean 4.2% decrease in body weight after 12 months of treatment. Eating behaviour was assessed by the German modification of Stunkard and Messick's Three Factor Eating Questionnaire (TFEQ) at baseline, and after 20 and 52 weeks of DIAMOND treatment in 10 type 2 diabetic patients inadequately managed with oral antihyperglycaemic agents [31]. The results of the metabolic effects of DIAMOND treatment in these patients and their change in eating behaviour are shown in Table 14.4. DIAMOND treatment increased cognitive restraint of eating, reduced disinhibition and reduced hunger. The weight loss associated with DIAMOND treatment is most likely due to these changes in eating behaviour and to an increase in satiety.

Table 14.4 DIAMOND treatment and changes in eating behaviour. Ten obese patients with type 2 diabetes inadequately controlled on oral agents were evaluated by the German edition of the Stunkard and Messick three-factor eating questionnaire at baseline, and after 20 weeks and 52 weeks of treatment by the DIAMOND non-excitatory gastric contractility modulation (GCM) device [31,32]

	Baseline	**20 weeks**	**52 weeks**
Age (years)	52.9 ± 1.9		
BMI (kg/m²)	44.6 ± 1.2		
Waist circumference (cm)	136.6 ±2.9		
HbA1c (%)	8.3 ± 0.2		
Decrease in HbA1c (%)		−1.5 ± 0.2*	−0.9 ± 0.3*
Weight (kg)	132.4 ± 6.7		
Decrease in weight (kg)		−7.4 ± 1.6*	−6.3 ± 3.4*
Percentage decrease in body weight		−5.6%	−4.7%
Cognitive restraint of eating	11.2 ± 1.7	14.0 ± 1.2*	13.7 ±1.3*
Disinhibition	9.8 ±1.3	5.9 ± 1.0*	Same as 20 weeks
Hunger	6.5 ±1.4	3.8 ± 1.2*	4.3 ±1.5*

*$p < 0.05$.

DIAMOND: safety issues

The relevant safety issues with the DIAMOND II are device- implantation related. In the 134 patients implanted there were 12 device-related adverse events, including three cases of vibration sensation when the device was activated requiring the current to be reduced, two lead impedance inconsistencies, five events of device down mode transiently, one case of pressure pain from the impulse generator, and one episode of hyperglycaemia when the device was transiently turned off. There were 27 implantation-related adverse events: nine events of postoperative pain at the laparoscopic insertion site, eight short-term episodes of abdominal pain, five cases of non-infectious inflammation around the pocket, two cases of gastro-oesophageal efflux, two episodes of postoperative vomiting, and one event of scarring and oedema around the pocket. All events were mild to moderate in severity and were resolved easily. Three patients who were on sulphonylureas had mild hypoglycaemia when the DIAMOND was activated and the sulphonylurea dose was decreased or discontinued.

Aspects of DIAMOND treatment that might be beneficial in treating comorbid diabetes and depression

DIAMOND treatment of type 2 diabetes has several features that make it an attractive option to treat comorbid diabetes and depression. The device automatically detects food ingestion [33]. The current device can detect up to five meals per day with approximately an 85% accuracy. The meal detection triggers a 75-minute postprandial stimulation. The DIAMOND has a central nervous system effect that changes eating behaviour and increases satiety so that it is easier for many patients to comply with their dietary management. DIAMOND treatment is associated with modest short-term side effects that are transient and minimal long-term side effects. The device can be used as an alternative to the addition of insulin since it does not cause hypoglycaemia and is associated with weight loss rather than weight gain. Finger sticks for blood glucose measurements can be minimized. The patient's burden of diabetes management is significantly reduced by the DIAMOND device and this is of significant benefit in improving compliance particularly in diabetic patients who are depressed.

Potential issues in the DIAMOND treatment of diabetic patients with depression are the lack of clinical trial data. The data indicating that the best response to the DIAMOND is in those with normal triglyceride levels may initially limit the use of the DIAMOND device to that population but since the linear correlation between triglyceride levels and improvement in HbA1c has a correlation coefficient of 0.341, $p = 0.002$ (unpublished data) it may be possible to improve the response of hypertriglyceridemic patients by treatments that decrease triglyceride levels. A clinical trial to test this hypothesis is ongoing.

Summary

Comorbid diabetes and depression presents a major clinical challenge. Each component of the comorbid condition has detrimental effects on the other condition. Clinical data suggest that depression increases the incidence of diabetes mellitus and in those who already have diabetes mellitus, it worsens metabolic control and increases chronic diabetic complications. Diabetes creates a huge burden for the depressed patient and worsens the clinical course and the response to therapy. The DIAMOND device is an interventional treatment for overweight and obese patients with type 2 diabetes. It minimizes non-adherence, reduces the burden of diabetes management in patients, improves glycaemic control, causes modest weight loss and reduces systolic blood pressure. It is a treatment worth considering in some patients with concomitant diabetes and depression.

References

1. **Kessler RC, Bromet EJ.** The epidemiology of depression across cultures. *Annual Review of Public Health* 2013; **34**:119–38.

2. **Lustman PJ, Penckofer SM, Clouse RE.** Recent advances in understanding depression in adults with diabetes. *Current Psychiatry Reports* 2008;**10**:495–502.

3. **Holt RIG, de Groot M, Golden SH.** Diabetes and depression. *Current Diabetes Reports* 2014;**14**:491.

4. **Eaton WW, Armenian HA, Gallo J, Pratt L, Ford DE.** Depression and risk of for onset of type II diabetes: a prospective population based study. *Diabetes Care* 1996;**19**:1097–102.

5. **Kawakami N, Takatsuka N, Shimizu H, Ishibashi H.** Depressive symptoms and occurrence of type 2 diabetes among Japanese men. *Diabetes Care* 1999;**22**:1071–6.

6. **Knol MJ, Twisk JW, Beekman AT,** et al. Depression as a risk factor for the onset of type 2 diabetes mellitus. A meta-analysis. *Diabetologia* 2006;**49**:837–45.

7. **Rotella F, Mannucci E.** Depression as a risk factor for diabetes: a meta-analysis of longitudinal studies. Journal of *Clinical Psychiatry* 2013;**74**:31–7.

8. **Yu M, Zhang X, Lu F, Fang L.** Depression and risk for diabetes: a meta-analysis. *Canadian Journal of Diabetes* 2015;**39**:266–72.

9. **Ali S, Stone MA, Peters JL,** et al. The prevalence of co-morbid depression in adults with type 2 diabetes: a systemic review and meta-analysis. *Diabetic Medicine* 2006;**23**:1165–73.

10. **Anderson RJ, Freedland KE, Clouse RE, Lustman PJ.** The prevalence of comorbid depression in adults with diabetes: a meta-analysis. *Diabetes Care* 2001;**24**:1069–78.

11. **Rotella F, Manmucci E.** Diabetes as a risk factor for depression. A meta-analysis of longitudinal studies. *Diabetes Research and Clinical Practice* 2013;**99**:98–104.

12. **Vancampfort D, Mitchell AJ, De Hert M,** et al. Type 2 diabetes in patients with major depressive disorder: a meta-analysis of prevalence estimates and predictors. *Depress Anxiety* 2015;**32**:763–73.

13. **Bogner HR, de Vries HE, O'Donnell AJ, Morales KH.** Measuring concurrent oral hypoglycemic and antidepressant adherence and clinical outcomes. *American Journal of Managing Care* 2014;**19**:e85–e92.

14. **Gonzalez JS, Peyrot M, McCarl LA,** et al. Depression and diabetes treatment nonadherence: a meta-analysis. *Diabetes Care* 2008;**31**:2398–403.

15. **Krass I, Schieback P, Dhippayom T.** Adherence to diabetes medication: a systemic review. *Diabetic Medicine* 2015;**32**:725–37.

16. **Lustman PJ, Anderson RJ, Freedland KE, de Groot M, Carney RM, Clouse RE.** Depression and poor glycemic control. A meta-analytic review of the literature. *Diabetes Care* 2000;**23**:934–42.

17. **Polonsky WH, Henry RR.** Poor medication adherence in type 2 diabetes: recognizing the scope of the problem and its key contributors. *Patient Preference and Adherence* 2016;**10**:1299–307.

18. **Bogner HR, Morales KH, Post ER, Bruce MI.** Diabetes, depression and death. *Diabetes Care* 2007;**30**:3005–10.

19. **De Groot M, Anderson R, Freedland KE, Clouse RE, Lustman PJ.** Association of depression and diabetes complications: a meta-analysis. *Psychosomatic Medicine* 2001;**63**:619–30.

20. **Egede LE, Nietert PJ, Zheng D.** Depression and all-cause and coronary heart disease mortality among adults with and without diabetes. *Diabetes Care* 2005;**28**:1339–45.

21. **Park M, Katon WJ, Wolf FM.** Depression and risk of mortality in individuals with: a meta-analysis and systemic review. *General Hospital Psychiatry* 2013;**35**:217–25.

22. **Scherrer JF, Garfield LD, Chrusciel T,** et al. Increased risk of myocardial infarction in depressed patients with type 2 diabetes. *Diabetes Care* 2011;**34**:1729–34.

23. **Lustman PJ, Griffith LS, Clouse RE.** Depression in adults with diabetes. Results of 5-yr follow-up study. *Diabetes Care* 1988;**11**:605–12.

24. **Anderson RJ, Gott BM, Sayuk GS,** et al. Antidepressant pharmacotherapy in adults with type 2 diabetes. Rates and predictors of initial response. *Diabetes Care* 2010;**33**:485–9.

25. **Lustman PJ, Griffith LS, Freedland KE,** et al. Cognitive behavior therapy for depression in type 2 diabetes mellitus. A randomized, controlled trial. *Annals of Intern Med* 1998;**129**:613–21.

26. **Georgiades A, Zucker N, Friedman KE,** et al. Changes in depressive symptoms and glycemic control in diabetes mellitus. *Psychosomatic Medicine* 2007;**69**:235–41.

27. **Huang Y, Wei X, Wu T, Chen R, Guo A.** Collaborative care for patients with depression and diabetes mellitus: a systematic review and meta-analysis. *BMC Psychiatry* 2013:**13**:260.

28. **Lebovitz HE, Ludvik B, Yaniv I,** et al. Treatment of patients with obese type 2 diabetes with Tantalus-DIAMOND gastric electrical stimulation: normal triglycerides predict durable effects for at least 3 years. *Hormone and Metabolic Research* 2015;**47**:456–62.

29. **Lebovitz HE.** Interventional treatment of obesity and diabetes: an interim report on gastric electrical stimulation. *Review of Endocrine and Metabolic Disorders* 2016;**17**:73–80.

30. **Wong SK, Kong AP-S, Luk AO-Y,** et al. A pilot study to compare meal-triggered gastric electrical stimulation and insulin treatment in Chinese obese type 2 diabetes. *Diabetes Technology and Therapeutics* 2015;**17**:283–90.

31. **Bohdjalian A, Prager G, Rosak C,** et al. Improvement in glycemic control in morbidly obese type 2 diabetic subjects by gastric stimulation. *Obesity Surgery* 2009; **19**:1221–7.

32. **Stunkard AJ, Messick S.** The three-factor eating questionnaire to measure dietary restraint, disinhibition and hunger. *Journal of Psychsometric Research* 1985;**29**:71–83.

33. **Policker S, Lu H, Haddad W,** et al. Electrical stimulation of the gut for the treatment of type 2 diabetes: the role of automatic eating detection. *Journal of Diabetes Science and Technology* 2008; **2**:906–12.

Chapter 15

Current and emerging psychological models

Christopher Garrett

Introduction

Comorbid depression and type 2 diabetes are associated with glycaemic control and advanced complications [1,2]. The co-existence of the two conditions and increased morbidity and mortality inclines clinicians and researchers to treat both conditions together. Pharmacological co-treatment is discussed elsewhere; however, psychosocial interventions also attempt to improve mood and anxiety symptoms as well as directly or indirectly address glycaemic control in type 2 diabetes. This chapter critiques the current models for psychological interventions and suggests that we may need to take a more lifespan perspective when developing non-pharmacological interventions to support self-care.

Rationale for co-treatment

Before attempting to treat diabetes and depression using a single psychosocial intervention one must first understand the psychosocial elements of the two conditions.

Psychosocial perspective of type 2 diabetes

Glucose control in type 2 diabetes is connected to three key behavioural elements namely diet, exercise, and use of prescribed medications.

- Diet: food habits evolve through the life cycle and are constituted by personal tastes, family heritage, cost, and convenience. Diet is also affected by use of food as a method of emotion regulation, which is particularly relevant for certain psychiatric conditions including depression.
- Exercise: use of one's body for work and play is affected by long-term habits, work conditions, and social norms.

◆ Medication use: intellectual understanding of condition including future impact of complications, emotional burden of condition, and support in close relationships are important factors in treatment concordance.

These factors are underpinned by psychological, socioeconomic, and cultural elements, the complexity of which has led to the use of health psychology models including the Theory of Planned Behaviour and the Theory of Reasoned Action, which attempt to understand the constituent health behaviours through underlying intentions. These ideas have been used to shape psychosocial interventions to varying levels of success. A recent published example of such an intervention was a randomized controlled trial using motivational techniques delivered by practice nurses trained in psychological techniques [3]. A key active ingredient in such an intervention is a clinician's ability to evoke a desire to change diabetes behaviours in individuals with the condition. Once such a desire has been elicited, the clinician's role is to help the patient to understand what aspects of their character and life circumstances will help them to make changes in diet, exercise, or medication use or conversely hinder such changes.

Psychosocial perspective of depression

Depression is a mental health condition characterized by pervasive low mood, lack of enjoyment, and low energy levels as well as negative ideas about oneself, one's environment or future, and biological symptoms such as early morning wakening and poor concentration. It can be described across four interconnecting mental health domains: cognitions, affect, behaviour, and relationships; through these the effect on type 2 diabetes can be illustrated.

• Cognitions: thoughts and ideas are typically negative in depression and experienced concretely, that is with little possibility that they are incorrect or arise because of the depression itself. Engaging with a condition such as diabetes while overwhelmed by negative ideas is continually difficult. For example, if blood glucose testing is necessary for monitoring, negativity can affect the purpose of testing ('why should I bother'), the experience of testing ('it should hurt, I deserve to be hurt'), and the result ('I'm failing at diabetes, I fail at everything'). A further example might include a profound over-inclusive experience of guilt or blame associated with acquiring type 2 diabetes ('I have brought this upon myself').

• Affect: mood is continually low in depression and punctuated by periods of tearfulness or disconnectedness or numbness, with little or no enjoyment. Such chronic levels of sadness can cause apathy and lack of motivation and might lead to a failure to initiate changes that might benefit future health such as increasing exercise or a beneficial change in diet.

- Behaviour: the actions of a depressed person are directed and shaped by the cognitions and affect as previously described. For example, low self-esteem and self-loathing driving self-destructive behaviours that range from poor self-care in the form of non-adherence [1], to self-harm and suicide, which has increased incidence in diabetes [4]. An additional common behaviour seen in depression is episodic dysregulated eating or so-called binge eating, which can lead to profound weight gain and treatment failure in patients with diabetes.
- Relationships: connectedness to family and friends during depression is markedly reduced. The affected person becomes more withdrawn, guarded, and less trustful in those around them, including clinicians. This inevitably leads to patients being less likely to attend appointments or to follow a clinician's advice [5].

Current psychological or psychosocial interventions

This section sets out the evidence base for current psychological interventions used to treat diabetes with depression or improve glucose control. They fall broadly into 2 categories, those specifically treating depression (cognitive behavioural therapy (CBT) and counselling and supportive psychotherapy) with the premise that it will also improve diabetes behaviours or those approaching diabetes behaviours (psychological and educational and motivational interviewing and other interventions) and a by-product will be an improvement in symptoms of depression. A third category combines elements of both depression treatment and diabetes behavioural approaches within a diabetes and mental health interdisciplinary service.

Cognitive behavioural therapy

CBT has been a long-established treatment for psychological disorders and is recommended by many national and international bodies as first-line treatment for depression and anxiety disorders. In type 2 diabetes research it is the most commonly used psychological intervention [1,6]. CBT interventions are generally one to one, but can be delivered in a group setting or online. They are short, lasting 6 to 12 sessions, though more complex presentations can be treated over a longer time period. The central focus is the interconnecting aspects of thoughts, feelings, behavioural responses, and bodily experiences in the here and now. Patients will often be asked to keep a mood or thoughts diary, which will be referred to during sessions to investigate how a thought has arisen and help increase a patient's level of self-knowledge and rebalance away from more negative interpretations. Much of the work is about reframing or questioning of negative cognitions. Is a particular self-critical idea correct? A diabetes example might be to address a negative cognition, which has arisen from a high blood glucose reading after an enjoyable, but high glucose meal. The individual might become particularly self-critical and catastrophize the one-off glucose and convince themselves that they have completely failed at diabetes. Cognitive reframing would therefore consist of a reassessment of the evidence and attempt to neutralize the experience of self-blame that is common in depressed states. A more complex behavioural example for diabetes might be the attribution of sweating to hypoglycaemia (with subsequent requirement of testing) rather than anxiety. In such an example, a so-called positive behaviour (i.e. testing) is actually a manifestation of a mental health presentation and without careful elucidation might not be realized as such.

Counselling and supportive psychotherapy

Counselling or supportive psychotherapy is a short, semi-structured exploratory intervention, normally lasting less than 6 months and can be as time limited as six sessions. Its theoretical background is a mosaic of different theoretical models, with different geographical areas favouring different approaches though most would have features of Adlereian Individual Psychology [7] and Gestalt, that is considering the whole person [8]. At its core it provides a safe place with a reflective thoughtful therapist, where the patient's complete concerns are at the centre of things. This less clearly defined approach makes reproducibility through a manualized intervention more difficult though efficacy is comparable with CBT [9]. Though infrequently used in type 2 diabetes and depression research, after CBT it is one of the most commonly used interventions for depression within primary care. An advantage in diabetes practice over a more structured intervention such as CBT is an ability to explore how diabetes affects the person as an individual and also through providing support while the person strives for resilience to adjust and cope with the condition.

Psychological and educational interventions

Although essential as an adjunct to most psychotherapeutic interventions, psychoeducational interventions have limited efficacy on their own, particularly in moderate to severe mental health presentations. They consist of an educational programme and/or material on mental health, which are designed to improve an individual's understanding of their mind or of a particular psychiatric condition and often are delivered to groups or increasingly as online modules. As an adjunct they are often used in preparation, prior to starting a more in-depth, supportive intervention. In diabetes self-management education, there is an expectation that a psychoeducational intervention is part of a comprehensive diabetes educational package [10]. This would likely take the form of an exploration of the impact of type 2 diabetes and its affect on emotional well-being and associated behaviours.

Motivational interviewing and other interventions

MI is not specifically indicated in treatment of depression. However, it is increasingly used by non-mental health professionals in diabetes services and primary care as a behaviour change tool aiming to alter diet, increase exercise, and stop cigarette smoking. However, although popular, research interventions for MI have produced mixed outcomes in type 2 diabetes [11] and there is very little evidence for its effectiveness for depression [12]. MI is a brief intervention, sometimes with as few as one or two sessions with the aim to evoke a desire to change in an individual. Once a wish to change has been alighted upon, the person is guided through what would be the positives and pitfalls of change and supported in putting together plans to initiate and then maintain the changes in the person's life. Other types of psychological intervention used in diabetes research include 'problem focused' and 'behaviour change' approaches, often where delivery of an intervention is by a diabetes clinician, supervised by a clinical psychologist and where interventions are particularly focussed on specific diabetes behaviours.

Psychosocial interdisciplinary interventions

Psychosocial interventions might have CBT as a constituent part of a broader multidisciplinary intervention. Patients managed within such a service will be assessed by a mental health professional, for example a psychiatrist, and a treatment programme will be formulated depending on precipitating or perpetuating factors. Teams will consist of a psychiatrist and/or clinical psychologist, a social worker, and a diabetes clinician. The social intervention might consist of helping an individual to improve their living conditions through assistance in applying for increased social care benefits or improving access through translation services or support in returning to work. The 'psych' aspect of the intervention might consist of a psychopharmacological treatment of depression or a brief CBT package. In the UK, Doherty and colleagues described 'Three dimensions for diabetes (3DFD)' as an example of a successful psychosocial intervention in improving mental health and diabetes management [13]. Their programme used a case management approach and several different psychotherapeutic approaches including CBT, MI (see earlier), and family work, as well as social interventions such as debt advocacy, literacy, and support with accessing appropriate housing.

Limitations of current interventions

A meta-analysis and two systematic reviews have been conducted on psychosocial interventions in diabetes and depression over the last 5 years [6,14,15], and all concluded in their analyses of type 2 diabetes that although there is an improvement in depression outcomes, glucose control, the outcome measure for diabetes, does not improve. In their meta-analysis, Baumeister and colleagues [6] pooled findings from eight studies, five of which did not show a significant change in glycaemic control compared with their control group, resulting in a non-significant pooled effect size overall. Interestingly, in the same paper, a meta-analysis on pharmacological interventions for depression indicated an improvement in depression outcomes and a statistical improvement in glycaemic control.

Although these results are disappointing the findings suggest new directions for future research, both for the interventions used and in the fundamental theories that are being examined. There are two key questions to address. Is the link between depression and glucose control cause or association? Is it the lack of focus on diabetes in the interventions that must be resolved in future studies to harness the potential of a psychosocial intervention?

The association between depression and poor glycaemic control was initially assumed to be causal. However, the inconsistent findings on meta-analyses across pharmacological and psychological treatments for depression suggest that a causal link is too simplistic. In their review paper on depression in diabetes and diabetes distress, Fisher and colleagues [16] also refer to the variable association of depression symptoms and glycaemic control, pointing to the higher levels of depression in insulin using patients with type 2 and in patients with co-morbid physical health conditions. They infer from this that it is the emotional burden of diabetes *per se*, incrementally worsened by increased need for self-management or associated with other conditions, that is the context resulting in higher symptom scores for self-rated depression scales. This emotional burden, also referred to as diabetes distress, and codified by self-rating scales such as PAID or DDS17 [17,18], has itself been found to be associated with glycaemic control rather than depression [19,20,21], and another research group found that diabetes distress mediated the effect of depression on glycaemic control [22]. Key themes in diabetes distress are the social effect of the condition, relationship with clinicians, and regimen-related distress and one might envisage the interplay of these aspects with low mood and self-management. As yet though, the relative importance of each and other elements such as resilience and coping are yet to be defined.

With the diabetes component playing a key part in the potential severity of depression and a growing understanding of the role of diabetes distress, the lack of diabetes focus is a weakness in the psychological interventions that have been investigated to date. However, although tailoring the intervention so that it specifically addresses the interface of the two conditions and diabetes distress is a rational approach, the diversity of presentations might make a manualized CBT programme difficult. Superficially two patients might have high depression scores and poor glycaemic control, though clinically they might be very different, for example an obese patient with depression and dysregulated eating is likely to require a different approach from a depressed patient with no eating problems but severely non-adherent to medication. In comparison, an explorative intervention, which is able to adapt flexibly to the clinical setting, though keeping a focus on diabetes as a key component to the intervention, might be of greater advantage in this setting.

Personality, attachment, and type 2 diabetes

It is an important caveat to note the limited evidence for interventions attempting to impact behaviour change in type 1 and 2 diabetes in patients without depression [23,24]. This emphasizes the magnitude of the challenge involved and the ambition that will be necessary to significantly impact diabetes control.

The fact that diabetes behaviours are difficult to influence implies that either interventions are not efficacious or possibly that behaviours are linked to more stable aspects of human psychology, such as personality traits, which are much less susceptible to short-term psychological interventions. Within the field of psychological research, personality is defined as a group of characteristic behaviours and emotional responses that make up an individual. These characteristics or 'traits' are grouped together by some researchers into five main themes: conscientiousness, extroversion, neuroticism, agreeableness, and openness to experience. Using these so-called big five personality traits, several research groups have investigated the risk of type 2 diabetes and glycaemic control. In a large multinational longitudinal study of personality traits and type 2 diabetes, low conscientiousness was consistently associated with acquiring type 2, partially mediated through obesity and physical inactivity and, importantly, was also associated with subsequent mortality [25]. This finding has been replicated in two large national studies, which have suggested that low conscientiousness was mediating polygenic risk of type 2 diabetes [26,27].

A national cross-sectional study further defined tendency to 'order' as a key facet of conscientiousness in mitigating diabetes risk, mediated through BMI, alcohol intake, physical activity and diet, all behaviours associated with low impulse control [28]. Similarly, once diabetes is established, conscientiousness has been found to be associated with lower HbA1c in a type 1 diabetes setting [29], and a longitudinal study of personality traits in type 2 found higher altruism was positively associated with HbA1c, at baseline and follow-up [30]. Supporting this finding, Hyphantis and colleagues found that self-sacrificing traits, which are akin to altruistic traits, predicted higher HbA1c in a longitudinal study of type 2 diabetes, a finding that the authors linked to neglecting one's own self-care over the needs of others [31]. Interestingly, Hall and colleagues [32] found that higher tendency to anxious temperament appeared to lead to earlier detection of type 2 diabetes, presumably through anxiety driven higher vigilance and presentation to primary care, but that once detected, the anxiety did not aid self-management at follow-up. The effects of personality traits may be attenuated in a diabetes condition that is mostly symptomless and lacks the physiological reminders of a condition such as pain in osteoarthritis.

If certain personality characteristics are players in development of type 2 diabetes and subsequent outcomes, these traits will inevitably be more frequently seen in the type 2 diabetes population that is struggling to maintain good glycaemic control. It is also possible that these traits are predisposing to a subtype of depression less amenable to usual treatment. Therefore understanding personality maturation and its developmental links with the key diabetes behaviours referred to at the start of this chapter (diet, exercise, and adherence to medication) could lead to psychosocial interventions with a more sophisticated approach to treating diabetes adherence with or without depression.

Attachment theory is a biopsychosocial approach to development that attempts to explain key elements of personality development throughout the life cycle, including emotional and social development and has already been used in the study of health behaviours in children and with adults with type 2 diabetes. The central premise of attachment is that infants and young children require a stable relationship with a caregiver capable of mentalizing the child's experiences in order for normal psychological development to take place. Mentalization is an unconscious process, which consists of reading and interpreting the intentions and mental states of others, as well as an internal monitoring of ones own emotional states. In extreme situations, difficulties with mentalization present in psychiatric conditions, most frequently emotionally unstable personality disorder. In the parent and child dyad the process of mentalizing involves the caregiver thinking about, mirroring, and verbalizing the experiences of the child (discomfort, upset, anger, hunger) so that they develop a structure of thinking about emotion and learn the differences between the inner and outer world and the separateness of the self and other. It is well recognized that mentalizing aids the attachment process and that mother's that have high levels of mentalization are more likely to have securely attached children than mothers less able to mentalize [33]. Broadly speaking, securely attached children with higher levels of mentalization have greater ability to understand and tolerate their emotions, whereas insecurely attached children will struggle more with emotions and relationships, sometimes using other processes for emotion regulation, such as blame, avoiding close relationships or overeating. In a clinical setting, for disengaged, non-attending patients or patients that repeatedly re-present but with little clinical improvement, attachment insecurity is a primary differential. Such patients are more likely to struggle with establishing a therapeutic relationship primarily because of a lack of trust in all people, not only clinicians [34]. Affect regulation is more difficult with low levels of mentalization because the individual is less able to think about and represent what is going on in their mind or the mind of the other leading to higher levels of distress, and use of alternative methods to contain distress including poor health behaviours. In addition it also makes a consistent and coherent approach to living with type 2 diabetes less likely; with ever-changing mood comes an ever-changing mind set as to how one copes with the condition or the importance that one places on maintaining beneficial health behaviours. Where mentalizing is the ideal scenario, the three non-mentalizing states are more problematic and have a symbiotic relationship with affect regulation. Psychic equivalence is one of the non-mentalizing states and is a state of mind where internal and external reality are perceived as identical, i.e. what is imagined has to be true. For instance, an individual might believe that they are not able to alter diet because those around them would not be supportive or because a person like them isn't meant to use a gym. These ideas are experienced concretely and are hence less likely to be available to change. In addition to this, the inability to think about the self and mind as a construct and therefore to some extent malleable is likely to lead to an inability to imagine the self as different. For example, it might be difficult to imagine oneself as a non-smoker through difficulties in mentalizing. Another example of non-mentalizing states is pretend mode, whereby the individual can appreciate the difference between internal and external reality but only if an 'as if' 'this is not for real' quality can be maintained. In health behaviour terms, an example of pretend mode might be the person that constructs a complex reason as to why they are unable to change, while at the same time on an unconscious level are aware that this is not the reason why they cannot change.

An example of the potential links between secure and insecure attachment and future risk of type 2 diabetes is seen in two studies that illustrate the effect of attachment on eating and weight in young children. Bost and colleagues conducted a cross sectional study of 497 children, assessing their attachment relationships, ability to cope with negative affect and eating habits. Those children with insecure attachment relationships, struggled more with negative affect and used eating more frequently to regulate emotion [35]. In a longitudinal study of 8,750 children, Anderson and Whitaker assessed attachment security at 24 months and weight at 4.5 years, finding that insecure attachment was significantly associated with risk of obesity [36]. Although there is not complete continuity between child and adult attachment, strategies developed in childhood for coping with emotion are more likely to persist into adulthood. Researchers in Seattle, USA, studying the effect of adult attachment relationships on type 2 diabetes, conducted a large cross-sectional and subsequent, longitudinal study, finding that insecure attachment style was associated with weight, smoking history, poor exercise, and dietary habits as well as all-cause mortality at follow-up [5,37]. The same research group also found associations between attachment style, depression and non-attendance of diabetes appointments [38].

The future psychosocial interventions

There should not be a one-size fits-all approach to depression with type 2 diabetes. Personality characteristics and attachment appear to shape behaviours potentiating risk of type 2 diabetes and are important in how depression presents and its affect on self-management. They will also affect whether a patient attends appointments and whether a psychosocial intervention is successful. In some patients it must be recognized that type 2 diabetes is the end result of low-level long-term mental health problems in the dimension of emotion regulation and interpersonal difficulty, whereas in others it has resulted from chronic poor health choices leaving a person vulnerable to experiences of guilt and shame and susceptibility to depression. This long lead in is likely to require longer periods of mental health treatment and follow-up and possibly treatment within a service that has clinicians trained across the mental health and diabetes boundaries. Traditional mental health models tend to be recovery based, assuming mental health problems are episodic or transient in nature. However, the chronicity of type 2 diabetes requires a more nuanced long-term approach including the possibility of relapse, which is more frequently seen in more chronic presentations. In addition, even if a period of depression ends, the person still has to contend with life long restrictions on diet and lifestyle.

An intervention able to take into account long-term aspects of personality and attachment and recognize the diversity of presentation under the umbrella of 'depression and type 2 diabetes' should therefore have several key components. Interventions should be stratified and be appropriate for degree of psychopathology and level of glycaemic control. Detailed assessment is therefore required at entry into a treatment programme to aid diagnosis of comorbid mental health conditions (e.g. personality disorder), and in order to guide appropriate level of intervention and experience of treating clinicians. For example, mild episodes of depression with diabetes distress might be seen to improve through a low intensity diabetes-focused educational intervention either in a group setting or online, whilst moderately severe episodes of depression could be more appropriately treated with a CBT type intervention that addresses depression *and* diabetes behaviours. Lastly, more severe episodes of depression will require longer periods of treatment using a longer term explorative style intervention with a diabetes focus, with or without additional psychopharmacological co-treatment. Whatever the level of intervention, however, the emotional and behavioural elements of type 2 diabetes must be a principle focus of the intervention and not be approached as secondary to depression; previous studies oversimplify the connection between glycaemic control and depression, assuming that improved mood automatically leads to improvement in the diabetes behaviours. Following on from this, treatment for depression and diabetes behaviours should in some cases be decoupled so that patients that show improvements in depression symptoms can continue an intervention that focuses more on diet, exercise and/or adherence to treatment and thus be cognoscente of the long-term nature of these behaviours. Goals should be calibrated to the context of severity of presenting mental health difficulty and prior achievements in diabetes management. Patients should not be set up to fail by clinicians expecting quick, unachievable results.

All interventions should be guided by the principles of attachment theory. The central themes of trust and continuity in attachment potentiate an intervention even if not overtly using an attachment orientated psychological intervention, particularly given the difficulties of withdrawal and loss of trust in states of depression. Case management interventions where one or two clinicians have responsibility for managing a patient could easily be adapted to be specifically attachment focused, particularly for the disengaged subgroup of patients that repeatedly non-attend despite evidence of a mental health problem and poor glycaemic control. This would likely require greater effort on the part of the clinician in order to establish trust because of underlying insecure attachment. This might include the option of home visits in the initial stages of engagement and repeated attempts to engage and re-engage the patient to emphasize the availability of the service and the importance that the service places on the therapeutic relationship.

Therapies specifically using attachment theory and mentalization are currently mainly focussed on treatment of emotionally unstable personality disorder [39], although there have also been innovative uses in the adolescent mental health setting with young people that are 'hard to reach' where case workers use mentalizing in order to create a trusted environment and a place for new learning [40]. Mentalization therapy aims to help individuals to coherently understand themselves, regulate emotions and be able to make better life choices that they can consistently adhere to, and broadening this approach to type 2 diabetes would have a logical rationale. Better regulated emotion and thereby less day-to-day stress and distress has a multilayered benefit, both psychologically so that the person copes better with managing diabetes, but also physiologically from hypothalamic–pituitary–adrenal axis responses to stress activation. A tiered format whereby those with least difficulty could be treated using a group psychoeducational intervention, whilst those most impaired might require a group intervention over a time-frame of 18–24 months.

It should be noted that the slowness of therapeutic change, even long after the end of therapy requires extended length of follow-up to establish whether there has been a definitive benefit from an intervention.

Conclusions

Non-pharmacological treatment should be able to aid remission of a depressive episode and improve glycaemic control. However, interventions must take into account other elements including diabetes distress, prior personality characteristics and attachment security, which require careful assessment in the first instance. In the clinical and the research setting, this requires clinicians able to work across the diabetes and mental health setting, with an understanding of their complex psychological and biological interplay.

References

1. **Gonzalez JS, Peyrot M, McCarl LA**, et al. Depression and diabetes treatment nonadherence: a meta-analysis. *Diabetes Care* 2008;**31**:2398–403.
2. **Lin EHB, Rutter CM, Katon W**, et al. Depression and advanced complications of diabetes. *Diabetes Care* 2010;**33**:264–9.
3. **Graves H, Garrett C, Amiel SA**, et al. Psychological skills training to support diabetes self-management: Qualitative assessment of nurses' experiences. *Primary Care Diabetes* 2016;**10**:376–82.
4. **Wang B, An X, Shi X, Zhang J.-A.** Management of endocrine disease: suicide risk in patients with diabetes: a systematic review and meta-analysis. *European Journal of Endocrinology* 2017;**177**:R169–R181.

5. **Lin EHB, Katon W, Von Korff M**, et al. Relationship of depression and diabetes self-care, medication adherence, and preventive care. *Diabetes Care* 2004;**27**:2154–60.

6. **Baumeister H, Hutter N, Bengel J.** Psychological and pharmacological interventions for depression in patients with diabetes mellitus: an abridged Cochrane review. *Diabetic Medicine* 2014;**31**:773–86.

7. **Miller R, Dillman Taylor D.** Does Adlerian theory stand the test of time? Examining individual psychology from a neuroscience perspective. *Journal of Humanistic Counseling* 2016;**55**:111–28.

8. **Fogarty M, Bhar S, Theiler S, O'Shea L.** What do Gestalt therapists do in the clinic: the expert consensus. *British Gestalt Journal* 2016;**25**:32–41.

9. **Cuijpers P, Karyotaki E, Weitz E**, et al. The effects of psychotherapies for major depression in adults on remission, recovery and improvement: a meta-analysis. *Journal of Affective Disorders* 2014;**159**:118–26.

10. **Powers MA, Bardsley J, Cypress M**, et al. Diabetes self-management education and support in type 2 diabetes: a joint position statement of the American Diabetes Association, the American Association of Diabetes Educators, and the Academy of Nutrition and Dietetics. *Diabetes Educator* 2017;**43**:40–53.

11. **Ekong G, Kavookjian J.** Motivational interviewing and outcomes in adults with type 2 diabetes: a systematic review. *Patient Education and Counseling* 2016;**99**:944–52.

12. **Westra HA, Aviram A, Doell FK.** Extending motivational interviewing to the treatment of major mental health problems: current directions and evidence. *Canadian Journal of Psychiatry* 2011;**56**:643–50.

13. **Doherty AM, Britneff E, Gayle C, Ismail K.** Improving outcomes and reducing healthcare costs in diabetes by integrating psychosocial care with medical care: three dimensions of care for diabetes (3dfd). *Diabetic Medicine* 2015;**32**:185.

14. **Kok JLA, Williams A, Zhao L.** Psychosocial interventions for people with diabetes and co-morbid depression. A systematic review. *International Journal of Nursing Studies* 2015;**52**:1625–39.

15. **Markowitz SM, Gonzalez JS, Wilkinson JL, Safren SA.** A review of treating depression in diabetes: emerging findings. *Psychosomatics* 2011;**52**:1–18.

16. **Fisher L, Gonzalez JS, Polonsky WH.** The confusing tale of depression and distress in patients with diabetes: a call for greater clarity and precision. *Diabetic Medicine* 2014;**31**:764–72.

17. **Polonsky WH, Anderson BJ, Lohrer PA**, et al. Assessment of diabetes-related distress. *Diabetes Care* 1995;**18**:754–60.

18. **Polonsky WH, Fisher L, Earles J**, et al. Assessing psychosocial distress in diabetes. *Diabetes Care* 2005;**28**:626–31.

19. **Asuzu CC, Walker RJ, Williams JS, Egede LE.** Pathways for the relationship between diabetes distress, depression, fatalism and glycemic control in adults with type 2 diabetes. *Journal of Diabetes and Its Complications* 2017;**31**:169–74.

20. **Fisher L, Mullan JT, Arean P**, et al. Diabetes distress but not clinical depression or depressive symptoms is associated with glycemic control in both cross-sectional and longitudinal analyses. *Diabetes Care* 2010;**33**:23–8.

21. **Tsujii S, Hayashino Y, Ishii H.** Diabetes distress, but not depressive symptoms, is associated with glycaemic control among Japanese patients with type 2

diabetes: Diabetes Distress and Care Registry at Tenri (DDCRT 1). *Diabetic Medicine* 2012;**29**:1451–5.

22. **Van Bastelaar KMP, Pouwer F, Geelhoed-Duijvestijn P**, et al. Diabetes-specific emotional distress mediates the association between depressive symptoms and glycaemic control in type 1 and type 2 diabetes. *Diabetic Medicine* 2010;**27**:798–803.

23. **Ismail K, Winkley K, Rabe-Hesketh S**. Systematic review and meta-analysis of randomised controlled trials of psychological interventions to improve glycaemic control in patients with type 2 diabetes. *Lancet* 2004;**363**;1589–97.

24. **Winkley K, Landau S, Eisler I, Ismail K**. Psychological interventions to improve glycaemic control in patients with type 1 diabetes: systematic review and meta-analysis of randomised controlled trials. *British Medical Journal* 2006;**333**:65.

25. **Jokela M, Elovainio M, Nyberg ST**, et al. Personality and risk of diabetes in adults: Pooled analysis of 5 cohort studies. *Health Psychology* 2014;**33**:1618–21.

26. **Cheng H, Treglown L, Montgomery S, Furnham A**. Associations between familial factor, trait conscientiousness, gender and the occurrence of type 2 diabetes in adulthood: Evidence from a British cohort. *PloS One*, 2015l10:e0122701.

27. **Čukić I, Mõttus R, Luciano M**, et al. Do personality traits moderate the manifestation of type 2 diabetes genetic risk? *Journal of Psychosomatic Research* 2015;**79**:303–8.

28. **Čukić I, Mõttus R, Realo A, Allik J**. Elucidating the links between personality traits and diabetes mellitus: Examining the role of facets, assessment methods, and selected mediators. *Personality and Individual Differences* 2016;**94**:377–82.

29. **Waller D, Johnston C, Molyneaux L**, et al. Glycemic control and blood glucose monitoring over time in a sample of young Australians with type 1 diabetes: the role of personality. *Diabetes Care* 2013;**36**:2968–73.

30 **Lane JD, McCaskill CC, Williams PG**, et al. Personality correlates of glycemic control in type 2 diabetes. *Diabetes Care* 2000;**23**:1321–5.

31. **Hyphantis T, Kaltsouda A, Triantafillidis J**, et al. Personality correlates of adherence to type 2 diabetes regimens. *International Journal of Psychiatry in Medicine* 2005;**35**:103–7.

32. **Hall PA, Rodin GM, Vallis TM, Perkins BA**. The consequences of anxious temperament for disease detection, self-management behavior, and quality of life in Type 2 diabetes mellitus. *Journal of Psychosomatic Research* 2009;**67**:297–305.

33. **Fonagy P, Steele H, Steele, M**. Maternal representations of attachment during pregnancy predict the organization of infant-mother attachment at one year of age. *Child Development* 1991;**62**:891–905.

34. **Fonagy P, Allison E**. The role of mentalizing and epistemic trust in the therapeutic relationship. *Psychotherapy*, 2014;**51**:372.

35. **Bost K, Wiley A, Fiese B**. associations between adult attachment style, emotion regulation, and preschool children's food consumption. *Journal of Developmental and Behavioral Pediatrics* 2014;**35**:50–61.

36. **Anderson S, Whitaker R**. Attachment security and obesity in US preschool-aged children. *Archives of Pediatrics* 2011;**165**:235–42.

37. **Ciechanowski P, Russo J, Katon,WJ**, et al. Relationship styles and mortality in patients with diabetes. *Diabetes Care*, **33**:539–44.

38. **Ciechanowski P, Russo J, Katon W**, et al. Where is the patient? The association of psychosocial factors and missed primary care appointments in patients with diabetes. *General Hospital Psychiatry* 2006;**28**:9–17.

39. **Bateman A, Fonagy P.** 8-year follow-up of patients treated for borderline personality disorder: mentalization-based treatment versus treatment as usual. *American Journal of Psychiatry* 2008;**165**:631–8.

40. **Bevington D, Fuggle P, Fonagy P.** Applying attachment theory to effective practice with hard-to-reach youth: the AMBIT approach. *Attachment & Human Development* 2015;**17**:157–74

Chapter 16

Targeting the circadian system

Gregory D. M. Potter and Eleanor M. Scott

The circadian system

Life evolved in the presence of the daily light/dark (LD) cycle. To maximize survival in this temporal environment, most species have evolved circadian (approximately 24-hour) rhythms in biology and behaviour. In humans, these rhythms are coordinated by a system of oscillators primarily regulated by a central clock in the suprachiasmatic nuclei (SCN) of the hypothalamus. The SCN comprise autonomous, self-sustaining, single-cell oscillators coupled to form networks that produce stable circadian rhythms [1]. Without sufficient zeitgebers (time cues), the most important of which is clear 24-hour LD cycles, circadian rhythm periods are typically not precisely 24 hours and may hence lose appropriate timing relationships with each other. The circadian system must therefore be entrained (synchronized) every day with the LD cycle.

Entrainment to the LD cycle occurs by way of melanopsin-containing intrinsically photosensitive retinal ganglion cells (ipRGCs) that relay information about the photoperiod from the eyes to the SCN via the retinohypothalamic tract. The SCN then convey temporal information to synchronize clocks in peripheral tissues throughout the body, primarily through the autonomic nervous system, humoral signalling, and temperature mechanisms [2,3]. Whereas the SCN are principally entrained by the LD cycle, peripheral clocks are particularly responsive to changes in energy and nutrient availability resulting from eating/fasting cycles [4]. Therefore, mistimed eating relative to the LD cycle (night eating) can disrupt the normal timing relationships between central and peripheral clocks.

The molecular clock

Although the main entraining stimuli for SCN and peripheral clocks differ, cellular clocks throughout the body share a common molecular basis. This molecular clockwork consists of 'clock' genes that form transcriptional/translational feedback loops. The positive arm of the core clock loop comprises circadian locomotor output cycles kaput (CLOCK, replaced by its paralogue neuronal period-aryl hydrocarbon receptor nuclear translocator single-minded protein 2 in some tissues) and brain and muscle aryl hydrocarbon receptor nuclear translocator-like 1 (BMAL1), the products of which stimulate the transcription of the genes of the negative arm. The negative arm comprises cryptochrome (CRY) 1, CRY2, Period (PER) 1, PER2, and PER3, the products of which inhibit CLOCK/BMAL1 transcription, thus closing the feedback loop and permitting a new cycle to begin the next day. Auxiliary loops add robustness to the core loop and couple the molecular clock with nutritional status [4]. As transcription factors, clock genes regulate daily changes in expression of numerous 'clock controlled' genes, temporally optimizing cellular functions. Non-transcriptional oscillators involving redox-sensitive peroxiredoxin proteins have also recently been identified [5]. These pervade all kingdoms of life, but how these oscillators interact with clock genes is not well understood.

Maintaining circadian system order

The endocrine system is an important means by which the SCN regulate the timing of peripheral clocks, with preeminent roles played by melatonin and cortisol. Photic information is relayed from ipRGCs to the SCN, which project to the pineal gland. This gland synthesizes melatonin during darkness, making the melatonin rhythm the most reliable marker of the timing of the circadian system. As melatonin receptors are distributed both in the SCN and widely in peripheral tissues, melatonin helps synchronize clocks throughout the body [6]. Cortisol is another hormone with a high amplitude circadian rhythm and pivotal synchronizing roles in peripheral clocks [7].

When entrained to the LD cycle, internal temporal order optimizes our bodies for activity and feeding during the day, and resting and fasting at night. In anticipation of the stressors of daytime activity, the circadian system ensures daytime peaks in catecholamines, cortisol, and heart rate [8]. The circadian system also produces timely changes to aid digestion and favour energy storage during daylight: insulin secretion and sensitivity peak during the day [9], for example, and the circadian system shapes daily alterations in the gut microbiota and nutrient transport [10,11]. In the presence of strong zeitgebers (aligned LD, activity/rest, and eating/fasting cycles), the entrained circadian system is a cornerstone of health. Nowadays, however, artificial lighting and heating, social clock demands (such as shifting work schedules), inactivity because of modern transportation means, and around-the-clock food access can weaken entrainment and disrupt the circadian system (Fig. 16.1).

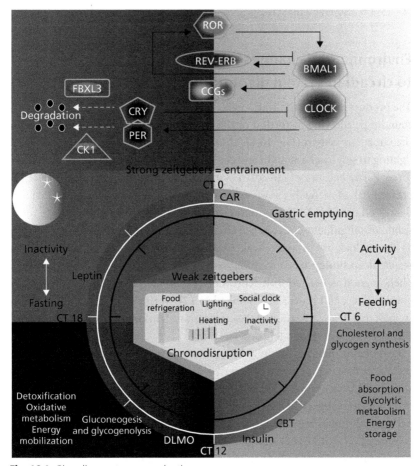

Fig. 16.1 Circadian system organization.

Upper segment: During the day, BMAL1 and CLOCK proteins form a complex that activates the transcription of clock-controlled genes (CCGs) including *CRY1-2* and *PER1-3*. CRY and PER proteins then form complexes that repress the transcription of CLOCK and BMAL1, ending the feedback loop before another cycle starts the next day. CK1 and FBXL3 influence degradation of PER and CRY and thereby help regulate the period of this feedback loop. In the best characterized auxiliary feedback loop, ROR stimulates *BMAL1* transcription and REV-ERB represses it.

Lower segment: Strong zeitgebers (sufficient light exposure and eating during the day, and minimal light exposure and fasting at night) ensure that the circadian system is synchronized to the solar day. Nowadays, however, artificial lighting and heating, social clock demands (like shifting work schedules), inactivity because of modern transportation means, and around-the-clock food access can weaken entrainment and disrupt the circadian system.

When entrained, the cortisol awakening response (CAR) around waking increases alertness and blood pressure and mobilizes energy reserves in anticipation of activity. A peak in core body temperature (CBT) in the afternoon maximizes physical capacities such as neuromuscular function. During the day, the body is therefore primed for activity and feeding. In the early evening, dim-light melatonin onset (DLMO) is an endogenous signal of night time that relays this information throughout the body. Peak leptin levels at night may help consolidate sleep by blunting appetite while energy availability falls as the night progresses.

Environmental changes now predispose us to circadian system disruption

The products of industrialization give us unprecedented control over our surroundings, allowing distortion of the daily environmental cycles that entrain the circadian system (Fig. 16.1). Shift workers, for example, rely on artificial lighting to stay awake at night and constitute about 20% of the European workforce. Partly because of circadian system disruption, these workers are at increased risk of many diseases, including type 2 diabetes mellitus (T2DM) and depressed mood [12,13]. Common working schedules can also produce more subtle misalignment between the circadian system and environmental cycles, as alarm clock use produces waking when sleep would otherwise occur. As a result, sleep timing tends to differ between work days and work-free days, a phenomenon associated with depression [14]. Widespread alarm clock use also curtails sleep, and short sleep is linked to T2DM risk [15]. These observations suggest that disorganization of the circadian system contributes to the development of T2DM and mood disorders.

Loss of circadian system organization is common in organisms with existing metabolic diseases. Some circadian rhythm amplitudes are blunted in humans with T2DM, for example [16]. Although observational studies have repeatedly shown relationships between circadian system disruption and T2DM risk, experimental studies are required to determine whether such associations reflect causality [17]. Studies of clock gene disruption in other animals and circadian system misalignment in humans provide evidence that circadian system disruption is indeed likely to be a key contributor to impaired glucose metabolism and T2DM development.

Circadian system genes and diabetes

Studies of rodents have been integral to demonstrating the effects of disruption of the molecular clock on glucose and adipose tissue metabolism. Homozygous CLOCK mutant mice have blunted daily feeding rhythms and become obese. Of particular relevance to T2DM, these animals produce insufficient insulin to compensate for their hyperglycaemia [18]. BMAL1 disruption produces perhaps the most severe consequences of all clock genes studied, nullifying most circadian rhythms in physiology and behaviour and producing premature mortality [19].

Studies of clock gene disruption in model organisms support human studies that have linked polymorphisms in clock genes with diabetes [20]. Nevertheless, larger, unbiased genome-wide association (GWA) studies are required to support or refute these observations. A common variant of one particular circadian system gene has consistently been shown to be associated with T2DM risk in GWA studies, however, namely the melatonin receptor gene *MNTR1B* [21]. This may be related to inhibition of glucose-mediated insulin secretion by MNTR1B [22], although roles of MTNR1B in glucose metabolism are contentious.

Diabetogenic effects of circadian system disruption

The deleterious effects of sleep disruption on glucose metabolism are beyond the scope of this chapter and have been reviewed elsewhere [23]. However, while sleep restriction alone reduces insulin sensitivity, these impairments are nearly doubled when circadian misalignment is concurrently imposed [24]. Enforcing environmental cycles outside the range of human entrainment is often used to induce misalignment. When such misalignment and sleep restriction occur over longer periods, insulin secretion is impaired, suggesting pancreatic dysfunction [25]. Notably, long-term shift workers remain susceptible to detrimental effects of circadian system misalignment on metabolic health [26].

Circadian system disorganization and depression

As is true of T2DM, individuals with depression often experience abnormal circadian rhythms, one of which is different diurnal variations in symptom severity. This may be related to altered temporal changes in regional brain glucose metabolism in comparison to healthy controls [27]. Furthermore, time-of-death analysis of brains of deceased individuals has shown that the pervasiveness of brain gene transcripts with 24-hour expression profiles is reduced in depressed patients, among whom timing relationships between circadian genes also differ in comparison to controls [28].

Depression is associated with widespread changes in rhythmic physiological processes. Depression is frequently characterized by increased mean body temperature and diminished temperature rhythm amplitude [29]. Cortisol has pivotal roles in stress responses, and dysregulated cortisol rhythms, including hypercortisolaemia and reduced cortisol rhythm amplitude, are typically evident in depression [30]. Similarly, melatonin rhythm amplitudes are commonly smaller in depressed individuals [31]. Whereas higher body temperature and cortisol levels are alerting, melatonin is somewhat hypnogenic. Therefore, changes in these three rhythms may all impair sleep. Up to 90% of depressed patients report sleep disturbances such as early awakening and insomnia, and sleep problems often precede depression, suggesting reciprocity between sleep disruption and depression [32]. Furthermore, changes in sleep architecture, including shortened latency of rapid-eye-movement sleep onset and reduced slow-wave sleep, are common in depression [33].

One form of depression also characterized by disrupted circadian rhythms is seasonal affective disorder (SAD) [34]. SAD entails periods of depression coinciding with seasonal transitions, most frequently with episodes during autumn and winter that pass on transition to the longer photoperiods of spring and summer [35]. SAD affects perhaps 2–5% of individuals in temperate regions, but a larger proportion of people may be affected further north. Although abnormalities in the circadian systems of patients with SAD are well documented (particularly delays in circadian timing [36]), SAD aetiology is poorly understood.

The development of models of depression in other animals poses many difficulties. However, findings from studies of model organisms support roles of circadian system disorganization in depression. The monoaminergic hypothesis of depression focuses on roles of monoamines such as dopamine in depression. Activity in dopaminergic brain structures is temporally regulated by clock genes, as is *monoamine oxidase A* (MAO-A), the gene encoding the rate-limiting enzyme in dopamine deamination [37]. The SCN contribute to dopamine transport regulation, and SCN lesions produce depressive behaviours in rats [38]. Like the SCN, the olfactory bulb is a self-sustained pacemaker with roles in regulation of circadian rhythms, and its destruction also produces depression-like behaviour in rats [39,40].

Dysregulated dopamine signalling is also apparent in *Clock*Δ19 mutant mice [41], which show reward-seeking (manic) behaviour [18]. Other clock genes appear to have important roles in mood disorders. Glycogen synthase kinase-3β (GSK-3β) phosphorylates PER2 and promotes PER2 nuclear translocation. Transgenic mice that overexpress GSK-3β show mania-like behaviour [42], and lithium, a medication commonly prescribed for mood disorders, phosphorylates and thus inhibits GSK-3β [43]. Studies linking genetic modifications of the circadian system to mood disorders support human studies that have associated single nucleotide polymorphisms in circadian system gene variants with depression [44]. Again, candidate gene studies require support from GWA studies, however, a small proportion of individuals with hereditary circadian system gene mutations experience mood issues.

Together, it appears that circadian system disorganization and depression are intertwined, although our understanding of the nature of this interaction is incomplete and many questions remain. Nevertheless, as circadian system disorganization appears to contribute to the risk of depression and diabetes, therapies targeting circadian system function are a promising means of reducing the burden of both diseases.

Chronotherapies to counter diabetes and depression

Both depression and T2DM are often characterized by circadian system dysfunction. Chronotherapies aimed at restoring appropriate timing relationships between oscillator subsystems and alignment between circadian timing and the 24-hour day may therefore benefit individuals affected by these diseases.

Over 50% of the best-selling drugs in the USA target products of genes with 24-hour transcription profiles [45], and, under the control of the circadian system, drug absorption, distribution, metabolism, and elimination all vary in a 24-hour manner [46]. Therefore, pharmaceuticals must be appropriately timed to optimize their therapeutic effects and minimize toxicity.

Antidepressants

Commonly prescribed antidepressants, including MAO inhibitors, selective serotonin reuptake inhibitors (SSRIs), and lithium, exert chronobiotic effects (changing the amplitude, period, or timing of circadian rhythms), from *in vitro* studies of the molecular clock to *in vivo* studies of humans [47]. Although these drugs are often efficacious, they can disrupt the circadian system and sleep: SSRIs, for example, may disturb slow-wave sleep [48]. Furthermore, some of these pharmaceuticals may be linked to diabetes, although there is contradictory evidence [49].

Melatonin and its analogues

Melatonin and melatonin analogues have well-documented chronobiotic effects. Exogenous melatonin has antidepressant-like effects in mice but does not appear to be an effective antidepressant in humans [50]. It is possible that melatonin could be a useful adjunct to traditional antidepressant treatment, however, and a slow-release melatonin formulation has also been shown to improve sleep and glycated haemoglobin in people with insomnia and T2DM [51].

Similar to other melatonin analogues, agomelatine has few documented side-effects. Owing to its unique actions as both an agonist at both melatonin receptors and an antagonist at serotonin receptors 5-HT_{2B} and 5-HT_{2C} [52], Agomelatine is a particularly promising antidepressant and anxiolytic [53]. Novel clock-enhancing small molecules intended to improve circadian system resilience are also in development, but none has proven efficacy and safety in humans yet.

Light

Like melatonin, non-pharmaceutical means of restoring circadian system organization may enhance antidepressive effects of pharmaceutical treatments and can be particularly effective at improving glucose regulation and metabolic health. First used effectively in SAD [35], daytime bright-light therapy sometimes improves mood in non-seasonal mood disorders such as major depression [54], perhaps partly through suppressive effects of bright light exposure on cortisolaemia [55]. Furthermore, melatonin has roles in glucose homeostasis. As the duration, intensity, timing, and wavelength of light all influence melatonin regulation and the circadian system [56], tailoring an individual's light exposure is also important in treating diabetes. Recent developments in 'smart' lighting are especially promising in this respect, as are orange-tinted glasses and apps that modify light emitted from electronic device screens.

Sleep

Appropriate sleep interventions can both improve mood in people suffering from depression and also enhance glucose and insulin metabolism. Sleep deprivation (SD), for example, has potent antidepressive effects in ~60% of people with major depression [57]. However, these effects are generally transient, and SD exerts many adverse metabolic consequences, including reduced glucose tolerance and insulin sensitivity [23]. In contrast to the beneficial effects of SD on mood, sleep extension improves many aspects of health in short-sleeping individuals, such as glucose metabolism, insulin sensitivity, and appetite [58,59]. Therefore, it is important to consider the positive effects on mood and the negative metabolic effects of periodic SD, and an emphasis should be placed on improving sleep hygiene and maintaining consistent bed times that permit complete sleep, minimizing the use of alarms where possible.

Exercise

The favourable effects of exercise on glycaemic control in diabetes and mood in depression are without contention [60,61], and some evidence indicates that exercise influences the circadian system [62]. The extent to which the benefits of exercise on metabolism and mood are mediated by chronobiotic actions is unclear, but personalized physical activity interventions remain integral to the prevention and management of both depression and diabetes. By combining appropriate light exposure and physical activity, exercise outdoors may be a particularly effective treatment.

Diet

Nutrition is a potent zeitgeber for peripheral clocks and is a foundation of T2DM management [63]. Time -restricted eating, where caloric events are typically confined to a consistently timed period of <12 hours daily (during the active period), has many positive metabolic consequences in animal models of metabolic disease. Whether the same is true in humans is not yet clear, however [64], and effects of these schedules on mood are little understood.

Summary

Circadian system organization is important to metabolic and cognitive health and disrupting this system contributes to the development of T2DM and depression. Interventions to enhance or restore circadian system entrainment may therefore be valuable countermeasures against both T2DM and depression. Optimizing time cues such as LD, eating/fasting, and activity/rest cycles should be a commonality in promoting health in all individuals. Ultimately, a better understanding of the circadian system in the pathogenesis of T2DM and depression may help to develop novel therapeutic approaches to prevent and treat both diseases.

References

1. Mohawk JA, Green CB, Takahashi JS. Central and peripheral circadian clocks in mammals. *Annual Review of Neuroscience* 2012;**35**:445–62.
2. Buhr ED, Yoo SH, Takahashi JS. Temperature as a universal resetting cue for mammalian circadian oscillators. *Science* 2010;**330**:379–85.
3. Buijs RM, Scheer FA, Kreier F, et al. Organization of circadian functions: interaction with the body. *Progress in Brain Research* 2006;**153**:341–60.
4. Ribas-Latre A, Eckel-Mahan K. Interdependence of nutrient metabolism and the circadian clock system: Importance for metabolic health. *Molecular Metabolism* 2016;**5**:133–52.
5. Edgar RS, Green EW, Zhao Y, et al. Peroxiredoxins are conserved markers of circadian rhythms. *Nature* 2012;**485**:459–64.
6. Zawilska JB, Skene DJ, Arendt J. Physiology and pharmacology of melatonin in relation to biological rhythms. *Pharmacological Reports* 2009;**61**:383–410.
7. Sujino M, Furukawa K, Koinuma S, et al. Differential entrainment of peripheral clocks in the rat by glucocorticoid and feeding. *Endocrinology* 2012;**153**:2277–86.
8. Scheer FA, Hu K, Evoniuk H, et al. Impact of the human circadian system, exercise, and their interaction on cardiovascular function. *Proceedings of the National Academy of Sciences of the United States of America* 2010;**107**:20541–6.
9. Scheer FA, Hilton MF, Mantzoros CS, Shea SA. Adverse metabolic and cardiovascular consequences of circadian misalignment. *Proceedings of the National Academy of Sciences of the United States of America* 2009;**106**:4453–8.

10. **Hussain MM, Pan X.** Circadian regulation of macronutrient absorption. *Journal of Biological Rhythms* 2015;**30**:459–69.

11. **Zarrinpar A, Chaix A, Yooseph S, Panda S.** Diet and feeding pattern affect the diurnal dynamics of the gut microbiome. *Cell Metabolism* 2014;**20**:1006–17.

12. **Driesen K, Jansen NW, Kant I, Mohren DC, van Amelsvoort LG.** Depressed mood in the working population: associations with work schedules and working hours. *Chronobiology International* 2010;**27**:1062–79.

13. **Knutsson A, Kempe A.** Shift work and diabetes—a systematic review. *Chronobiology International* 2014;**31**:1146–51.

14. **Levandovski R, Dantas G, Fernandes LC,** et al. Depression scores associate with chronotype and social jetlag in a rural population. *Chronobiology International* 2011;**28**:771–8.

16. **Mantele S, Otway DT, Middleton B,** et al. Daily rhythms of plasma melatonin, but not plasma leptin or leptin mRNA, vary between lean, obese and type 2 diabetic men. *PloS One* 2012;**7**:e37123.

15. **Shan Z, Ma H, Xie M** et al. Sleep duration and risk of type 2 diabetes: a meta-analysis of prospective studies. *Diabetes Care* 2015;**38**:529–37.

17. **Tan E, Scott EM.** Circadian rhythms, insulin action, and glucose homeostasis. *Current Opinion in Clinical Nutrition and Metabolic Care* 2014;**17**:343–8.

18. **Turek FW, Joshu C, Kohsaka A,** et al. Obesity and metabolic syndrome in circadian Clock mutant mice. *Science* 2005;**308**:1043–5.

19. **Kondratov RV, Kondratova AA, Gorbacheva VY,** et al. Early aging and age-related pathologies in mice deficient in BMAL1, the core component of the circadian clock. *Genes & Development* 2006;**20**:1868–73.

20. **Scott EM, Carter AM, Grant PJ.** Association between polymorphisms in the Clock gene, obesity and the metabolic syndrome in man. *International Journal of Obesity* 2008;**32**:658–62.

21. **Lyssenko V, Nagorny CL, Erdos MR,** et al. Common variant in MTNR1B associated with increased risk of type 2 diabetes and impaired early insulin secretion. *Nature Genetics* 2009;**41**:82–8.

22. **Peschke E, Frese T, Chankiewitz E,** et al. Diabetic Goto Kakizaki rats as well as type 2 diabetic patients show a decreased diurnal serum melatonin level and an increased pancreatic melatonin-receptor status. *Journal of Pineal Research* 2006;**40**:135–43.

23. **Alnaji A, Law GR, Scott EM.** The role of sleep duration in diabetes and glucose control. *Proceedings of the Nutrition Society* **2016**:1–9.

24. **Leproult R, Holmback U, Van Cauter E.** Circadian misalignment augments markers of insulin resistance and inflammation, independently of sleep loss. *Diabetes* 2014;**63**:1860–9.

25. **Buxton OM, Cain SW, O'Connor SP,** et al. Adverse metabolic consequences in humans of prolonged sleep restriction combined with circadian disruption. *Science Translational Medicine* 2012;**4**:129ra43.

26. **Morris CJ, Purvis TE, Mistretta J, Scheer FA.** Effects of the internal circadian system and circadian misalignment on glucose tolerance in chronic shift workers. *Journal of Clinical Endocrinology and Metabolism* 2016;**101**:1066–74.

27. **Germain A, Nofzinger EA, Meltzer CC,** et al. Diurnal variation in regional brain glucose metabolism in depression. *Biological Psychiatry* 2007;**62**:438–45.

28. **Li JZ, Bunney BG, Meng F,** et al. Circadian patterns of gene expression in the human brain and disruption in major depressive disorder. *Proceedings of the National Academy of Sciences of the United States of America* 2013;**110**:9950–5.

29. **Avery DH, Wildschiodtz G, Rafaelsen OJ.** Nocturnal temperature in affective disorder. *Journal of Affective Disorders* 1982;**4**:61–71.

30. **Pariante CM, Lightman SL.** The HPA axis in major depression: classical theories and new developments. *Trends in Neurosciences* 2008;**31**:464–8.

31. **Claustrat B, Chazot G, Brun J,** et al. A chronobiological study of melatonin and cortisol secretion in depressed subjects: plasma melatonin, a biochemical marker in major depression. *Biological Psychiatry* 1984;**19**:1215–28.

32. **Ford DE, Kamerow DB.** Epidemiologic study of sleep disturbances and psychiatric disorders. An opportunity for prevention? *Journal of the American Medical Association* 1989;**262**:1479–84.

33. **Riemann D, Berger M, Voderholzer U.** Sleep and depression—results from psychobiological studies: an overview. *Biological Psychology* 2001;**57**:67–103.

34. **Lewy AJ, Sack RL, Miller LS, Hoban TM.** Antidepressant and circadian phase-shifting effects of light. *Science* 1987;**235**:352–4.

35. **Rosenthal NE, Sack DA, Gillin JC,** et al. Seasonal affective disorder. A description of the syndrome and preliminary findings with light therapy. *Archives of General Psychiatry* 1984;**41**:72–80.

36. **Dahl K, Avery DH, Lewy AJ,** et al. Dim light melatonin onset and circadian temperature during a constant routine in hypersomnic winter depression. *Acta Psychiatrica Scandinavica* 1993;**88**:60–6.

37. **Hampp G, Ripperger JA, Houben T,** et al. Regulation of monoamine oxidase A by circadian-clock components implies clock influence on mood. *Current Biology* 2008;**18**:678–83.

38. **Sleipness EP, Sorg BA, Jansen HT.** Diurnal differences in dopamine transporter and tyrosine hydroxylase levels in rat brain: dependence on the suprachiasmatic nucleus. *Brain Research* 2007;**1129**:34–42.

39. **Abraham U, Prior JL, Granados-Fuentes D,** et al. Independent circadian oscillations of Period1 in specific brain areas in vivo and in vitro. *Journal of Neuroscience* 2005;**25**:8620–6.

40. **Vinkers CH, Breuer ME, Westphal KG,** et al. Olfactory bulbectomy induces rapid and stable changes in basal and stress-induced locomotor activity, heart rate and body temperature responses in the home cage. *Neuroscience* 2009;**159**:39–46.

41. **Spencer S, Torres-Altoro MI, Falcon E** et al. A mutation in CLOCK leads to altered dopamine receptor function. *Journal of Neurochemistry* 2012;**123**:124–34.

42. **Prickaerts J, Moechars D, Cryns K,** et al. Transgenic mice overexpressing glycogen synthase kinase 3beta: a putative model of hyperactivity and mania. *Journal of Neuroscience* 2006;**26**:9022–9.

43. **Jope RS.** Lithium and GSK-3: one inhibitor, two inhibitory actions, multiple outcomes. *Trends in Pharmacological Sciences* 2003;**24**:441–3.

44. Etain B, Milhiet V, Bellivier F, Leboyer M. Genetics of circadian rhythms and mood spectrum disorders. *European Neuropsychopharmacology* 2011;**21**(Suppl. 4):S676–82.

45. Zhang R, Lahens NF, Ballance HI, et al. A circadian gene expression atlas in mammals: implications for biology and medicine. *Proceedings of the National Academy of Sciences of the United States of America* 2014;**111**:16219–24.

46. Levi F, Schibler U. Circadian rhythms: mechanisms and therapeutic implications. *Annual Review of Pharmacology and Toxicology* 2007;**47**:593–628.

47. Kronfeld-Schor N, Einat H. Circadian rhythms and depression: human psychopathology and animal models. *Neuropharmacology* 2012;**62**:101–14.

48. Dumont GJ, de Visser SJ, Cohen AF, van Gerven JM, Biomarker Working Group of the German Association for Applied Human P. Biomarkers for the effects of selective serotonin reuptake inhibitors (SSRIs) in healthy subjects. *British Journal of Clinical Pharmacology*. 2005;**59**:495–510.

49. Hennings JM, Schaaf L, Fulda S. Glucose metabolism and antidepressant medication. *Current Pharmaceutical Design* 2012;**18**:5900–19.

50. Dalton EJ, Rotondi D, Levitan RD, et al. Use of slow-release melatonin in treatment-resistant depression. *Journal of Psychiatry & Neuroscience* 2000;**25**:48–52.

51. Garfinkel D, Zorin M, Wainstein J, et al. Efficacy and safety of prolonged-release melatonin in insomnia patients with diabetes: a randomized, double-blind, crossover study. *Diabetes, Metabolic Syndrome and Obesity: Targets and Therapy* 2011;**4**:307–13.

52. Millan MJ, Gobert A, Lejeune F, et al. The novel melatonin agonist agomelatine (S20098) is an antagonist at 5-hydroxytryptamine2C receptors, blockade of which enhances the activity of frontocortical dopaminergic and adrenergic pathways. *Journal of Pharmacology and Experimental Therapeutics* 2003;**306**:954–64.

53. Taylor D, Sparshatt A, Varma S, Olofinjana O. Antidepressant efficacy of agomelatine: meta-analysis of published and unpublished studies. *British Medical Journal* 2014;**348**:g1888.

54. Goel N, Terman M, Terman JS, et al. Controlled trial of bright light and negative air ions for chronic depression. *Psychological Medicine* 2005;**35**:945–55.

55. Jung CM, Khalsa SB, Scheer FA, et al. Acute effects of bright light exposure on cortisol levels. *Journal of Biological Rhythms* 2010;**25**:208–16.

56. Duffy JF, Czeisler CA. Effect of light on human circadian physiology. *Sleep Medicine Clinics* 2009;**4**:165–77.

57. Wirz-Justice A, Van den Hoofdakker RH. Sleep deprivation in depression: what do we know, where do we go? *Biological Psychiatry* 1999;**46**:445–53.

58. Killick R, Hoyos CM, Melehan KL, et al. Metabolic and hormonal effects of 'catch-up' sleep in men with chronic, repetitive, lifestyle-driven sleep restriction. *Clinical Endocrinology* 2015;**83**:498–507.

59. Leproult R, Deliens G, Gilson M, Peigneux P. Beneficial impact of sleep extension on fasting insulin sensitivity in adults with habitual sleep restriction. *Sleep* 2015;**38**:707–15.

60. Cooney GM, Dwan K, Greig CA, et al. Exercise for depression. *Cochrane Database of Systematic Reviews* 2013:CD004366.

61. Umpierre D, Ribeiro PA, Kramer CK, et al. Physical activity advice only or structured exercise training and association with HbA1c levels in type 2 diabetes: a

systematic review and meta-analysis. *Journal of the American Medical Association* 2011;**305**:1790–9.

62. **Youngstedt SD, Kline CE, Elliott JA**, et al. Circadian phase-shifting effects of bright light, exercise, and bright light + exercise. *Journal of Circadian Rhythms* 2016;**14**:2.

63. **Evert AB, Boucher JL, Cypress M**, et al. Nutrition therapy recommendations for the management of adults with diabetes. *Diabetes Care* 2013;**36**:3821–42.

64. **Potter GD, Cade JE, Grant PJ, Hardie LJ.** Nutrition and the circadian system. *British Journal of Nutrition* 2016;**116**:434–42.

Chapter 17

Cultural and global perspectives

Kirsty Winkley, Ebaa Al-Ozairi,
and Boon-How Chew

Introduction

The global view of the relationship between diabetes and depression appears to have been generated primarily from research conducted in high-income countries (HIC) such as North America and Western Europe [1]. However, there is growing interest in the association between diabetes and depression on other continents. One of the main reasons for this increased awareness is the potential public health impact on low- to middle-income countries (LMIC) as their health services adapt from the challenge of communicable disease to the epidemic of type 2 diabetes mellitus (T2DM). The general agreement is that depression is common in T2DM and the prevalence of comorbidity is around twice that of people without T2DM: 18% versus 10% [2]. Although the available literature is sparse, a recent systematic review of the prevalence of depression and diabetes in LMIC suggests the average prevalence is 36% [3]. Related to this challenge is the shortage of specialists, including psychiatrists and psychologists, to cope with the number of people requiring treatment for depressive symptoms (DS). In addition, training mid-level health professionals such as nurses to provide specialized mental health and diabetes care (known as 'task-shifting') may not yet have happened [4]. This chapter will examine whether there are global or cultural variations in depression and T2DM and also diabetes distress (DD) which may account for sub-clinical depression in diabetes populations.

How culture impacts reporting, assessment, diagnosis, and help-seeking in depression and type 2 diabetes

Large population-based observational studies mostly rely on self-reported assessment of depressive symptoms. Cultural differences with regard to how depression is reported in self-report measures may lead to underdiagnosing depression in some cultures. For example, some argue that in Chinese society the word 'depression' is not in common usage and that it is usual for people to report physical symptoms, such as pain, dizziness, and fatigue [5]. This denial of emotional problems in favour of physical illness reporting is often referred to as the somatization hypothesis [6]. Another issue that may affect reporting is the stigmatization of mental illness in some cultures. In Turkey, for example, a cross-sectional study to determine public views of depression in Istanbul ($N = 161$) reported that depression was viewed negatively and depressed people were viewed as dangerous [7]. It therefore follows that depression in Istanbul is under-reported for fear of social exclusion, a common finding in north-western Europe from where there is more research evidence [8]. A final example for potential reporting problems might be that people from different socio-economic groups may hold different conceptual models of depression, which may affect both reporting and help seeking [9]. A qualitative approach to assess whether conceptual models of depression varied in European Americans (EA) and South Asian (SA) immigrants in New York City (USA) found that EAs had a more biological and medical explanation of depression whereas SAs viewed it more as a response to a difficult situation, which they were more likely to refer to as 'tension' [9].

Similarly, research into diabetes in LMIC also often relies on self-reported diabetes symptoms and therefore the potential for underdiagnosis of the population affected is great [10].

T2DM is also associated with stigma and help seeking. A qualitative study conducted in south London, UK, with people with T2DM who had not attended group structured education found that shame and stigma of diabetes and not wanting others to know of their diagnosis discouraged attendance. For the most part these respondents were of West African ethnicity and one of the issues was the perception that people with T2DM have fertility or virility problems [11]. In Western HIC, such as in Australia, stigma of T2DM is also an issue but usually because of the perception that people have brought it on themselves because of their lifestyle and being overweight or obese [12]. Other examples from the qualitative research literature in LMIC such as Malaysia suggest that diabetes stigma prevents people from monitoring their blood glucose when they are treated with insulin [13].

Despite potential issues with under-reporting of diabetes and depression due to cultural factors a recent study of a large cohort of people in urban and rural China with T2DM ($N = 25,000$) demonstrated that those who had a clinical rather than screen-detected diagnosis of T2DM had an odds ratio of 1.75 of major depression, although the overall prevalence of major depression was fairly low around 1% [14]. Similarly, somatization is thought to occur in HIC. For example, diabetes-related symptom distress is associated with depression in The Netherlands [15].

Factors such as religion may shape the culture of the individual and impact psychological functioning and subsequent help seeking. Furthermore, it may have both positive and negative impact on the health of the individual. In Malaysia adults with T2DM who self-reported to have no specific religion or those who were not sure of their adherence to religion (religiosity) compared with those who self-reported themselves as religious had more DD [16]. In Kuwait, religion and belief in God's power to heal, 'fatalism', may be psychologically protective, although, this is balanced by also being a factor affecting compliance to medication [17]. In general it is widely believed that religious involvement is an effective means of coping in response to life's stressors. For example, active social networks, access to crisis intervention resources and counselling, and quicker recovery [18,19].

The relationship between depression and diabetes distress in T2DM and global variation

DD can be defined as the patient's concerns about his/her diabetes management, social support, emotional burden, and access to diabetes care [20]. DD and psychological (general) stress could be considered similar as there was no specific measure for DD in the diabetes literature prior to 1995 [21,22]. T2DM patients with DD may find diabetes self-management difficult [23], leading to poor glycaemic control and increased morbidity and mortality [24,25]. Fisher et al. use the term 'emotional distress' to represent DD and depression [26] because according to them what has been widely defined as 'depression' among T2DM patients in the literature may really be either a major depressive disorder and/or DD, with only the latter displaying significant relationships with glycaemic control (HbA1c) [27]. It is argued that depression is at the more severe end of emotional distress, whereas DD measures provide the diabetes-specific content of psychological distress [28]. Many people with T2DM are likely to experience DS after the onset of T2DM but not before or at the time of screen-detected T2DM [29]. This demonstrates how T2DM might change life experiences, alter self-esteem, and increase uncertainty about the future [30–35]. There is cross-sectional evidence to suggest an association between DD and DS [36], and prospectively there appears to be a bidirectional relationship. DD predicts more DS 6 months to 2 years later [37,38] and vice versa. This evidence in the West on the positive longitudinal relations between DD and DS has not been seen in the East or LMIC [39]. Differences in culture and social values such as in living conditions, healthcare systems, life priorities, family and personal beliefs may lead to different experiences of emotional distress [16,32,40,41]. Qualitative research illustrates how this relationship unfolds. Mendenhall et al. [42] conducted a mixed methods study with urban Indians in Delhi. There was a high prevalence of DS, 55% in the lowest income group (former slum dwellers living in resettlement areas) and qualitative interviews with participants demonstrated that people in this group were more likely to report comorbid DS and DD as they were unable to afford diabetes treatment [42]. This delay in accessing diabetes treatment might therefore mean they are more symptomatic and at risk of diabetes complications.

The global prevalence of depression and diabetes distress

The largest international study examining the prevalence of DD is almost certainly the DAWN2 study covering 17 countries and five continents (see Table 17.1). Algeria had the highest prevalence at 65% and the lowest level of DD was in the Netherlands (21%). The main limitation of DAWN2 is that this was a highly selected group of participants who were likely to be high functioning individuals throughout the countries involved as most participants were recruited via the internet rather than face to face in a clinic [43,44]. Not all studies of comorbid diabetes and depression also measure DD. In Malaysia, the combination of both DD and depression was found in ~30% of the patients (Fig. 17.1). And even though the DAWN2 study measured both, the association between the two conditions was not investigated. Self-reported DS from the 17 participating countries suggest rates between 6% and 24%; Mexico and Algeria were the lowest and highest respectively [43]. However, prevalence differs substantially across settings and studies (Table 17.1), but there is a tendency for higher rates in LMIC than HIC [16,45–57].

Do T2DM and depression have the same causal pathways, risk factors, and outcomes across countries?

Causal pathways

The move from the biomedical to the biopsychosocial model in diabetes care and increasing evidence of the relationship between psychological manifestations and objective biomarkers has stimulated discussion regarding the possible causal relationship between diabetes and depression. Although much

Table 17.1 Global prevalence of co-morbid depression and diabetes distress

Author, country	Study design, setting	Sample size	Measures used	Depression (%)	Diabetes distress (%)
Agbir et al. 2010, Nigeria	Cross-sectional, secondary care	160	SCID	19.4	n/a
Chew et al. 2016, Malaysia	Cross-sectional, urban and rural primary care	700	PHQ-9 DDS-17	41.7 (PHQ ≥ 5) 11.0 (PHQ ≥ 10)	49.2
Chong et al. 2009, Singapore	Cross-sectional, in a hospital	537	CES-D	31.1	n/a
Ganasegeran et al. 2014, Malaysia	Cross-sectional, secondary care	169	HADS	40.3	n/a
James et al. 2010, Nigeria	Cross-sectional, secondary care	200	SCAN	30	n/a
Jie et al. 2013, China	Cross-sectional, in two hospitals	200	ZSDS DDS	24	64
Kaur et al. 2013, Malaysia	Cross-sectional, urban primary care	2508	DASS	11.5	n/a
Lee et al. 2006, Hong Kong	Cross-sectional, urban primary care	333	DSQ	33.6 as being anxious-depression	n/a
Mezuk et al. 2013, China	Cross-sectional, urban and rural primary care	15,981 (clinically identified T2DM) 10,528 (screen-detected T2DM)	CIDI-SF	0.9% clinically diagnosed 0.6% screen detected	n/a
Mier et al. 2008, USA and Mexico	Cross-sectional, primary care	172	CES-D	39-40.5	n/a
DAWN2, Nicolucci et al. 2013, 17 countries	Cross-sectional, online questionnaire	8,596	WHO-5 PAID 5	6.5-24.1	21-65
Sasi Sekhar et al. 2013, India	Cross-sectional, outpatients at a diabetes centre	546	DDS	n/a	40
Sulaiman et al, 2010, United Arab Emirates	Cross-sectional, primary care	347	K6	n/a	12.5

(continued)

Table 17.1 Continued

Author, country	Study design, setting	Sample size	Measures used	Depression (%)	Diabetes distress (%)
Tellez-Zenteno et al. 2002, Mexico	Cross-sectional, secondary care	189	Beck	39%	n/a
Tsujii et al. 2012, Japan	Cross-sectional, in a hospital	3,305	CES-D PAID	27.8	12.0
Yang et al. 2009, China	Cross-sectional, urban primary care	148	ZSDS	39.2	n/a
Zhu et al. 2016, China	Cross-sectional, in a hospital	397	DDS	n/a	33.8

CIDI-SF, Composite International Diagnostic Interview (CIDI) Short-Form; WHO-5, World Health Organization Well-being Questionnaire; Beck, Beck depression Inventory; SCAN, Schedules for Clinical Assessment in Neuropsychiatry; SCID, Structured Clinical Interview for DSM-III-R (SCID); CES-D= Center for Epidemiologic Studies Depression Scale; DASS, the Depression; Anxiety and Stress Scale 21-item questionnaire; DDS= 17-item Diabetes Distress Scale; DSQ, 57-item Diabetes Stress Questionnaire; HADS, Hospital Anxiety and Depression Scale; PAID= Problem Areas in Diabetes scale; PHQ, 9-item Patient Health Questionnaire; ZSDS, Zung Self-Rating Depression Scale; K6, mental health assessment tool.

of the evidence has been generated from HIC it may not necessarily relate to LMICs because the social and economic conditions are different [58]. However, some argue that similar effects may be scientifically applicable to Asian populations [36]. Stress response has been implicated to be the underlying pathophysiological mechanism between T2DM and depression [59]; psychological factors such as anxiety, depression, and hostility can alter DNA methylation to produce immune/inflammatory system markers [60]; unattended DD progresses to depression [61]; unresolved psychological distress leads to increased disability, health decline [62], increased healthcare utilization [63], poor treatment adherence [48], decreased quality of health [64], and premature mortality [65]; even after adjustment for demographic variables and micro- and macrovascular complications, depression was associated with an increased risk of all-cause mortality (HR = 1.46, 95% CI 1.29–1.66), and cardiovascular mortality (HR = 1.39, 95% CI 1.11–1.73) [66].

There also lies another possible explanation from a more sociological perspective. Mendenhall argues that social and economic factors cluster with diabetes and depression [67]. She says 'social conditions contribute significantly to a biosocial negative feedback loop wherein social and economic inequalities are both a cause and consequence of disease interactions and associated morbidities and mortalities' [42]. This underpins the theory of 'syndemics',

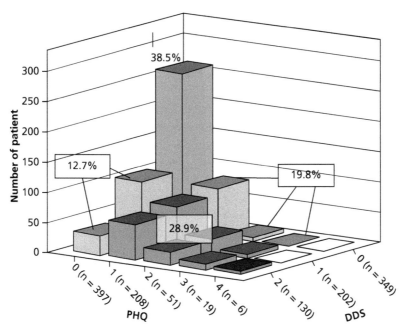

Fig. 17.1 Prevalence of depression and diabetes-related distress among 684 adult Malaysians with type 2 diabetes mellitus at primary care.

Adapted from *PLoS ONE*, 11, 3, Chew B. H., Vos R., Mohd-Sidik S., Rutten G.E.H.M., Diabetes-Related Distress, Depression and Distress-Depression among Adults with Type 2 Diabetes Mellitus in Malaysia. © 2016 Chew et al. This is an open access article distributed under the terms of the Creative Commons Attribution License (https://creativecommons.org/licenses/by/4.0/), which permits unrestricted use, distribution, and reproduction in any medium, provided the original author and source are credited.

which integrates social, cultural, psychological, and biological factors. Syndemics involves (1) the clustering of two or more diseases within a specific population; (2) specific contextual and social factors within this cluster of diseases; and (3) this clustering of disease and interaction creates hardship for those affected [42,67]. She argues that it is necessary to understand the specific social and cultural context of the diabetes–depression link; therefore, how their manifestation in one population or group is different from that of another. Qualitative research of Mexican immigrant women with T2DM in the USA led to a complex dynamic between violence, immigration, depression, diabetes, and abuse [68]. A diabetes and depression study in urban Delhi, India, revealed more depression in lower income groups and these were more likely to be distressed because of less access to diabetes care [42]; in Soweto, South Africa, where one in four are HIV positive, diabetes, depression, and HIV/AIDS are intertwined with many people confused as to which, diabetes or HIV, is most serious and stigma is attached to both [69]. Meanwhile, in south London, the stigma of having T2DM has reportedly had a huge psychological impact and prevented people of Nigerian origin from attending diabetes education because of the shame associated with the condition and the idea that it affects fertility and virility [11].

How T2DM is viewed through different lenses across the world warrants further research. Mendenhall has given us examples from South Africa, India, and Mexican immigrants in the USA, and another region that may benefit from this type of close scrutiny is the UAE. This area has seen the fastest change in economy from LMIC to HIC brought about by the discovery of oil in the 1960s. The wealth accrued by many of the population coupled with the climate and the avoidance of travelling on foot and reliance on cars has led to a rapid rise in obesity; current figures suggest a prevalence of 75% [70] and the associated rise in T2DM [71]. Traditional perceptions of wealth and the fuller figure have been the norm, although increasingly among the urban elite the Western image of beauty and the desire to be slim is becoming more apparent. This change in attitude towards body image has received some investigation with a case study centred on young women at university in Dubai and Al Ain, where there was less overweight and obesity than in the background population, particularly among young women in Dubai [72]. Whether this attitude favouring being slim will filter down towards the less well educated and/or young male populations remains to be seen. The rate of gestational diabetes (GDM) in Emirati women is one of the highest in the world and although this population has access to free healthcare there is a lack of obesity prevention. Women at risk of T2DM cite issues preventing them from exercising such as wearing traditional dresses, having nowhere to walk, childcare, having maids doing the cleaning and cooking, and exercise being frowned upon by their husbands unless it is in a women-only gym, of which there are few [73,74]. Hospitality centres on the giving and receiving of food, often sweet things, and it is difficult to avoid excessive consumption at social or family engagements without causing offence [75]. Women are fearful of becoming overweight following pregnancy and there is a tendency that women with T2DM are more likely to experience depression than their male counterparts [75]. Therefore, there is something about the experience of being female in the UAE that makes T2DM more likely and the experience of coping with the disease more difficult and it is cultural factors such as these that need to be considered when developing interventions to reduce T2DM and psychological distress.

Risk factors of depression and distress in different cultures

At the epidemiological level there are similarities and differences in terms of risk factors for DD and depression in people with T2DM across cultures and geographical regions in terms of socio-demographic and clinical characteristics. For example in Australia, Malaysia, and Kuwait, female gender [31,50,76] was associated with general stress, whereas younger age groups were more likely to have DD [77,78], and in other Asian populations DD and older age were associated with depression [52,55,79]. However, the association between depression, DD and socio-economic status appears to be prevalent across LMIC because of the lack of access to T2DM treatment [42].

Inconstancy in the availability diabetes treatment can also be a risk factor for depression and DD. For example, this is true in Malaysia where the clustering of symptoms is associated with particular clinics [16]. The reasons for this may be twofold: first the quality of the health/medical services and doctor–patient communication at the clinic level; and, second, the patients' 'neighbourhood culture', which influences their perception of the clinical care, social, and physical environment where the patient lives when comparing these personal situations with others within the similar neighbourhood but experiencing something better [80]. The mismatch between expectations and experiences may predispose individuals to emotional distress and the loss of trust in the clinical care that they receive at the clinics may lead to experimentation with complementary and alternative medicine [81].

Outcomes

Past studies have shown distinctive effects of DD and DS on different aspects of diabetes care, although these have generally been conducted in HIC [66]. In the USA [27,82] research suggests that DD is prospectively associated with glycaemic control, compared with DS. In Germany, a study of adults with T2DM in primary care demonstrated that baseline depression predicted medication non-adherence, problems with health-related behaviours (poor diet and physical inactivity), and unsatisfactory glycaemic control (HbA1c $\geq$7%) at the 12-month follow-up [83]. The US REGARDS (REasons for Geographic And Racial Differences in Stroke) [84] showed that among those with diabetes and median follow-up of 6 years, the combination of both elevated stress and DS in subjects with diabetes was associated with a higher incidence of cardiovascular death (HR = 2.15, 95% CI 1.33–3.47) than with either stress or DS alone (HR = 1.53, 95% CI 1.08–2.17). This Western evidence of negative effects of DD and DS on outcomes has not been seen in the East, a contradictory observation has even been reported [41]. An increase in DD may be expected along with patient empowerment programmes such as educational or psychological interventions if they do not improve resilience or self-efficacy; at the same time, higher DD was associated with lower systolic blood pressure and triglycerides [85]. It is likely that these are early and preliminary indications that DD and DS do not have straightforward effects on diabetes self-care and outcomes [86], and complex influences from the culture, social values, and personal perceptions of illness could be expected. However, it is important to note that there is a growing body of evidence to support the use of psychological and pharmacological interventions for people with T2DM with DD or depression [87–92].

Summary

T2DM and depression are costly in terms of morbidity and mortality and are likely to have a greater economic impact on LMIC than HIC as T2DM disproportionately affects the economically active in these countries and there is less availability of specialist care. The scale of the problem is not known because of the paucity of data from LMIC and the likelihood that both conditions are underdiagnosed. Also, research into causal pathways, risks and consequences is generally conducted in HIC and potential interventions may or may not be applicable to LMIC [58]. The inconsistency of factors that are associated with DD or depression in T2DM may be due to different settings, psychological measures used, or real differences in the cultural background of the population. Further research is needed to determine the exact nature of the diabetes and depression link across cultures and to investigate the relationship between psychological status, self-care behaviour, and clinical outcomes, so that culturally appropriate interventions can be developed.

References

1. Lloyd CE, Pambianco G, Orchard, TJ. Diabetes-related distress, depression and self-care in individuals with Type 1 diabetes. *Diabetes Care* (in press).
2. Ali S, Stone MA, Peters JL, et al. The prevalence of co-morbid depression in adults with Type 2 diabetes, a systematic review and meta-analysis. *Diabetic Medicine* 2006;**23**:1165–73.
3. Mendenhall E, Norris SA, Shidhaye R, et al. Depression and type 2 diabetes in low- and middle-income countries, a systematic review. *Diabetes Research and Clinical Practice* 2014;**103**:276–85.
4. Lekoubou A, Awah A, Fezeu L, et al. Hypertension, diabetes mellitus and task shifting in their management in sub-Saharan Africa. *International Journal of Environmental Research and Public Health* 2010;7:353–63.

5. **Kleinman A.** Culture and depression. *New England Journal of Medicine* 2004;**351**:951–53.

6. **Ryder AG, Yang J, Heine SJ.** Somatization vs. psychologization of emotional distress, a paradigmatic example for cultural psychopathology. *Online Readings in Psychology and Culture* 2002;**10**:article 3.

7. **Ozmen E, Ogel K, Aker T,** et al. Public attitudes to depression in urban Turkey. *Social Psychiatry and Psychiatric Epidemiology* 2004;**39**:1010–16.

8. **Evans-Lacko S, Courtin E, Fiorillo A,** et al. The state of the art in European research on reducing social exclusion and stigma related to mental health. A systematic mapping of the literature. *European Psychiatry* 2014;**29**:381–89.

9. **Karasz A.** Cultural differences in conceptual models of depression, *Social Science & Medicine* 2005;**60**:1625–35.

10. **Egede LE, Ellis C.** Diabetes and depression, global perspectives. *Diabetes Research in Clinical Practice* 2010;**87**.

11. **Winkley K, Evwierhoma C, Amiel SA,** et al. Patient explanations for non-attendance at structured diabetes education sessions for newly diagnosed Type 2 diabetes. A qualitative study. *Diabetic Medicine* 2015;**32**:120–28.

12. **Browne JL, Ventura A, Mosely K,** et al. I call it the blame and shame disease, a qualitative study about perceptions of social stigma surrounding type 2 diabetes. *BMJ Open* 2013;**3**:11.

13. **Ong WM, Chua SS, Ng CJ.** Barriers and facilitators to self-monitoring of blood glucose in people with type 2 diabetes using insulin, a qualitative study, *Patient Preference and Adherence* 2014;**8**, 237–46.

14. **Mezuk B, Chen Y, Yu C,** et al. Depression, anxiety, and prevalent diabetes in the Chinese population, findings from the China Kadoorie Biobank of 0.5 million people, *Journal of Psychosomatic Research* 2013;**75**:511–17.

15. **Adriaanse MC, Pouwer F, Dekker JM,** et al. Diabetes-related symptom distress in association with glucose metabolism and comorbidity the Hoorn study. *Diabetes Care* 2008;**31**:2268–70.

16. **Chew BH, Vos R, Mohd-Sidik S, Rutten GEHM.** Diabetes-related distress, depression and distress-depression among adults with type 2 diabetes mellitus in Malaysia. *PLoS ONE* 2016;**11**:e0152095.

17. **Jeragh-Alhaddad FB, Waheedi M, Barber N, Brock T.** Barriers to medication taking among Kuwaiti patients with type 2 diabetes, a qualitative study. *Patient preference and adherence* 2015;**9**:1491–503.

18. **Levin JS.** Religion and health, is there an association, is it valid, and is it causal? *Social Science and Medicine* 1994;**38**:1475–82.

19. **Van Olphen J, Schulz A, Israel B,** et al. Religious involvement, social support, and health among African-American women on the east side of Detroit. *Journal of General Internal Medicine* 2003;**18**:549–57.

20. **Polonsky WH, Fisher L, Earles J,** et al. Assessing psychosocial distress in diabetes, development of the diabetes distress scale. *Diabetes Care* 2005;**28**:626–31.

21. **Lloyd C, Smith J, Weinger K.** Stress and diabetes. A review of the links. *Diabetes Spectrum* 2005;**18**:121–27.

22. **Polonsky WH, Anderson BJ, Lohrer PA,** et al. Assessment of diabetes-related distress. *Diabetes Care* 1995;**18**:754–60.

23. **Ogbera A, Adeyemi-Doro A.** Emotional distress is associated with poor self care in type 2 diabetes mellitus. *Journal of Diabetes* 2011;**3**:348–52.

24. **Gallo JJ, Bogner HR, Morales KH**, et al. Depression, cardiovascular disease, diabetes, and two-year mortality among older, primary-care patients. *American Journal of Geriatric Psychiatry* 2005;**13**:748–55.

25. **Nozaki T, Morita C, Matsubayashi S**, et al. Relation between psychosocial variables and the glycemic control of patients with type 2 diabetes, a cross-sectional and prospective study. *Biopsychosocial Medicine* 2009;**3**:4.

26. **Fisher L, Gonzalez JS, Polonsky WH.** The confusing tale of depression and distress in patients with diabetes, a call for greater clarity and precision. *Diabetic Medicine* 2014;**31**:764–72.

27. **Fisher L, Mullan JT, Arean P**, et al. Diabetes distress but not clinical depression or depressive symptoms is associated with glycemic control in both cross-sectional and longitudinal analyses. *Diabetes Care* 2010;**33**:23–8.

28. **Das-Munshi J, Stewart R, Ismail K**, et al. Diabetes, common mental disorders, and disability, findings from the UK National Psychiatric Morbidity Survey. *Psychosomatic Medicine* 2007;**69**:543–50.

29. **Aujla N, Abrams KR, Davies MJ**, et al. The prevalence of depression in white-European and South-Asian people with impaired glucose regulation and screen-detected type 2 diabetes mellitus. *PLoS One* 2009;**4**:e7755.

30. **Hinder S, Greenhalgh T.** This does my head in. Ethnographic study of self-management by people with diabetes. *BMC Health Service Research* 2012;**12**:83.

31. **Koch T, Kralik D, Sonnack D.** Women living with type II diabetes, the intrusion of illness. *Journal of Clinical Nursing* 1999;**8**:712–22.

32. **Low LL, Tong SF, Low WY.** Mixed feelings about the diagnosis of type 2 diabetes mellitus, a consequence of adjusting to health related quality of life. *Collegium Antropologicum* 2014;**38**:11–20.

33. **Schabert J, Browne JL, Mosely K, Speight J.** Social stigma in diabetes, a framework to understand a growing problem for an increasing epidemic. *Patient* 2013;**6**:1–10.

34. **Stuckey HL, Mullan-Jensen CB, Reach G**, et al. personal accounts of the negative and adaptive psychosocial experiences of people with diabetes in the second Diabetes Attitudes, Wishes and Needs (DAWN2) study. *Diabetes Care* 2014;**37**:2466–74.

35. **Weaver RR, Lemonde M, Payman N, Goodman WM.** Health capabilities and diabetes self-management, the impact of economic, social, and cultural resources. *Social Science and Medicine* 2014;**102**:58–68.

36. **Chew BH, Shariff-Ghazali S, Fernandez A.** Psychological aspects of diabetes care, Effecting behavioral change in patients. *World Journal of Diabetes* 2014;**5**:796–808.

37. **Burns RJ, Deschenes SS, Schmitz N.** Cyclical relationship between depressive symptoms and diabetes distress in people with type 2 diabetes mellitus, results from the Montreal Evaluation of Diabetes Treatment Cohort study. *Diabetic Medicine* 2015;**32**:1272–8.

38. **Ehrmann D, Kulzer B, Haak T, Hermanns N.** Longitudinal relationship of diabetes-related distress and depressive symptoms, analysing incidence and persistence. *Diabetes Medicine* 2015;**32**:1264–71.

39. **Chew BH, Vos RC, Stellato RK, Rutten GEHM.** Diabetes-related distress and depressive symptoms are not merely negative over a 3-year period in Malaysian adults

with Type 2 diabetes mellitus receiving regular primary diabetes care. *Frontiers in Psychology* 2017;**8**:1834.

40. **Lee YK, Low WY, Ng CJ.** Exploring patient values in medical decision making, a qualitative study. *PLoS One* 2013;**8**: e80051.

41. **Wang RH, Hsu HC, Kao CC,** et al. Associations of changes in psychosocial factors and their interactions with diabetes distress in patients with type 2 diabetes, a longitudinal study. *Journal of Advanced Nursing* 2017;**73**;1137–46.

42. **Mendenhall E, Shivashankar R, Tandon N,** et al. Stress and diabetes in socioeconomic context, a qualitative study of urban Indians. *Social Science & Medicine* 2012;**75**:2522–29.

43. **Nicolucci A, Kovacs Burns K, Holt RI,** et al. Diabetes attitudes, wishes and needs second study (DAWN2™), cross-national benchmarking of diabetes-related psychosocial outcomes for people with diabetes. *Diabetic Medicine* 2013;**30**:767–77.

44. **Peyrot M, Burns KK, Davies M,** et al. Diabetes Attitudes Wishes and Needs 2 (DAWN2), A multinational, multi-stakeholder study of psychosocial issues in diabetes and person-centred diabetes care. *Diabetes Research and Clinical Practice* 2013;**99**:174–84.

45. **Agbir TM, Audu MD, Adebowale TO,** et al. Depression among medical outpatients with diabetes, a cross-sectional study at Jos University Teaching Hospital, Jos, Nigeria. *Annals of African Medicine* 2010;**9**:5–10.

46. **Chong SA, Subramaniam M, Chan YH,** et al. Depressive symptoms and diabetes mellitus in an Asian multiracial population. *Asian Journal of Psychiatry* 2009**2**:66–70.

47. **Ganasegeran K, Renganathan P, Manaf RA,** et al. Factors associated with anxiety and depression among type 2 diabetes outpatients in Malaysia, a descriptive cross-sectional single-centre study. *BMJ Open* 2014;**4**:e004794.

48. **James BOO, Omoaregba JO, Eze, Morakinyo O,** et al. Depression among patients with diabetes mellitus in a Nigerian teaching hospital. *South African Journal of Psychology* 2010;**16**;61–4.

49. **Zhang J, Xu CP, Wu HX,** et al. Comparative study of the influence of diabetes distress and depression on treatment adherence in Chinese patients with type 2 diabetes, a cross-sectional survey in the Peoples Republic of China. *Neuropsychiatric Disease and Treatment* 2013;**9**:1289–94.

50. **Kaur G, Tee GH, Ariaratnam S,** et al. Depression, anxiety and stress symptoms among diabetics in Malaysia, a cross sectional study in an urban primary care setting. *BMC Family Practice* 2013;14, 69.

51. **Mier N, Bocanegra-Alonso A, Zhan D,** et al. Clinical depressive symptoms and diabetes in a binational border population. *Journal of American Board of Family Medicine* 2008;**21**:223–33.

52. **Sasi STVD, Kodali M, Burra KC,** et al. Self care activities, diabetic distress and other factors which affected the glycaemic control in a tertiary care teaching hospital in South India. *Journal of Clinical and Diagnostic Research* 2013;**7**:857–60.

53. **Sulaiman N, Aisha Hamdan, Hani Tamim,** et al. The prevalence and correlates of depression and anxiety in a sample of diabetic patients in Sharjah, United Arab Emirates. *BMC Family Practice* 2010;**11**:1–7.

54. **Tellez-Zenteno JF, Cardiel MH.** Risk factors associated with depression in patients with type 2 diabetes mellitus. *Archives of Medical Research* 2002;**33**:53–60.

55. **Tsujii S, Hayashino Y, Ishii H.** Diabetes distress, but not depressive symptoms, is associated with glycaemic control among Japanese patients with type 2 diabetes, Diabetes Distress and Care Registry at Tenri (DDCRT 1). *Diabetic Medicine* 2012;**29**:1451–5.

56. **Yang J, Li S, Zheng Y.** Predictors of depression in Chinese community-dwelling people with type 2 diabetes. *Journal of Clinical Nursing* 2009;**18**:1295–304.

57. **Zhu Y, Fish AF, Li F,** et al. Psychosocial factors not metabolic control impact the quality of life among patients with type 2 diabetes in China. *Acta Diabetologica* 2016;**54**:535–41.

58. **Leone T, Coast E, Narayanan S,** et al. Diabetes and depression comorbidity and socio-economic status in low and middle income countries (LMICs), a mapping of the evidence. *Globalization and Health* 2012;**8**:1–10.

59. **Berge LI, Riise T.** Comorbidity between type 2 diabetes and depression in the adult population, directions of the association and its possible pathophysiological mechanisms. *International Journal of Endocrinology* 2015;164760.

60. **Kim D, Kubzansky LD, Baccarelli A,** et al. Psychological factors and DNA methylation of genes related to immune/inflammatory system markers, the VA Normative Aging Study. *BMJ Open* 2016;**6**:e009790.

61. **Skinner TC, Carey ME, Cradock S,** et al. Depressive symptoms in the first year from diagnosis of Type 2 diabetes, results from the DESMOND trial. *Diabetic Medicine* 2010;**27**:965–7.

62. **Nakaya N, Kogure M, Saito-Nakaya K,** et al. The association between self-reported history of physical diseases and psychological distress in a community-dwelling Japanese population, the Ohsaki Cohort 2006 study. *European Journal of Public Health* 2014;**24**:45–9.

63. **Callahan CM, Hui SL, Nienaber NA,** et al. Longitudinal study of depression and health services use among elderly primary care patients. *Journal of American Geriatric Society* 1994;**42**:833–8.

64. **Egede LE, Hernandez-Tejada MA.** Effect of comorbid depression on quality of life in adults with Type 2 diabetes. *Expert Review of Pharmacoeconomics & Outcomes Research* 2013;**13**:83–91.

65. **Kawamura T, Shioiri T, Takahashi K,** et al. Survival rate and causes of mortality in the elderly with depression, a 15-year prospective study of a Japanese community sample, the Matsunoyama-Niigata suicide prevention project. *Journal of Investigative Medicine* 2007;**55**:106–14.

66. **van Dooren FE, Nefs G, Schram MT,** et al. Depression and risk of mortality in people with diabetes mellitus, a systematic review and meta-analysis. *PLoS One* 2013;**8**:e57058.

67. **Mendenhall E.** Beyond comorbidity, a critical perspective of syndemic depression and diabetes in cross-cultural contexts. *Medical Anthropology Quarterly* 2016;**30**:462–78.

68. **Mendenhall E,** et al. Speaking through diabetes. *Medical Anthropology Quarterly* 2010;**24**:220–39.

69. **Mendenhall E, Norris SA.** Diabetes care among urban women in Soweto, South Africa, a qualitative study. *BMC Public Health* 2015;**15**:1300.

70. **Malik M, Bakir A, Saab BA,** et al. Glucose intolerance and associated factors in the multi-ethnic population of the United Arab Emirates, results of a national survey. *Diabetes Research and Clinical Practice* 2005;**69**:188–95.

71. **Shaw JE, Sicree RA, Zimmet PZ.** Global estimates of the prevalence of diabetes for 2010 and 2030. *Diabetes Research and Clinical Practice* 2010;**87**:4–14.

72. **Trainer S.** Negotiating weight and body image in the UAE, Strategies among young emirati women, *American Journal of Human Biology* 2012;**24**:314–24.

73. **Ali HI, Baynouna LM, Bernsen RM.** Barriers and facilitators of weight management, perspectives of Arab women at risk for type 2 diabetes. *Health & Social Care in the Community* 2010;**18**:219–28.

74. **Baglar R.** 'Oh God, save us from sugar', an ethnographic exploration of diabetes mellitus in the united arab emirates. *Medical Anthropology* 2013;**32**:109–25.

75. **AL-Baik MZ, Moharram MM, Elsaid T,** et al. Screening for depression in diabetic patients. *International Journal of Medical Science and Public Health* 2014;**3**:156–60.

76. **Aiash HM, Al-Abbasi A, Haji H,** et al. Prevalence of depressive disorder in diabetic patients in Kuwait Oil Company (Al-Ahmadi Hospital). *Medical Journal of Cairo University* 2011;**79**:67–72.

77. **Lee S, Shiu ATY, Wong RYM.** Treatment-related stresses and anxiety-depressive symptoms among Chinese outpatients with type 2 diabetes mellitus in Hong Kong. *Diabetes Research & Clinical Practice* 2006;**74**:282–8.

78. **Li C, Ford ES, Zhao G,** et al. Association between diagnosed diabetes and serious psychological distress among U.S. adults, the Behavioral Risk Factor Surveillance System, 2007. *International Journal of Public Health* 2009;**54**(Suppl. 1):43–51.

79. **Zhang J, Xu CP, Wu HX,** et al. Comparative study of the influence of diabetes distress and depression on treatment adherence in Chinese patients with type 2 diabetes, a cross-sectional survey in the Peoples Republic of China. *Neuropsychiatric Disease and Treatment* 2013;**9**:1289–94.

80. **Gariepy G, Smith, Kimberley J, Schmitz, N.** Diabetes distress and neighborhood characteristics in people with type 2 diabetes. *Journal of Psychosomatic Research* 2013;**75**:147–52.

81. **Low LL, Tong SF, Low WY.** Selection of treatment strategies among patients with type 2 diabetes mellitus in Malaysia, a grounded theory approach. *PLoS One* 2016;**11**:e0147127.

82. **Aikens JE.** Prospective associations between emotional distress and poor outcomes in type 2 diabetes. *Diabetes Care* 2012;**35**:2472–8.

83. **Dirmaier J, Watzke B, Koch U,** et al. Diabetes in primary care, prospective associations between depression, nonadherence and glycemic control. *Psychotherapy and Psychosomatics* 2010;**79**:172–8.

84. **Cummings DM, Kirian K, Howard G,** et al. Consequences of comorbidity of elevated stress and/or depressive symptoms and incident cardiovascular outcomes in diabetes, results from the REasons for Geographic And Racial Differences in Stroke (REGARDS) study. *Diabetes Care* 2016 **39**:101–9.

85. **Chew BH, Sherina MS, Hassan NH.** Association of diabetes-related distress, depression, medication adherence, and health-related quality of life with glycated hemoglobin, blood pressure, and lipids in adult patients with type 2 diabetes, A cross-sectional study. *Therapeutics and Clinical Risk Management* 2015;**11**:669–81.

86. **Devarajooh C, Chinna K.** Depression, distress and self-efficacy. The impact on diabetes self-care practices. *PLoS One* 2017;**12**:e0175096.

87. **Anonymous**. Behavioural interventions for type 2 diabetes, an evidence-based analysis. *Ontario Health Technology Assessment Series* 2009;**9**: 1–45.

88. **Baumeister H, Hutter N, Bengel J.** Psychological and pharmacological interventions for depression in patients with diabetes mellitus and depression, *Cochrane Database of Systematic Reviews* 2012;**12**:008381.

89. **Chew BH, Vos RC, Metzendorf MI**, et al. Psychological interventions for diabetes-related distress in adults with type 2 diabetes mellitus. *Cochrane Database of Systematic Reviews* 2017;**9**:011469.

90. **Harkness E, Macdonald W, Valderas J**, et al. Identifying psychosocial interventions that improve both physical and mental health in patients with diabetes, a systematic review and meta-analysis. *Diabetes Care* 2010;**33**:926–30.

91. **Safren SA, Gonzalez JS, Wexler DJ**, et al. A randomized controlled trial of cognitive behavioral therapy for adherence and depression (CBT-AD) in patients with uncontrolled type 2 diabetes. *Diabetes Care* 2014;**37**:625–33.

92. **Sturt Jackie, Dennick K, Hessler D**, et al. Effective interventions for reducing diabetes distress, systematic review and meta-analysis. *International Diabetes Nursing* 2015;**12**:40–55.

Chapter 18

National and international policy initiatives on multimorbidity

Peter E. H. Schwarz and Patrick Timpel

What we know

An increasing number of people are affected by multimorbidity. Estimations suggest that 50 million European citizens suffer from two or more chronic health conditions [1]. In particular, diabetes patients often suffer from more than one disease. Epidemiological studies indicate that patients with diabetes mellitus have a higher risk for hypertension [2], cardiovascular disease [3–5], and mental disorders [6]. Comorbidities can have profound effects on the professional care, case management, and individual self-management of patients leading to competing demands [7–9]. Diabetes care as an example is costly for both individuals and health systems. It requires an efficient management of professionals, informal caregivers, and the patients' expertise and involvement at a certain point in time [10–12]. The increasing number of people with chronic and multiple illnesses like diabetes is putting high burdens on health systems, society, and individuals [13,14]. This rising number of people with complex care needs requires the development of delivery systems that bring together a range of professionals and competences from health care, long-term care, social care, rehabilitation, and public health and prevention sectors. This underlines how important it will be for health policy makers, insurers, and providers to create a framework that enables all patients to manage their conditions effectively as part of a coordinated strategy. One important tool to prepare for this challenge is policy development.

Although evidence supports that individualized chronic care management is an effective strategy to provide patient-centred care, professionals are still struggling to find the right strategies to support its implementation [15]. While self-management support is recognized as an important element of chronic care, only a few countries seem to be developing or implementing systematic strategies to promote this support. However, if the intervention is shown to be effective in the respective ongoing feasibility and pilot work, scaling-up of the intervention will require greater consideration of the external context of healthcare policy and widespread implementation.

Adequate policies are the essence of implementing a population-wide health strategy into the healthcare system. Inadequate policies can lead to a failure of the strategy implementation. Politicians, researchers, and healthcare stakeholders always call for policy development but what makes the difference between relevant and irrelevant policies? Which policy is having an impact and how to identify impacting strategies and policies making a difference for people with chronic diseases? Developing the right policy framework and interventions for multimorbid patients therefore means to ask, which policy options are the most effective for the relevant target group and which benefit the relevant health system. This chapter will highlight some policies, discuss how to learn from international examples, give recommendations on how to develop policies, and describe how to point out imbalances in recent policy environment. The chapter shall motivate to rethink existing policies and to foster the development of adequate population-wide health policies.

Policies between ambitions and reality

Public policies are the means by which a government maintains order or addresses the needs of its citizens through actions defined by its constitution [16]. Although this definition sounds rather vague, a policy is more than a term to describe a collection of laws, mandates, or regulations established through a political process. Taking the above described definition, a health policy covers not only the insurance mandates, but also refers to all policies related to the health of a particular group. This includes the treatment of diseases as well as the education of citizens according to their specific needs [17].

The question is, however, do we need government protection from foods and beverages whose long-term consumption will inevitably cause health problems? In this respect, it is undisputed that it is the responsibility of a state to protect citizens from health threats an individual cannot control. According to article 25 (1) of the Universal Declaration of Human Rights:

> Everyone has the right to a standard of living adequate for the health and well-being of himself and of his family, including food, clothing, housing and medical care and necessary social services, and the right to security in the event of unemployment, sickness, disability, widowhood, old age or other lack of livelihood in circumstances beyond his control. [18]

Looking at this human right given to everybody, we have to admit that everybody has the right to live in a healthy (food) environment.

According to the definition used by the WHO, 'health policy' refers to

> decisions, plans, and actions that are undertaken to achieve specific health care goals within a society.… It defines a vision for the future which in turn helps to establish targets and points of reference, … outlines priorities and the expected roles of different groups; and it builds consensus and informs people. [19]

In 2013, the American Medical Association (AMA) recognized obesity as a disease. This marked a key milestone in progress towards advancing evidence-based approaches for its prevention and treatment. The review of these concepts underlines that there is a responsibility of (health) policy to protect citizens from becoming sick by reducing health risks, support the adoption of healthy behaviours and adequately treat patients with (multiple) conditions according to their individual needs.

Can we learn from international examples?

To answer this question with an unbiased focus, individualized pragmatic approaches should be taken into account next to evidence-based practices [20]. Policy development can substantially benefit from translational science [21]. There are a few examples where single scientific projects used simple interventions on national and regional levels to deliver significant effects in prevention [22].

A tax on saturated fat in Denmark led to a lower consumption of costly unhealthy products [23]. Although it was an effective strategy of diabetes prevention, it did not survive because of lobby interests of the food industry [23,24]. A national competition in Canadian schools supported children to be more physically active and improve their coordination skills with the help of computer animated games [25]. The level of physical activity of some children increased up to three times. The question, however, is whether there is a need for randomized controlled trials to test the evidence of these approaches. Is it not enough to know that a reduction of saturated fat and an improvement of physical activity are effective ways to prevent diabetes and other chronic diseases? This first selection of approaches shows that policies on multimorbidity start with the prevention of health risks in early childhood and the promotion of healthy environments. This therefore combines both individual level as well as population-based prevention initiatives.

Looking at campaigns and policies targeting diabetes, the situation in the EU seems nationally and regionally fragmented [13]. As the burden of diabetes continues to grow throughout Europe, many EU member states have developed national diabetes plans or policy frameworks. The most successful of these frameworks go beyond medical needs, address psychosocial needs and encourage patient autonomy through disease education and self-management

[13]. Diabetes self-management education is effective and widely recommended [26]. However, questions remain with respect to the cost-effectiveness, the best delivery strategy, and the impact of patient and provider characteristics on self-management education effectiveness [27,28].

Currently, there are no Europe-wide and only few national policies implemented, which address the need for more integrated care for people with multimorbidity [29]. The WHO also noted that a lack of interventions is not the primary obstacle for inadequate progress in prevention and control of non-communicable diseases (NCDs) [30]. Therefore, the next question is, how these successful programmes can be scaled up and adapted to the regional and national requirements of the different health and community systems.

The EU project IMAGE

The European project IMAGE is an excellent example of how a research project can translate evidence-based and practice-based recommendations into policy development [31,32]. The IMAGE project consisted out of more than 100 experts in Europe and abroad who dedicated themselves to develop practical tools for diabetes prevention based on the results learned from scientific studies [31,33,34]. A very active discussion took place about the relevance of scientific evidence and practicability. The IMAGE consortium finally tried to address all levels necessary for diabetes prevention including policy development, education, and practical implementation. A practical toolkit for prevention of type 2 diabetes was developed together with an evidence-based guideline in the field. In addition, a curriculum for the training of prevention managers, who can spread and scale up diabetes prevention activities, was released, including an outline on how to perform and measure the quality of management in diabetes prevention. These tools were presented in 2010 at the 6th World Congress for the Prevention of Diabetes and its Complications and have spread into more than 50 countries ever since. There, they have initiated translation, further development, and policy development in diabetes prevention. Then, an interesting process took place: based on the same tools from the IMAGE project, significantly different policies and strategies were developed in different countries. For example, screening approaches used in clinical practice in Germany, Portugal, Australia, Finland, and other countries [31,32,34,35] were based on the IMAGE recommendation, but with locally adapted approaches [36]. The IMAGE project used a consensus of international experts and initiated a global policy development for diabetes prevention, creating a variety of applications out of a standardized product. The IMAGE project is a good example of how cooperation between stakeholders from different backgrounds can address all different levels of strategy and policy development, including basic science in diabetes prevention, efficacy, effectiveness, efficiency, and also affordability of diabetes prevention programmes. What is still missing is a bigger effort in developing affordable programmes and distributing and scaling up diabetes prevention on a population-wide level.

The EU project Feel4Diabetes

In the European project Feel4Diabetes, policies on diabetes prevention and care in the early childhood of six low- and middle-income countries (Belgium, Bulgaria, Finland, Greece, Hungary, and Spain) were investigated [37]. Although all countries had developed diabetes plans, the situation differed considerably among them and even among regions in a single country. The first results of the analysis and discussions with representatives of the countries show that the six countries have different treatment methods for Diabetes care and prevention but, in general, the majority of approaches do not target children. Practical guidelines for supporting diabetes prevention especially in children only exist in Finland, Greece, and Spain. Except Hungary, all countries acknowledge the possibility of improvements in terms of access to care and the availability of human resources. This might be due to the excessively hospital-centred care delivery system of Hungary and also be supported by high outpatient contacts per person in 2012 and 2013 [38,39]. It is well-known that patients' access to healthcare in rural and remote areas is determined by the geographical distance and shortage of services. These limitations may lead to unhealthy behaviours and reduced willingness to seek care and have the potential to further increase patients' vulnerability [40]. Such system-related aspects of chronic care require policy improvements and systematic innovation.

A role model for the prevention and care of diabetes is seen in Finland. Children at high risk for diabetes are identified by using screening tools and specific intervention programmes. Finland offers a variety of prevention activities such as a diabetes telephone helpline, a national diabetes campaign, a media campaign targeting a healthy lifestyle, education programmes in schools about a healthy lifestyle, and food labelling. Evidence shows that the effects of prevention initiatives increase whenever multiple interventions are combined [41]. Moreover, it is well known that people who are in need for prevention programmes tend not to be reached by them (prevention dilemma) [42]. To overcome this gap, targeted interventions for these (mostly) vulnerable groups (minorities, disabled, etc.) have to be implemented. These actions also have to be accompanied by setting interventions, continuously improving the environment of people to support healthier lifestyles, and reducing risks [43]. There is robust evidence that school-based diet and physical activity interventions with a home component or school-based combination interventions with a home and community component prevent obesity or overweight. At the same time, the literature on interventions to prevent obesity and diabetes that take place in settings other than schools is limited [44].

These insights underline that policies are not stand-alone or one-size-fits-all approaches. They need to be nationally developed, regionally adapted, and accompanied by the establishment of prevention initiatives on different levels. This needs to be done using the given resources and responsible stakeholders within concerted actions [45].

The EU project MANAGE CARE

The EU-funded project MANAGE CARE aims to prevent costly complications and frailty in elderly with type 2 diabetes, enabling them to live independent, healthy, and active lives as long as possible. Driving innovation and change in the current treatment approach is supported by shifting the focus from diabetes management (disease-specific care trajectory) to chronic care management (non-disease-focused model). The project combines applicable approaches through change in care delivery and partnering for change, addressing particularly older patients with multiple chronic conditions and using innovative business modelling. Diabetes is used as a 'test case' for developing this innovative model.

One result of the project is a new chronic care model based on Wagner et al.'s [46] fundamental framework invented in 1996. The new MANAGE CARE Model tackles challenges of today's healthcare systems and addresses upcoming needs. It includes health promotion, prevention, and aspects of the social system without being limited to medical conditions or citizens who have risk factors [42]. A roadmap for implementation of the model has been developed, also providing guidelines for the development of chronic care models in a broader context. Current research projects targeting public health topics often struggle to translate important findings into applicable changes [20,47]. Although they provide effective tools, they fail in terms of applying these findings under real-life conditions or when the project-based strategies need to be scaled up to other environments. To tackle this barrier, MANAGE CARE also developed 11 care recommendations designed as measurable, feasible, and adaptable requirements to provide a roadmap for a stepwise development of modern chronic care programmes. These 11 recommendations target the following topics of chronic care management and facilitate policy management discussed in Table 18.1.

The recommendations were developed to support the reception of findings applicable to health care management organizations, scientific and medical associations, and insurance and payer stakeholders as well as political partners.

Table 18.1 Care recommendations to facilitate development of innovative chronic care programmes

11 Care recommendations	
1	Education
2	Individual needs
3	Prevention and health promotion
4	Social support and community engagement
5	Accessibility
6	Cooperation/coordination
7	Sharing information
8	eHealth
9	Fairness
10	Business
11	Evaluation

Policy actions in Germany

In the past 15 years, much has been done to respond to the increasing number of chronically ill citizens and especially people with multimorbidity. To improve the German health system and service delivery according to the specific needs of these people on a basic scale, new policies were formulated and measures have been introduced. The new care programmes aim at a reduction of costs, decrease of service utilisation, and improved quality and outcomes of care.

In general, the policy initiatives focus on three major developments:

- closing the gap between sectors by promoting intersectoral care (e.g. promoting disease management programmes and contracts on integrated care, developing standards for hospital discharges, implementing a legal right for care management)
- providing incentives to boost collaboration (financial support system for integrated care physician networks)
- broaden the starting points of prevention (promoting the collaboration of institutions covering all stages of live from kindergarten to long-term care).

Most of the major laws invented since 1988 were adopted to improve the quality of health care and to innovate the structural division of delivery, administration, and financing. These laws and initiatives have led to an increase of integrated care contracts and have attracted substantial interest among hospitals, which had been hesitant until then [48]. In conclusion, outcomes of the care programmes and policies addressing patients with multiple (chronic) conditions seem to be positive, but long-term evaluation is needed.

To boost research and innovation, an 'Innovation Fund' has been invented, spending up to €225M annually from 2016 to 2019. In addition, €75M are allocated to project evaluation annually. The intention of the fund is to support new forms of health care, which are going beyond current traditional care. The fund is supposed to favour projects that further develop cross-sector care. One of the four funding topics is directly designed for the development and expansion of geriatric healthcare, taking into account the challenges of multimorbidity. Projects funded under this topic are supposed to improve networking of ambulatory and hospital-centred geriatric care, support coordinated care, and develop integrated strategies to provide interface management between prevention, treatment, rehabilitation, and care. The example of the 'Innovation Fund' is seen as a research policy with huge potential aimed at supporting innovative cross-sectoral types of healthcare and healthcare research.

Strategic policy development is also supported by a process of developing national health goals. With the collaboration of the Federal Government, the Federal States, the statutory health insurance, the pension insurance, private health insurances, doctors, patient organizations, self-help groups, and additional service providers in the healthcare system, eight national health goals have been agreed on. In 2003, the target 'Type 2 diabetes mellitus: reduction of disease risk, early recognition, and treatment of patients' was invented.

We need policies tackling the toxic food environment

The toxic food environment impedes a sustainable health strategy. To date, we have gained a lot of evidence about the benefits and effects of a healthy lifestyle as well as the disadvantages of unhealthy eating behaviour and physical inactivity. Parallel to this, eating behaviour has changed not only in Western countries but more dramatically in Gulf States and Asian countries, including many low-income countries. The prevention paradox: parallel to the gain of knowledge and evidence in prevention of chronic diseases, morbidity, and mortality based on individual lifestyle increases. Today's recommendations for a healthy lifestyle are based on study evidence planned 20 years ago [45]. However, these decade-old suggestions cannot compensate for the unhealthy behaviour in today's eating and activity environment. They generate a continuous disconnection between behaviour and policy recommendation for prevention. We are living in a so called 'toxic food environment', surrounded by cheap, energy-rich food, provided in high quantities, available 24/7 in our living environment. Marketing provides emotional incentives to promote exhaustive food consumption, sometimes even suggesting health benefits for large portions of energy-overloaded, cheap food. Children and adolescents are in the focus of targeted marketing campaigns for unhealthy food and false health promises. Looking at this from a non-consumer perspective opens a substantial dilemma: the consumer gets attracted by emotionally driven, targeted marketing campaigns and feels 'healthy' by consuming promoted health products.

Prevention campaigns and health policies often use rational arguments and by doing so, are totally failing to attract consumers on an emotional level. The risk of losing the battle against large food companies' marketing campaigns is real and evidence-based policies are missing [45]. As a consequence, government, policy-makers, and public health experts have to unify in a concerted action to confine the toxic food environment and to develop health determinants targeted policies to protect the citizens from common unhealthy choices.

Health policies in the Arab world

The fastest increase in incidence and prevalence of chronic diseases, especially diabetes mellitus, is currently experienced in the Arab world, specifically the Gulf States. The prevalence of diabetes in Saudi Arabia will rise very fast and, including those with disease risk, reach a 50% level within the next two decades. A similar scenario can be found in the neighbouring Arabic states driven by the very fast change of culture, environment, and lifestyle. Parallel to this development, healthcare professionals and politicians call for sustainable diabetes strategies and policy development. Often, international experts are hired to develop local and national Arab health policies, increasing the challenge and the need for cultural and regional adaptation. Each policy that is developed has to strategically address the individual need of a person or the target group. External experts have to carefully develop a policy for another country, especially if the cultural, religious, and environmental surroundings differ significantly. The State of Qatar has recently released a Qatar National Diabetes Strategy, which was predominantly developed by external consulting firms, but using interviews of national and local stakeholders. The remaining policy contains a stepwise procedure identifying strategic pillars with the most relevant need for diabetes policy. Furthermore, recommendations for implementations are given. Reviewing the strategy in detail reveals an inadequate copy of national policies from Westernized countries. The cultural adaptation is missing and concrete recommendations how to tackle the diabetes epidemic are not addressed. The policy development looks like a strategic business plan for consulting firms to develop further business. Even if this statement sounds critical, the development of such a policy is basically good because activities have started. Politicians have recognized the need for a relevant policy. Having a strategic business plan will subsequently lead to activities facilitating the policy.

This will benefit the population but also contains a high risk of failure, as a sustainable and coherent strategic policy is missing.

Diabetes prevention and global health policies

Effective global public health policies are crucial for addressing diabetes and other NCDs, especially as these account for a majority of deaths worldwide and constitute a 'slow-motion disaster' [49]. Although NCDs are by definition non-infectious, type 2 diabetes has also been elegantly characterized as an infectious disease by Matthews and Matthews in their 2010 Banting Memorial Lecture [50] and as such might be 'eradicated' in the same fashion. Calorie excess serves as a transmissible agent, propagated by inadequate food labelling and poorly regulated advertising vectors in a reservoir of fast-food outlets providing cheap calories. Sedentary lifestyles provide a predisposing toxic milieu in which limited physical activity works in concert with consumption of excess calories, ultimately leading to weight gain, obesity, and increased risk of diabetes [51]. Analogous to an infectious pandemic, breaking the cycle of transmission in the diabetes outbreak must involve political will, a decisive legislation, and support by the medical community [47,51].

Regardless of whether or not diabetes is characterized as communicable or non-communicable, both perspectives commonly point to the critical need for action. Thus, the increasing toll associated with NCDs led to a 2-day meeting of the UN General Assembly in September 2011, creating awareness for the enormity of the global problem culminating in the adoption of a political declaration. While recognizing the NCD epidemic, the conference did not set deadlines, targets, or a system of accountability, and no funding was allocated for treatment or prevention. Although the UN summit did not address all expectations, it provided diabetes and NCDs with a global platform [52]. It was left to governments to 'customize the implementation' of their commitments [47].

The International Diabetes Federation (IDF) has been instrumental in providing an overall framework representing the global diabetes community [52]. In addition to improving the health outcomes of individuals with diabetes and addressing discrimination of individuals with diabetes, prevention of type 2 diabetes constitutes a key objective of the plan. Prevention and treatment are not considered alternative options, as they are both equally important. The UN and its agencies are advised to work with national governments to reorient health systems to a preventative model, addressing health in all policies such as urban design and housing, workplace design, food production, healthy nutrition, and physical activity. Concerted action at the international and national policy levels will therefore be required to advance science-driven health initiatives in these areas and translation into practice [50,53], while meticulously avoiding over-zealous and well-meaning policy initiatives of hitherto unproven benefit. These recommendations are congruous with the three pivotal levers of change described by Yach et al. [54]:

1. raising profile of chronic disease in the mind and on the agenda of policy makers;

2. providing policy-makers with evidence to support the case for prevention;

3. advocate the need for widespread health system change.

These should include entire government systems beyond healthcare and involve global corporations, labour unions, and non-governmental organizations. Furthermore, chronic disease alliances need to be formulated including industry and academia [45,54,55,56], such as the Oxford Health Alliance, the Global Alliance for Chronic Diseases, and the Global Partnerships Forum. Political commitment and action are critically required at high global and national levels, particularly as prevention of diabetes and its complications are dramatically underfunded and major gaps exist between findings from clinical trials and their implementation in clinical and public health practice [47,49,57].

Conclusion

To prevent multimorbidity, sustainable liability-oriented health policies for local, national, and international levels, but especially for globally acting companies, have to be developed. There is a strong need to develop modern health policies that take into account the mid-term and long-term health effect of food and beverage products. These policies provide the frame in which business models can be developed to strategically orient the business on healthy lifestyle products. The outcome should be increasingly related to a sustainable health outcome using this strategy in a policy and legal environment. Following the policy will give entrepreneurs the power and safety to invest in healthy prevention businesses [45].

Since the focus on individual approaches has not led to improvements in diabetes prevalence on a public health level, a strategy shift from individual to shared responsibility, as well as a combination of strategies forming multi-level approaches is needed. The combination of science and prevention business leads to new insights in terms of access to target groups, quality management, and evaluation. New developments in telemedicine and low-resource initiatives in communities show encouraging results. They appear to have a high potential to reach target groups who are out of scope when traditional prevention campaigns are applied. As researchers, we have to pass the baton to entrepreneurs, policy makers, and tax lawyers. Implementation, scalability, and sustainable business must become a shared action with business partners to finally halt the rising prevalence of type-2-diabetes [45]. Action at the policy level is urgently needed. To put this claim in concrete terms, we would like to present a selection of fields of action which have a high potential of scalability on national levels.

Prevention policies

- Liability for adverse effects with food consumption—food and beverage industry should be made responsible for mid-term (obesity) and long-term (heart attack, diabetes, and metabolic syndrome) side-effects of consumption of their products.
- Food labelling—food and beverage industry should be obliged to print easy-to-read labels on pre-packed foods to facilitate choosing healthy and avoiding unhealthy products (i.e. traffic light system).
- Health tokens, a currency for health increasing liquidity in the prevention market—health tokens are an incentive for consuming health products or performing a healthy lifestyle, collected health tokens can be used as a currency but only to consume health products.
- Tax exemption for sustainable business models in diabetes prevention—tax exemption for prevention services and products in the healthcare sector, together with tax increase for energy-dense foods, could speed up the development of prevention businesses (i.e. reg. chronic disease services) and healthy products for consumers.
- Support preventive initiatives in the embryonic stage and early childhood [45].

Targeting the threats of multimorbidity by developing more effective, affordable, and sustainable care has gained in importance on the political agenda at an international, European, and national level. Today's healthcare systems seem inadequately adapted to deal with the challenges of patients with multimorbidity. First of all, evidence on the epidemiology and pathogenetic mechanisms of multimorbidity is limited. Second, clinical guidelines do not always meet the individual needs relevant to this target group. Third, care delivery systems and financial resources have not been sufficiently developed to assess quality and performance of new care models. To overcome these challenges, we have formulated further recommendations.

General recommendations

- Overcoming the silo mentality in research and policy: policies on lifestyle risks and unhealthy behaviours are often compartmentalized. Additionally, separate policy leads and teams are focusing on single issues with a limited focus instead of concrete risks in real-life settings. On the other hand, individual lifestyle policies have been developed in silos and behaviour change policies were produced separately from inequalities policy [58]. Policymakers and researchers have the power and the evidence-based arguments to jointly develop strategies. This would help to form an alliance against food industry lobbying and on the other hand support implementation research on a new level.

- Focus on practical instead of evidence-based approaches: randomized controlled trials mostly do not cover the real life settings of different target groups. Furthermore, it takes a long time to put research into practice, especially when evidence-based recommendations are intended. One reason for this circumstance is that research and policy development have been using different and often contradictory strategies to tackle chronic conditions for many years. Another reason is the system of funding research on a short term.

- We need policies tackling (health) inequalities: there is a lack of effort to understand how the population, and especially the vulnerable patient groups, actually experience lifestyle risks and unhealthy behaviours in their social context, and to relate to these perceptions within inequality policies. We have to overcome policies designed for the whole population that primarily work for those groups with a considerable level of health literacy.

- There is a need for reliable, appropriate, and comparable data to inform local and national initiatives, and to develop national and even European policies.

- Systematically assess and delete false and unintended incentives in health systems: A continuous adaption of the quality and financial systems is needed to further improve integrated and patient-centred care going beyond short episodes of care visits.

References

1. **Lam DW, Leroith D.** The worldwide diabetes epidemic. *Current Opinions in Endocrinology Diabetes and Obesity* 2012;**19**:93–6.
2. **Schutta MH.** Diabetes and hypertension: epidemiology of the relationship and pathophysiology of factors associated with these comorbid conditions. *Journal of Cardiometabolic Syndrome* 2007;**2**:124–30.
3. **Chiha M, Njeim M, Chedrawy EG.** Diabetes and coronary heart disease: a risk factor for the global epidemic. *International Journal of Hypertension* 2012;**2012**:697240.
4. **Matheus AS, Tannus LR, Cobas RA,** et al. B. Impact of diabetes on cardiovascular disease: an update. *International Journal of Hypertension* 2013;**2013**:653789.

5. **Meigs JB.** Epidemiology of type 2 diabetes and cardiovascular disease: translation from population to prevention: the Kelly West award lecture 2009. *Diabetes Care* 2010;**33**:1865–71.

6. **Freitas C, Deschenes S, Au B,** et al. Risk of diabetes in older adults with co-occurring depressive symptoms and cardiometabolic abnormalities: prospective analysis from the English longitudinal study of ageing. *PLoS One* 2016;**11**:e0155741.

7. **Chernof B, Sherman SE, Lanto AB,** et al. Health habit counseling amidst competing demands: effects of patient health habits and visit characteristics. *Medical Care* 1999 **37**:738–47.

8. **Jaen CR, Stange KC, Nutting PA.** Competing demands of primary care: a model for the delivery of clinical preventive services. *Journal of Family Practice* 1994;**38**:166–71.

9. **McEwen LN, Kim C, Ettner SL,** et al. Competing demands for time and self-care behaviors, processes of care, and intermediate outcomes among people with diabetes: Translating Research Into Action for Diabetes (TRIAD). *Diabetes Care* 2011;**34**:1180–2.

10. **Handelsman Y, Bloomgarden, Z. T, Grunberger G,** et al. American association of clinical endocrinologists and American college of endocrinology—clinical practice guidelines for developing a diabetes mellitus comprehensive care plan—2015—executive summary. *Endocrine Practice* 2015;**21**:413–37.

11. **International Diabetes Federation.** IDF Diabetes Atlas—7th Edition. N. Cho, International Diabetes Federation. 2015.

12. **Muller G, Weser G, Schwarz PE.** The European perspective of diabetes prevention: the need for individualization of diabetes prevention. *Journal Endocrinologic Investigation* 2013;**36**:352–7.

13. **European Coalition for Diabetes.** *Diabetes in Europe: Policy Puzzle. The State We Are In.* 2014; 4th edition.

14. **Schofield D, Cunich MM, Shrestha RN,** et al. The economic impact of diabetes through lost labour force participation on individuals and government: evidence from a microsimulation model. *BMC Public Health* 2014;**14**:1–8.

15. **Yeoh EK,** et al. Benefits and limitations of implementing chronic care model (CCM) in primary care programs: a systematic review. *International Journal of Cardiology* 2018;**258**:279–88.

16. **Kilic B, Kalaca S, Unal B,** et al. Health policy analysis for prevention and control of cardiovascular diseases and diabetes mellitus in Turkey. *International Journal of Public Health* 2015;**60**(Suppl. 1):S47–53.

17. **Timpel P, Lang C, Wens J,** et al. **on behalf of the MANAGE CARE Study Group.** Individualising chronic care management by analysing patients needs—a mixed method approach. *International Journal of Integrated Care* 2017;**17**:2.

18. **United Nations.** Universal Declaration of Human Rights. 1948. www.un.org (accessed 13 March 2017).

19. **WHO.** Health policy' Definition. www.who.int (accessed 13 March 2017).

20. **Schwarz PE, Albright AL.** Prevention of type 2 diabetes: the strategic approach for implementation. *Hormone and Metabolic Research* 2011;**43**:907–10.

21. **Schwarz PE.** Public health implications: translation into diabetes prevention initiatives—four-level public health concept. *Med Clin North Am* 2011;**95**:397–407, ix.

22. **Tuomilehto J, Schwarz P.E.** Primary prevention of type 2 diabetes is advancing towards the mature stage in Europe. *Hormone and Metabolic Research* 2010;**42**(Suppl. 1):1–2.

23. **Vallgarda S, Holm L, Jensen J.D.** The Danish tax on saturated fat: why it did not survive. *European Journal of Clinical Nutrition* 2015;**69**:223–6.

24. **Sassi F, Cecchini M, Lauer J.** and **Chisholm D.** OECD health working papers No. 48, improving lifestyles, tackling obesity: the health and economic impact of prevention strategies. *Health Working Papers* 2009;**1**:107.

25. **Vander Ploeg KA, Wu B, McGavock J, Veugelers PJ.** Physical activity among Canadian children on school days and nonschool days. *Journal of Physical Activity and Health* 2012;**9**:1138–45.

26. **Van den Broucke S, Van der Zanden G, Chang P,** et al. Enhancing the effectiveness of diabetes self-management education: the Diabetes Literacy Project. *Hormone and Metabolic Research* 2014;**46**:933–8.

27. **Damery S, Flanagan S.** and **Combes G.** Does integrated care reduce hospital activity for patients with chronic diseases? An umbrella review of systematic reviews. *BMJ Open* 2016;**6**(11):e011952.

28. **de Bruin SR,** et al. Comprehensive care programs for patients with multiple chronic conditions: a systematic literature review. *Health Policy* 2012;**107**(2–3):108–45.

29. **Albreht T, Dyakova M, Schellevis F, Van den Broucke S.** Many diseases, one model of care? *Journal of Comorbidity* 2016;**6**:9.

30. **WHO.** Global Status Report on Noncommunicable Diseases 2014. www.who.int

31. **Lindstrom J, Neumann A, Sheppard K. E.** et al. Take action to prevent diabetes--the IMAGE toolkit for the prevention of type 2 diabetes in Europe. *Hormone and Metabolic Research* 2010;**42**(Suppl. 1):37–55.

32. **Schwarz PE, Lindstrom J.** From evidence to practice-the IMAGE project-new standards in the prevention of type 2 diabetes. *Diabetes Research and Clinical Practice* 2011;**91**:138–140.

33. **Pajunen P, Landgraf R, Muylle F,** et al. Quality Indicators for the Prevention of Type 2 Diabetes in Europe—IMAGE. *Hormone and Metabolic Research* 2010;**42**:S56–S63.

34. **Paulweber B, Valensi P, Lindström J,** et al. A European evidence-based guideline for the prevention of type 2 diabetes. *Hormone and Metabolic Research* 2010;**42**(Suppl. 1):3–S36.

35. **Pereira M, Carreira H, Lunet N, Azevedo A.** Trends in prevalence of diabetes mellitus and mean fasting glucose in Portugal (1987-2009): a systematic review. *Public Health* 2014;**128**:214–21.

36. **Schwarz PE, Li J, Lindstrom J, Tuomilehto J.** Tools for predicting the risk of type 2 diabetes in daily practice. *Hormone and Metabolic Research* 2009;**41**:86–97.

37. Feel4Diabetes. www.feel4diabetes.eu (accessed 13 March 2017).

38. **Health Consumer Powerhouse.** Euro Health Consumer Index 2014. 2015. www.healthpowerhouse.com (accessed 13 March 2017).

39. **Health Consumer Powerhouse.** Euro Health Consumer Index 2015. 2016. www.healthpowerhouse.com (accessed 13 March 2017).

40. **DeJean D, Giacomini M, Vanstone M, Brundisini F.** Patient experiences of depression and anxiety with chronic disease: a systematic review and qualitative meta-synthesis. *Ontario Health Technology Assessment Series* 2013;**13**:1–33.

41. Lindstrom J, Peltonen M, Eriksson JG, et al. Determinants for the effectiveness of lifestyle intervention in the Finnish Diabetes Prevention Study. *Diabetes Care* 2008;**31**:857–62.

42. Tuomilehto J, Schwarz PE. Preventing diabetes: early versus late preventive interventions. *Diabetes Care* 2016;**39**(Suppl. 2):S115–20.

43. Rothe U, Mueller G, Tselmin S, et al. Prevalence for the cluster of risk factors of the metabolic vascular syndrome in a working population in Germany. *Hormone and Metabolic Research* 2009;**41**:168–70.

44. Wang Y, Wu Y, Wilson RF, et al. *Childhood Obesity Prevention Programs: Comparative Effectiveness Review and Meta-Analysis.* Rockville: Agency for Healthcare Research and Quality (US), 2013.

45. Schwarz PE, Riemenschneider H. slowing down the progression of type 2 diabetes: we need fair, innovative, and disruptive action on environmental and policy levels! *Diabetes Care* 2016;**39**(Suppl. 2):S121–6.

46. Wagner EH, Austin BT, Von Korff M. Organizing care for patients with chronic illness. *Milbank Q* 1996;**74**:511–44.

47. Bergman M, Buysschaert M, Schwarz PE, et al. Diabetes prevention: global health policy and perspectives from the ground. *Diabetes Management (London)* 2012;**2**:309–21.

48. Busse R, Blümel M. Germany: health system review. *Health Systems in Transition* 2014;**16**:1–296.

49. Fox CS, Coady S, Sorlie PD, et al. Increasing cardiovascular disease burden due to diabetes mellitus: the Framingham Heart Study. *Circulation* 2007;**115**:1544–50.

50. Matthews DR, Matthews PC. Banting Memorial Lecture 2010. Type 2 diabetes as an infectious disease: is this the Black Death of the 21st century? *Diabetic Medicine* 2011;**28**:2–9.

51. Yach D, Stuckler D, Brownell KD. Epidemiologic and economic consequences of the global epidemics of obesity and diabetes. *Nature Medicine* 2006;**12**:62–6.

52. Rosenbaum L, Lamas D. Facing a 'slow motion disaster'—the UN meeting on noncommunicable diseases. *New England Journal of Medicine* 2011;**365**:2345–8.

53. Keeling A. World Diabetes Congress 2011: turning policy into action after the UN High-Level Summit on NCDS. *Diabetes Research and Clinical Practice* 2011;**94**:477–8.

54. Yach D, Hawkes C, Gould CL, Hofman KJ. The global burden of chronic diseases: overcoming impediments to prevention and control. *Journal of the American Medical Association* 2004;**291**:2616–22.

55. Hu FB. Globalization of diabetes: the role of diet, lifestyle, and genes. *Diabetes Care* 2011;**34**:1249–57.

56. Karve A, Hayward R. A. Prevalence, diagnosis, and treatment of impaired fasting glucose and impaired glucose tolerance in nondiabetic U.S. adults. *Diabetes Care* 2010;**33**:2355–9.

57. Narayan KM, Ali MK, Koplan JP. Global noncommunicable diseases—where worlds meet. *New England Journal of Medicine* 2010;**363**:1196–98.

58. Buck D, Frosini F. Clustering of unhealthy behaviours over time. Implications for policy and practice. *Kings Fund* 2012;**08**:1–24.

Index

Tables, figures, and boxes are indicated by an italic *t*, *f*, and *b* following the page number

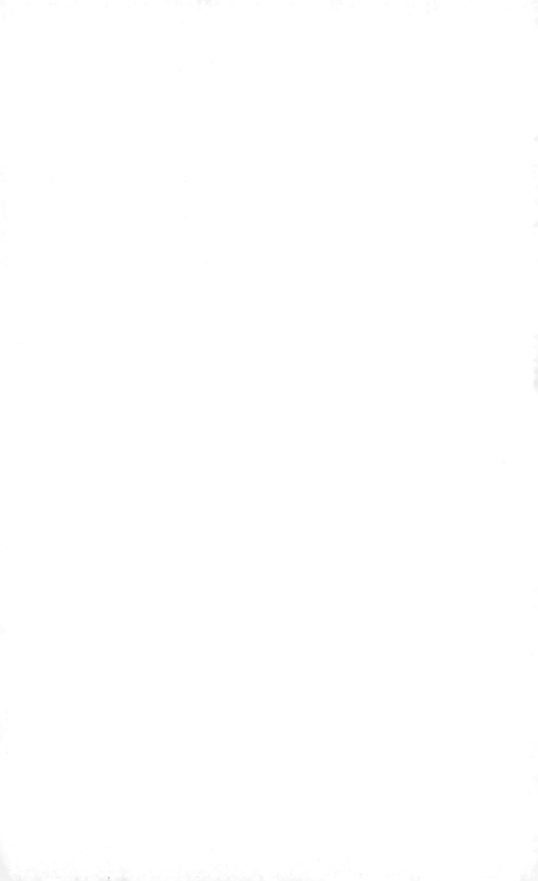